Natural Products and Therapeutics

Endocrinology Research and Clinical Developments

nova
Medicine & Health
New York

Natural Products and Therapeutics

Herbal Prescriptions for Signs and Symptoms: GMP Herbal Formulations for Treating Clinical Manifestations of Diseases
Sun-Chong Wang (Editor)
2023. ISBN: 979-8-88697-835-3 (Hardcover)
2023. ISBN: 979-8-88697-901-5 (eBook)

Health Benefits of Phenolic Antioxidants
Aman B. Upaganlawar, PhD (Editor)
Vipin V. Dhote, PhD (Editor)
M. K. Mohan Maruga Raja, PhD (Editor)
2022. ISBN: 979-8-88697-058-6 (Hardcover)
2022. ISBN: 979-8-88697-120-0 (eBook)

More information about this series can be found at
https://novapublishers.com/product-category/series/natural-products-and-therapeutics/

Endocrinology Research and Clinical Developments

The Biochemical Guide to Hormones
David Aebisher, PhD, DSc (Editor)
2023. ISBN: 979-8-88697-492-8 (Hardcover)
2023. ISBN: 979-8-88697-534-5 (eBook)

Natural Products for Treatment of Metabolic Syndrome
Ajmer Singh Grewal, PhD (Editors)
Ashwani Kumar Dhingra, PhD (Editors)
2022. ISBN: 979-8-88697-152-1 (Hardcover)
2022. ISBN: 979-8-88697-233-7 (eBook)

More information about this series can be found at
https://novapublishers.com/product-category/series/endocrinology-research-and-clinical-developments/

Yachana Mishra
and Vijay Mishra
Editors

Management of Diabetes Mellitus Based on Natural Products

nova
Medicine & Health
New York

https://doi.org/10.52305/JCWM1341

NOTICE TO THE READER

Library of Congress Cataloging-in-Publication Data

Names: Mishra, Yachana, editor. | Mishra, Vijay, Dr., editor.
Title: Management of diabetes mellitus based on natural products / Yachana Mishra, PhD (editor), Associate Professor, School of Bioengineering and Biosciences, Lovely Professional University, Phagwara, Punjab, India, Vijay Mishra, PhD (editor), Professor, School of Pharmaceutical Sciences, Lovely Professional University, Phagwara, Punjab, India.
Identifiers: LCCN 2023029998 (print) | LCCN 2023029999 (ebook) |
ISBN 9798886978537 (hardcover) | ISBN 9798886979701 (adobe pdf)
Subjects: LCSH: Diabetes--Alternative treatment | Hypoglycemic agents. | Medicinal plants.
Classification: LCC RC661.A47 M36 2023 (print) | LCC RC661.A47 (ebook) |
DDC 616.4/62--dc23/eng/20230630
LC record available at https://lccn.loc.gov/2023029998
LC ebook record available at https://lccn.loc.gov/2023029999

Published by Nova Science Publishers, Inc. † New York

Dedication

This book is dedicated to our adorable children,
Vidhi Mishra and Jay Mishra.

Contents

Preface ix

Acknowledgments xi

Chapter 1 **Diabetes Mellitus: Worldwide Statistics and Types** 1
Vijay Mishra, Aishwarya Joshi, Neha Shrivastava and Alaa A. A. Aljabali

Chapter 2 **The Pathophysiology of Diabetes Mellitus** 21
Yachana Mishra, Aditi Chattaraj and Kajal

Chapter 3 **The Social Determinants of Diabetes** 41
Yachana Mishra, Kajal and Aditi Chattaraj

Chapter 4 **Diabetes Mellitus in Pregnancy** 51
Yachana Mishra

Chapter 5 **Current Treatment Methods for Diabetes Mellitus** 63
Vijay Mishra and Abhigyan Ranjan

Chapter 6 **Oral Antidiabetic Agents** 105
Vijay Mishra, Abhigyan Ranjan and Murtaza M. Tambuwala

Chapter 7 **Molecular Targets and the Mechanisms of Antidiabetic Agents** 147
Sumit Roy, Archita Dutta, Paranjeet Kaur, Manish Vyas and Sanjeev Kumar Sahu

Chapter 8 **Sodium-Glucose Co-Transporter 2 Inhibitors in Diabetes** 175
Yachana Mishra and Vijay Mishra

Chapter 9 **Chemical Scaffolds as Antidiabetic Agents** 187
Charanjit Kaur and Sanjeev Kumar Sahu

Chapter 10 **Phytoconstituents as Antidiabetic Agents and Their Chemical Aspects** 235
Nancy Saini, Manish Vyas and Sanjeev Kumar Sahu

Chapter 11 **Natural Products in the Treatment of Diabetes: An Insight into the Mechanism of Action** 259
Pranav Kumar Prabhakar and Yachana Mishra

Chapter 12 **A Targeted Therapeutic Approach Based on Medicinal Plants in the Management of Diabetes Mellitus** 271
Pranav Kumar Prabhakar and Yachana Mishra

Index 287

About the Editors 291

Preface

The most prevalent endocrine condition, diabetes mellitus (DM), is characterized by underutilization of glucose, elevated blood sugar levels, and an ineffective or insufficient insulin secretory mechanism. DM is a severe health issue that affects 3% of the global population and 5% of the people in the US. Each year, it accounts for around 5% of all fatalities worldwide. Type 2 diabetes affects more than 90% of diabetic patients, whereas type 1 affects the remaining 10%. Today the management of diabetes without any side effects is still a challenge. Herbal medicines are prescribed widely because of their effectiveness, fewer side effects, and relatively low cost. Numerous active principles produced from plants have proven to have anti-diabetic properties. Herbal treatments for diabetes have been used in patients with insulin-dependent and non-insulin-dependent diabetes, diabetic retinopathy, diabetic peripheral neuropathy, etc. Various plants can lower glucose production, promote glucose utilization, and combat secondary complications.

This book will offer an updated, comprehensive resource of information on diabetes mellitus and its treatment by natural products. The book intends to provide a state-of-the-art collection of reports for primary and clinician investigators interested in treating diabetes mellitus. We believe this book will be of value to clinicians, biochemists, public health authorities, medical laboratory sciences technologists, biotechnologists, pharmaceutical and medical students, and fellows in training. Each chapter begins with a summary of the concepts so that those not actively working in the field can readily understand what follows. We have endeavored to provide this information in a style that is accessible to the broad community of persons who are concerned with the impact of diabetes in our clinics and across wider global communities.

Acknowledgments

We wish to sincerely thank the authors for offering to write comprehensive chapters on a tight schedule. We express our earnest gratitude to the reviewers, who provided their critical views for improving the book chapters. We would like to thank the reviewers of our book proposal for their suggestions in framing the chapters.

Dr. Yachana Mishra and Dr. Vijay Mishra
Editors

Chapter 1

Diabetes Mellitus: Worldwide Statistics and Types

Vijay Mishra[1,*]
Aishwarya Joshi[1]
Neha Shrivastava[1]
and Alaa A. A. Aljabali[2]
[1]School of Pharmaceutical Sciences,
Lovely Professional University, Phagwara (Punjab), India
[2]Department of Pharmaceutics and Pharmaceutical Technology,
Yarmouk University, Irbid, Jordan

Abstract

Diabetes mellitus, a metabolic disease, is characterized by persistently elevated blood sugar levels, i.e., hyperglycemia. The present chapter discusses the historical background of diabetes, its symptoms and consequences, different types, and worldwide statistics on diabetes.

Keywords: diabetes mellitus, hyperglycemia, blood sugar

1. Introduction

Diabetes mellitus (DM) is becoming more common, frequently leading to severe metabolic disorders and consequences. Additionally, various therapeutic objectives in diabetes patients affect both quality of life and

* Corresponding Author's Email: vijaymishra2@gmail.com.

In: Management of Diabetes Mellitus Based on Natural Products
Editors: Yachana Mishra and Vijay Mishra
ISBN: 979-8-88697-853-7

glycemic control. All medical personnel has difficulty when it comes to providing the best treatment for a patient who has diabetes mellitus. Frequently, the diagnosis is made as soon as symptoms appear. Early diagnosis is made possible by screening individuals at high risk, which enables quick therapeutic start-ups and may help avoid long-term consequences. The most helpful diagnostic test is the fasting plasma glucose determination; however, in some cases, the oral glucose tolerance test and random plasma glucose are also used to identify diabetes. The effectiveness of existing treatment options for diabetes mellitus depends on proper individualization. The type and duration of diabetes, the patient's abilities and features, and the individual risk for acute and/or late-stage complications all influence the treatment goals. These complications include macrovascular and microvascular disease, which are defining characteristics of diabetes-related limitations; hypoglycemia, which can be severe and life-threatening; and hyperglycemia, a significant risk factor for the development of cardiovascular disease [1]. For individuals with insulin-dependent diabetes mellitus (IDDM) to achieve satisfactory glucose control, complicated insulin regimens and regular self-blood glucose monitoring are necessary. Several treatments may be used to treat non-insulin-dependent diabetes mellitus (NIDDM), including diet, sulfonylureas, insulin, and combinations. In addition to medicine, nutrition, monitoring, education, and ongoing care are necessary for the therapy to be successful.

2. Diabetes Mellitus and Its Historical Background

A series of metabolic diseases collectively referred to as diabetes, or DM, is characterized by persistently elevated blood sugar levels (hyperglycemia) [1]. The repercussions that DM has caused are social implications, economic, and health illnesses. It is a rapidly spreading global issue. Two major factors contributing to the rise are an aging population and obesity. Furthermore, research has revealed a high risk of increasing diabetes, due to which 50% of the population will not receive the treatment after ten years [2].

Weight loss and polyuria are hallmarks of diabetes, which the Egyptians first described. However, the Greek physician Aertaeus coined the phrase "diabetes mellitus." The words diabetes and mellitus come from the Greek meaning "to pass through." Aretaeus of Cappadocia's treatise is the oldest work (2nd or early 3rd Century CE) containing a specific mention of diabetes. According to his description of the sickness's signs and progression and his

"Pneumatic School" theories, the disease was brought on by dampness and cold. In addition to discussing the snakebite's alternative diagnoses, which also resulted in extreme thirst, he linked diabetes and other disorders hypothesis. His writing was unknown in the West until the first Latin edition was printed in Venice in 1552 [3]. Sushruta and Charaka, two Indian doctors who practiced in the 4th and 5th Centuries CE, distinguished for the first time two distinct forms of diabetes, one of which was linked to youth and the other to obesity. The development of a successful therapy did not occur before the invention of Insulin by Canadians Frederick Banting and Charles Herbert Best in 1921 and 1922, respectively [4]. From this, it has to be learned that the long history of the earliest accounts of diabetes emphasizes how crucial it is to track and observe medical issues as people develop. Early doctors relied on their senses, including smell and taste, to diagnose and gain knowledge. Langerhans produced a thesis pinpointing the cells that would later be recognized as the source of insulin production [5].

3. Prevalence of Diabetes: Worldwide Statistics

Diabetes, which is increasingly prevalent worldwide, is one of the significant and challenging health issues that the human population of the modern world must deal with. The prevalence of diabetes has increased throughout most of the world's regions due to rapid economic growth, urbanization, and the adoption of contemporary lifestyles. Diabetes contributes significantly to long-term sickness and early mortality, with one death occurring approximately every ten seconds. More people die from it annually than from HIV/AIDS. The onset of global industrialization and the incredible growth in obesity has made diabetes a global pandemic. Although it is challenging to determine prevalence due to two primary factors accurately—the vastly disparate criteria and methods of data collection—recent research revealed that the rate of diabetes in adults would increase between 4.4% in 1995 to 6.4% by 2025.

An estimated 463 million adults in the world, or 9.3% of all adults, have diabetes as of the year 2019. These adults range in age from 20 to 79. It is predicted that by 2030, this figure will rise from 578 million, or 10.2%, and by 2045, it will increase to 700 million, or 10.9% of the adult population globally. Estimates for 2019 show that men and women have a high prevalence of diabetes at 9.6% and 9.0% of the global population for each gender, respectively. Additionally, 4.2 million adults aged 20 to 99 died from diabetes-related problems in 2019. Pregnancy-related diabetes is thought to have affected more than 20 million live births (1 in 6 live births) in 2019. The cost of treating diabetes-related illnesses is estimated at least 760 billion USD, or 10% of all adult expenditures [6].

In addition to providing recommendations for decision-makers, people, members of civil society, and enterprises, the WHO Global Report on Diabetes provides an overview of the diabetes burden and a list of treatments that may be utilized to prevent and treat diabetes [7]. Among persons 18 and older in 2014, 8.5% had diabetes. About 1.5 million deaths in 2019 were directly related to diabetes, and 48% of all diabetes-related deaths occurred in those under 70. Diabetes also contributed to 460000 kidney disease fatalities, and elevated blood glucose is thought to be responsible for 20% of cardiovascular mortality. Age-standardized death rates from diabetes increased by 3% between 2000 and 2019 [8].

The death rate from diabetes climbed 13% in lower-middle-income nations. However, between 2000 and 2019, there was a 22% global decline in the likelihood of dying between the ages of 30 and 70 from any of the four major noncommunicable diseases like cancer, chronic respiratory diseases, diabetes, or cardiovascular disorders. The 219 data sources describing research carried out between 2005 and 2020, covering 215 countries and territories, defined quality requirements. Estimates from nations with comparable economies, ethnicities, geographies, and linguistics were extrapolated for nations whose data did not match quality standards. To produce smoothed age-specific diabetes prevalence estimates, logistic regression was utilized. An attributable fraction technique was used to quantify the costs associated with diabetes-related health care. In order to predict future prevalence, population projections for 2045 were combined with estimates of diabetes prevalence for 2021 [9].

The worldwide prevalence of diabetes among adults aged 20 to 79 was predicted to be 10.5% (536.6 million) in 2021 and 12.2% (783.2 million) in 2045. Diabetes prevalence was comparable between genders and was highest in people aged 75 to 79. In 2021, the prevalence was predicted to be higher in urban (12.1%) than rural (8.3%) locations and in high-income (11.1%) than low-income (5.5%) nations. Between 2021 and 2045, middle-income countries are predicted to experience the most significant relative increase in the prevalence of diabetes (21.1%), followed by high-income (12.2%) and low-income (11.9%) nations. The cost of treating diabetes-related illnesses worldwide was anticipated to be 966 billion USD in 2021 and is expected to rise to 1,054 billion USD by 2045 [10].

About 382 million individuals worldwide had diabetes in 2013, according to statistics, with type 2 diabetes accounting for 90% of cases. With equal rates for men and women, this equates to 8.3% of the adult population. Diabetes was the eighth most significant cause of death worldwide in 2012 and 2013, with a mortality rate of 1.5–5.1 million per year. By the year 2035, it is expected that 592 million people will have died from diabetes. The frequency of newly diagnosed cases of diabetes in the United States declined from 9.3 per 1,000 adults in 2009 to 5.9 per 1,000 adults in 2019, ending nearly two decades of steadily rising rates [11].

The proportion of US people with prediabetes stayed steady between 2005 and 2008, as well as between 2017 and 2020. The notification rate for prediabetes status, however, virtually quadrupled from 6.5% to 17.4%. The rates of diabetes diagnosis are greater among Hispanics than among non-Hispanic Whites, non-Hispanic Blacks, non-Hispanic Asians, and American Indians or Alaska Natives i.e., 14.5%, 12.1%, 11.8%, 9.5%, and 7.4%, respectively.

Globally, there will be 643 million diabetics by 2030 and 783 million by 2045. In low- and middle-income countries, three out of every four adults have diabetes. Adults with diabetes make up almost one in two people (240 million). The disease caused the deaths of nearly 6.7 million individuals. At least USD 966 billion, or 9% of all adult healthcare expenses, were related to diabetes.

Over 1.2 million children and adolescents have type 1 diabetes (T1DM) (0-19 years). Pregnancy-related diabetes affects 21 million live births (about 1 in 6). About 541 million people are at higher risk of developing type 2 diabetes (T2DM). Diabetes prevalence among adults is predicted to increase from 4.0% in 1995 to 5.4% by 2025. The developed world has a greater rate than the developing world. By 2025, there will be 300 million adults worldwide who have diabetes, up from 135 million in 1995. The majority of this numerical growth will take place in developing nations. From 51 to 72 million, there will be a 42% growth in wealthy countries and from 84 to 228 million in developing nations. By 2025, developing countries will host more than 75% of the world's diabetic population [10, 12-16].

4. Symptoms and Consequences of Diabetes

Unintentional weight loss, increased urination (polyuria), thirst (polydipsia), and hunger (polyphagia) are common indicators of uncontrolled diabetes

(Figure 1). In contrast to T2DM, where symptoms may not even occur, T1DM symptoms may appear suddenly (within weeks or months) [17]. Despite not being diabetes-specific, the onset of the illness might also be signaled by various additional indications and symptoms. They also consist of scratchy skin, impaired vision, lethargy, headaches, and slow wound healing may lead to glucose absorption in the eye's lens, which changes the lens's curvature and impacts vision. Long-term vision loss might also be a side effect of diabetic retinopathy. A range of skin rashes known as diabetic dermadromes can appear in patients with diabetes [18].

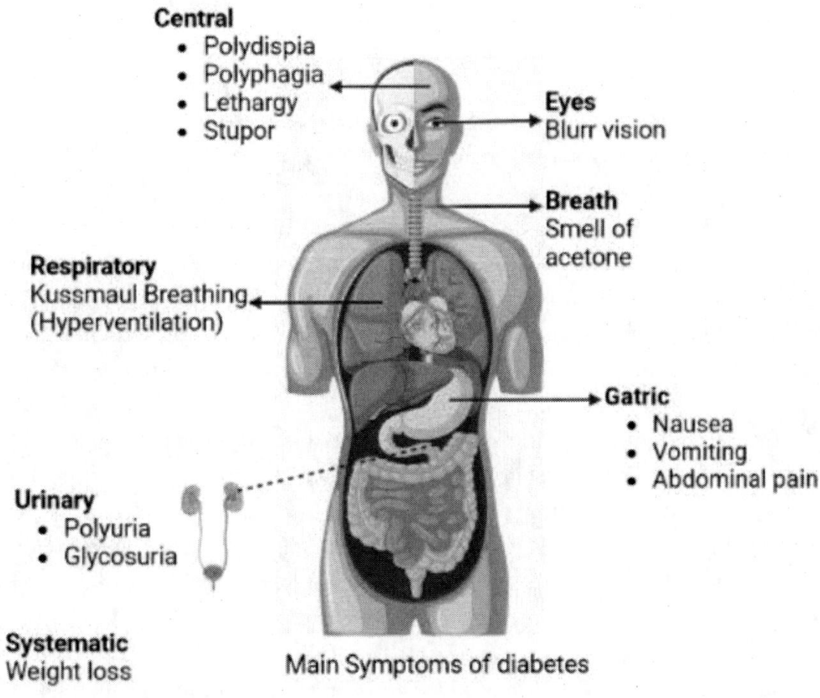

Figure 1. Symptoms of diabetes.

Additionally, diabetes patients may have Diabetic Ketoacidosis (DKA), a metabolic condition characterized by nausea, vomiting, and stomach pain, as well as the acetone odor on the breath, Kussmaul breathing, and in severe cases, a decreased level of consciousness. DKA requires immediate medical attention at a hospital. Dehydration is the primary cause of the hyperosmolar hyperglycemic condition (HHS), which is more common in T2DM. It is a relatively uncommon but severe illness [19].

Depending on the medicine used, hypoglycemia, a low blood sugar caused by treatment, can affect people with T1DM and T2DM. The majority of instances are minor and are not emergencies. In moderate situations, symptoms may include discomfort, shaking, sweating, and an increase in hunger; in severe cases, however, symptoms may include disorientation, violent behavior changes, seizures, unconsciousness, and, very rarely, death or irreversible brain damage [19, 20]. Long-term consequences are more likely in all types of diabetes and often appear after several years (10-20 years); however, they could be the initial symptom in those who haven't previously been diagnosed [21]. One of the primary long-term impacts is damage to blood vessel walls. Cardiovascular disease is two times more likely in those with diabetes, and coronary artery disease accounts for around 75% of those fatalities [22].

Peripheral artery disease and stroke are two examples of other macrovascular disorders [22, 23]. Eye, kidney, and nerve damage are among the most common consequences of diabetes brought on by tiny blood vessel damage. The condition known as diabetic retinopathy, which affects the eyes and can eventually lead to blindness, is brought on by damage to the blood vessels in the eye's retina. Glaucoma, cataracts, and other visual issues are all risk factors for diabetes. It is advised that people with diabetes consult an eye doctor once a year [1, 24].

Injuries to the kidneys from diabetes, known as diabetic nephropathy, can result in tissue damage, protein loss in the urine, and eventually, renal failure, which may necessitate dialysis or kidney transplanting. The most frequent side effect of diabetes is diabetic neuropathy, which causes damage to the body's nerves [1]. Numbness, tingling, sudomotor dysfunction, discomfort, and changed pain perception are some of the symptoms that might cause skin injury. It is possible for diabetes-related foot problems, such as diabetic foot ulcers, to develop, are occasionally challenging to treat, and occasionally require amputation. Cognitive decline is associated with diabetes [16, 25].

5. Diabetes and Its Types

Diabetes mellitus (DM) is a metabolic illness that occurs when the body cannot produce or utilize the hormone insulin, which is required to convert foods like sugar, starches, and other carbs into energy. In turn, a lack of insulin or decreased insulin results in persistently elevated blood sugar and tolerance to glucose. It is most likely the oldest sickness that exists for humans. The term "black death" dates back to the fourteenth century. Blood sugar levels continue to be elevated in those who have diabetes. Type 1 diabetes (T1DM), an autoimmune illness, affects 5% of diabetics; Type 2 diabetes (T2DM), which affects 95% of people with the disease, is most frequently brought on by obesity. Other types of diabetes, which are highly uncommon and brought on by a single gene mutation, include gestational diabetes.

4.1. Type 1 Diabetes Mellitus (T1DM)

Juvenile diabetes was previously referred to as type 1 diabetes (T1DM). It is a syndrome that manifests as an autoimmune disease when the immune system targets the beta cells, which are responsible for producing Insulin. Glucose levels in the blood are regulated by the hormone insulin. Frequent urination, increased hunger, thirst, and thirstiness are common signs of this raised blood sugar. Slow wound healing, fatigue, and blurred vision are possible additional symptoms. The fundamental mechanism entails an autoimmune attack on the pancreatic beta cells. Glycated hemoglobin (HbA1C) and blood sugar levels are used to diagnose diabetes. By checking for the presence of autoantibodies, T1DM can be separated from T2DM. T1DM cannot currently be prevented [26].

For survival, insulin therapy is necessary. Insulin is often administered via subcutaneous injection, however, an insulin pump can also be used. Exercise and a diabetic diet are crucial components of management. Diabetes can lead to a wide range of consequences if ignored. Nonketotic hyperosmolar coma and diabetic Ketoacidosis are complications with a reasonably quick onset. Long-term effects include eye damage, heart problems, renal failure, foot ulcers, and foot rashes. Additionally, if more insulin is given than it reduces blood sugar levels, issues from low blood sugar may result. T1DM is thought to account for 5 to 10% of all diabetes cases. The precise number of those afflicted is unknown, despite estimates that 80,000 children worldwide develop the sickness each year [27]. Affected individuals in the US are thought to number between one and three million.

The hallmark symptom of T1DM, which often manifests in children as a few days to weeks of very high blood sugar levels, is increased urination, thirst, and weight loss. Additional symptoms that kids may suffer include poor academic performance, increased appetite, blurry vision, bedwetting, recurrent skin infections, perineal candidiasis, irritability, and increased hunger. Symptoms for T1DM in adults generally last months instead of days or weeks, and they also encompass a greater spectrum of signs and symptoms. A sustained insulin deficit can also bring on diabetes ketoacidosis. This condition manifests as dry or flushed skin, stomach discomfort, nausea, or vomiting, disorientation, trouble breathing, and a fruity breath odor.

Geographically, in some parts of Europe and North America, the percentage of children whose T1DM is brought on by an episode of diabetic Ketoacidosis can be as low as 15%, whereas it can reach as high as 80% in developing nations. When a person has T1DM, only a small subset of their body's cells, called β-cells, produce Insulin leading to a gradual insulin shortage. Diabetics have continuous hyperglycemia because their bodies lack the hormone insulin, which allows them to respond to blood sugar increases effectively [28].

For unknown reasons normally, IA-2, IA-2, and/or ZNT8 proteins will eventually be the target of antibodies after IA-2, IA-2, and/or ZNT8 Insulin or the protein GAD65. People who produce more of these antibodies and who do so earlier in life have a higher chance of developing T1DM symptoms. What led to the development of these antibodies is yet unknown. It has been suggested that the reason might be a diabetogenic trigger, a genetic predisposition, or exposure to an antigen [29].

Idiopathic T1DM, which still has an unknown origin, has cell loss but no indication of autoimmune disease, and it affects the remaining 10–30% of T1DM. Numerous environmental risks have been investigated to understand what triggers cell autoimmunity. The relationship between each risk and diabetes is frequently unclear, although several environmental and life history factors are connected to modest increases in the risk of T1DM. Children whose mothers are overweight, older than 35, or born via cesarean section have a slightly greater risk of developing T1DM.

Small relationships between T1DM risk and dietary fiber or gluten intake have been reported in animal research. Numerous potential environmental factors, such as the length of breastfeeding, have been thoroughly investigated in human research and found to be unrelated to the incidence of T1DM, including the introduction of cow milk to the diet, vitamin D intake, blood levels of active vitamin D, and maternal intake of omega-3 fatty acids [30].

A condition resembling T1DM can be developed when certain drugs decrease the synthesis of insulin or harm β-cells. In 5 to 10% of people who use the antiviral drug didanosine, pancreatic inflammation develops, occasionally leading to long-lasting β-cell destruction. Similarly, diabetes and β-cell damage occur in up to 5% of those taking the anti-protozoal drug pentamidine. Other medications including statins (which may also harm beta cells), tacrolimus and cyclosporin A used to treat post-transplant immunosuppression, L-asparaginase used to treat leukemia, and gatifloxacin used to treat infection, all induce diabetes by reversibly lowering insulin secretion. T1DM develops as a result of accidental poisoning with the rodenticide Pyrinuron (Vacor). In 1979, the American market for pyrinuron was shut down [28, 29, 31].

T1DM is recognized from other forms of diabetes. Most commercially available tests search for antibodies to glutamic acid decarboxylase, the cytoplasm of beta cells, or Insulin, all of which are the targets of antibodies in roughly 80% of T1DM. IA-2 and ZnT8 are proteins found in beta cells, which are targeted by these antibodies in about 58% and 80% of T1DM, respectively. T1DM may be indicated by extremely low C-peptide levels [32].

The frequent administration of Insulin to control hyperglycemia is the cornerstone of treatment for T1DM. Numerous times each day, subcutaneous insulin injections with a syringe or an insulin pump are necessary, with doses altering to take into account changes in food consumption, blood glucose levels, and physical activity.

Maintaining blood sugar levels between 80 to 130 mg/dL before meals and 180 mg/dL after meals is the goal of therapy.To do this, diabetics frequently check their blood glucose levels at home. The American Diabetes Association (IDA) advises checking blood sugar six to ten times a day, ideally before each meal, before exercise, at sleep, sporadically after meals, and if hypoglycemia symptoms arise [30]. Hemoglobin A1C levels around 7% is the recommended target, according to the ADA [33-39].

4.2. Type 2 Diabetes Mellitus (T2DM)

Ketoacidosis is not common; however, abrupt onset of the hyperosmolar hyperglycemic condition is possible. 90% of diabetes cases are T2DM, while T1DM diabetes, and gestational diabetes make up the majority of the remaining 10%. In T1DM, there is a lower total level of Insulin needed to regulate blood glucose because an autoimmune-induced loss of insulin-producing beta cells in the pancreas. Diabetes is diagnosed using blood tests, such as those for glycated haemoglobin, the oral glucose tolerance test, and fasting plasma glucose (A1C).

The majority of T2DM may be prevented by eating sensibly (high in fruits and vegetables and low in sugar and saturated fats), staying at a healthy weight, and exercising often. The therapy includes dietary changes and exercise. If blood sugar levels are not appropriately controlled, the medication metformin is frequently suggested. In the future, a lot more people might also need insulin injections. Routine blood sugar monitoring is indicated for those on insulin but may not be necessary for those taking tablets. Diabetes is frequently improved with bariatric surgery in obese patients. Since 1960, both T2DM and obesity rates have sharply grown. Compared to about 30 million in 1985, there were approximately 392 million persons with the condition as of 2015. Although T2DM is increasingly prevalent in young individuals, it often manifests itself in middle or older age. Ten years less life expectancy are related to T2DM. One of the first diseases to be named was diabetes, which was originally mentioned in an Egyptian book from around 1500 BCE. In the 1920s, researchers discovered the significance of insulin in the condition [40].

In addition to these, peripheral neuropathy, itching, recurrent vaginal infections, weariness, and impaired vision are other symptoms frequently present at the time of diagnosis. Taste loss is one of the potential additional symptoms. However, many people get a diagnosis after routine testing since they show no symptoms for the first several years. A tiny percentage of individuals with T2DM may experience hyperosmolar hyperglycemia. A confluence of hereditary and lifestyle factors brings on T2DM. While some of these factors, like food and obesity, are under one's control, others, including advancing age, female sex, and heredity, are not. In many places of Africa, women are more likely than males to be obese. A potential contributing factor to the nutritional state of a woman during fetal development is DNA methylation, which has been hypothesized as one possible mechanism [41, 42].

TIDM and T2DM are defined by the WHO as elevated blood sugar reading along with symptoms. Another way to diagnose diabetes is to have a glycated haemoglobin (HbA1c) level less than 48 mmol/mol (less than 6.5 DCCT%) or a random blood sugar level of greater than 11.1 mmol/L (200 mg/dL) along with typical symptoms. ADA suggested a requirement of 48 mmol/mol (6.5 DCCT%), unless the patient exhibits specific symptoms and has blood sugar levels > 11.1 mmol/L (> 200 mg/dL). The threshold for diabetes diagnosis is based on the relationship between results of glucose tolerance tests, fasting glucose, or HbA1c, and repercussions such retinal problems. Since fasting or arbitrary blood sugar levels are more practical for people, the glucose tolerance test is not advised. HbA1c has the benefits of not requiring fasting and more reliable results, but it also has the drawback of being more expensive than measuring blood glucose. According to estimates, 20% of Americans with diabetes are unaware that they have the condition [43].

In contrast to T1DM, which causes an absolute lack of Insulin due to the destruction of islet cells in the pancreas, and gestational diabetes, which is characterized by a recent onset of high blood sugars associated with pregnancy, T2DM is characterized by high blood glucose in the context of insulin resistance and relative insulin deficiency. Antibody testing may be helpful in verifying the diagnosis of T1DM if there is any doubt about it, whereas C-peptide levels could be helpful in confirming T2DM, where C-peptide levels are low in T1DM and normal or high in T2DM [43-48].

4.3. Gestational Diabetes

A woman who does not already have diabetes can acquire gestational diabetes (GD) if she has high blood sugar levels while pregnant. There are typically few symptoms associated with GD, but it raises depression, pre-eclampsia risk, and the need for a Caesarean delivery are all factors. Babies delivered to mothers with GD untreated are more likely to experience macrosomia, postpartum hypoglycemia, and jaundice. Diabetes also increases the risk of stillbirth if left untreated. Children are more likely than adults to become overweight and at the first prenatal appointment for high-risk individuals. Pregnancy exercise and maintaining a healthy weight are preventative measures. Treatment for GD includes a diabetic diet, physical activity, drug (like metformin), and occasionally insulin injections. With diet and exercise, most women can control their blood sugar. Four times a day blood sugar testing is frequently advised for people who are impacted. As soon as possible after birth, breastfeeding is advised. Depending on the demographic examined, GD affects 3-9% of pregnancies. The third trimester is when it is most prevalent. 1% of people under the age of 20, and 13% of it affects persons above the age of 44 [49].

According to the official definition, GD is "any degree of glucose intolerance with onset or first detection during pregnancy." This concept recognizes the chance that a woman has DM, which may have developed while pregnant or previously undetected. Whether symptoms disappear after delivery has no bearing on the diagnosis; if pregnancy-related glucose intolerance lasts for longer than 24 to 28 weeks, a woman is identified as having GD. The White classification, named after Priscilla White, who initiated investigations on the effect of various kinds of diabetes on perinatal outcome, is commonly used to assess maternal and fetal risk.

According to this classification scheme, gestational diabetes has two subtypes:

Type A1 results on the oral glucose tolerance test (OGTT), but normal blood sugar levels when fasting and two hours after meals; only dietary changes are required to control blood sugar levels. Due to abnormal OGTT findings and abnormal glucose levels after meals or while fasting.

Type A2 requires further therapy with insulin or other medications. Reduced health issues for both mother and child due to GD treatment with diet and insulin. More labor inductions are also done in conjunction with GD treatment. The diabetes should be confirmed to be gone 6 weeks after delivery by performing another OGTT. After then, it is suggested to regularly screen for T2DM.

After giving delivery, women with GD who get lifestyle interventions seem to have less postpartum depressive symptoms and are more likely to reach their weight reduction objectives, who receive no therapies. Additionally, they have lower birthweight percentages and a lower likelihood of having kids who are large for gestational age. Which lifestyle modifications work best will require more investigation, though. Probiotics are used by certain GD patients, but it's unclear whether they have any advantages over conventional medicine for lowering blood sugar, treating hypertension, or starting labor early. Insulin therapy may be required if oral medications, exercise or diabetic diet are insufficient to regulate blood glucose levels [49-54].

Detecting GD is done with the O'Sullivan test. A patient who is fasting is given 50 g of glucose. A blood sample is taken every hour. Plasma values over 1500 mg/L suggest GD [55].

Treatment options include insulin therapy, medication, food, exercise, stopping cigarette smoking, weight reduction, dietary recommendations, a diabetic diet, and dietary fibre are all examples of self-care. Anti-diabetic drugs, blood thinners, statins, and insulin are some examples of medications [55, 56].

4.4. Miscellaneous Types of Diabetes

4.4.1. Latent Diabetes

It is becoming clear that certain individuals may have T1DM that develops slowly and is marked because of the existence of autoantibodies. T2DM who have been diagnosed quickly become insulin-dependent; Latent diabetes

(LADA), a T1DM variant that progresses gradually, may occur in these persons. Adult-onset autoimmune diabetes is distinguished from other types of autoimmune diabetes by the lack of a diabetes-related autoantibody and the presence of a need for insulin therapy for a certain amount of time following diagnosis [57].

4.4.2. Mature Onset Diabetes of the Young (MODY)

Mature onset diabetes of the young, often known as MODY, is an autosomal dominantly inherited variant of the condition brought on by heterozygous mutations in many transcription factors involved in the development and maturation of pancreatic beta-cells. Double diabetes is defined as the incidence of hyperglycemia in children and young adults with the concomitant presence of indicators common to both T1DM and T2DM.

4.4.3. Brittle Diabetes

T1DM is intrinsically unstable, which makes the disease fragile. A small percentage of T1DM, primarily young women, have persistently poor metabolic control, which is characterized by significant instability of glycemia readings and frequent, irregular hypoglycemia or diabetic ketoacidosis episodes that cannot be ascribed to other causes. These patients' quality of life is severely diminished, especially how frequently they experience acute episodes, hospital stays, and the rapid onset of chronic problems [58].

4.4.4. Diabetes Insipidus

Increased diluted urine output due to vasopressin deficiency, AVP resistance, or excessive water consumption characterizes diabetes insipidus. When the urine volume is greater than $21/m^2/24$ hours, which is around 150 mL/Kg/24 hours at birth, 100–110 mL/Kg/24 hours till the age of 2, and 40–50 mL/Kg/24 hours in older children and adults, polyuria is present. Neonatal DM is a single gene abnormality that manifests in the first six months of life. Not producing enough insulin, not gaining weight as soon as anticipated, and misdiagnosing T1DM with high plasma glucose [59]. Among the variables that cause diabetes are excessive growth hormone, polycystic ovarian disorders, insulin receptor abnormalities, lipodystrophy, obesity, and excessive glucocorticoids.

Conclusion

The prevalence of diabetes mellitus is rising globally, and females are more likely to develop it than males. Diabetes also has an impact on youngsters. Children with diabetes often exhibit symptoms of dehydration, chronic vomiting, metabolic disturbances, or major concurrent illnesses that call for appropriate therapy and intravenous rehydration. For the treatment of diabetes, there are many well-known treatments in the market, including Metformin, Insulin injection, and other medicines. The causes of diabetes mellitus include poor lifestyle choices, smoking, drunkenness, and other issues. For people with diabetes, blood sugar levels must be under control. The vast scope of the diabetes epidemic is highlighted in the WHO global report, as well as the opportunity to halt the current course of events. The UN Political Declaration on NCDs, the WHO NCD Global Action Plan, and the Sustainable Development Goals all provide the political framework for coordinated action to combat diabetes.

References

[1] He B, Shu K I, Zhang H. *Machine learning and data mining in diabetes diagnosis and treatment.* InIOP Conference Series: Materials Science and Engineering 2019;490(4): 042049.

[2] Kaul K, Tarr J M, Ahmad S I, Kohner E M, Chibber R. Introduction to diabetes mellitus. *Diabetes*. 2013:1-1.

[3] Laios K, Karamanou M, Saridaki Z, Androutsos G. Aretaeus of Cappadocia and the first description of diabetes. *Hormones*. 2012;11(1):109-13.

[4] Poretsky L, editor. *Principles of diabetes mellitus*. Springer Science & Business Media; 2010.

[5] Amitani M, Asakawa A, Amitani H, Inui A. The role of leptin in the control of insulin-glucose axis. *Frontiers in Neuroscience*. 2013;7:51.

[6] Saeedi P, Petersohn I, Salpea P, Malanda B, Karuranga S, Unwin N, Colagiuri S, Guariguata L, Motala A A, Ogurtsova K, Shaw J E. Global and regional diabetes prevalence estimates for 2019 and projections for 2030 and 2045: Results from the International Diabetes Federation Diabetes Atlas. *Diabetes Research and Clinical Practice*. 2019;157:107843.

[7] Tönnies T, Rathmann W, Hoyer A, Brinks R, Kuss O. Quantifying the underestimation of projected global diabetes prevalence by the International Diabetes Federation (IDF) Diabetes Atlas. *BMJ Open Diabetes Research and Care*. 2021;9(1):e002122.

[8] Gold J A, Wong K K, Szablewski C M, Patel P R, Rossow J, Da Silva J, Natarajan P, Morris S B, Fanfair R N, Rogers-Brown J, Bruce B B. Characteristics and clinical

outcomes of adult patients hospitalized with COVID-19—Georgia, March 2020. *Morbidity and Mortality Weekly Report*. 2020;69(18):545.

[9] Steinmetz J D, Bourne R R, Briant P S, Flaxman S R, Taylor H R, Jonas J B, Abdoli A A, Abrha W A, Abualhasan A, Abu-Gharbieh EG, Adal TG. Causes of blindness and vision impairment in 2020 and trends over 30 years, and prevalence of avoidable blindness in relation to VISION 2020: the Right to Sight: an analysis for the Global Burden of Disease Study. *The Lancet Global Health*. 2021;9(2):e144-60.

[10] Sun H, Saeedi P, Karuranga S, Pinkepank M, Ogurtsova K, Duncan B B, Stein C, Basit A, Chan J C, Mbanya J C, Pavkov M E. IDF Diabetes Atlas: Global, regional and country-level diabetes prevalence estimates for 2021 and projections for 2045. *Diabetes Research and Clinical Practice*. 2022;183:109119.

[11] Roth G A. Global Burden of Disease Collaborative Network. Global Burden of Disease Study 2017 (GBD 2017) Results. Seattle, United States: Institute for Health Metrics and Evaluation (IHME), 2018. *The Lancet*. 2018;392:1736-88.

[12] Hulbert L R, Zhang X, Ng B P, Nhim K, Khan T, Cannon M J. Health Care Providers' Knowledge, Attitudes, and Practices and the Association With Referrals to the National Diabetes Prevention Program Lifestyle Change Program. *American Journal of Health Promotion*. 2022;36(2):236-47.

[13] Steinmetz J D, Bourne R R, Briant P S, Flaxman S R, Taylor H R, Jonas J B, Abdoli A A, Abrha W A, Abualhasan A, Abu-Gharbieh E G, Adal T G. Causes of blindness and vision impairment in 2020 and trends over 30 years, and prevalence of avoidable blindness in relation to VISION 2020: the Right to Sight: an analysis for the Global Burden of Disease Study. *The Lancet Global Health*. 2021;9(2):e144-60.

[14] Tönnies T, Rathmann W, Hoyer A, Brinks R, Kuss O. Quantifying the underestimation of projected global diabetes prevalence by the International Diabetes Federation (IDF) Diabetes Atlas. *BMJ Open Diabetes Research and Care*. 2021;9(1):e002122.

[15] United States Renal Data System. 2018 USRDS annual data report: epidemiology of kidney disease in the United States. https://www. usrds. org/adr. aspx. 2018.

[16] Yang Y, Hu X, Zhang Q, Zou R. Diabetes mellitus and risk of falls in older adults: a systematic review and meta-analysis. *Age and Ageing*. 2016;45(6):761-7.

[17] Kamal W S, Abid A H. Metaphor in Political Discourse Press Articles By Louis Bassets As A Model: La metáfora en el discurso político. Los artículos de Lluís Bassets como ejemplo. *Journal of the College of Languages (JCL)*. 2021;(44):188-223.

[18] Rockefeller J D. *Diabetes: symptoms, causes, treatment and prevention*. JD Rockefeller; 2015.

[19] Kenny C. When hypoglycemia is not obvious: diagnosing and treating under-recognized and undisclosed hypoglycemia. *Primary Care Diabetes*. 2014;8(1):3-11.

[20] Verrotti A, Scaparrotta A, Olivieri C, Chiarelli F. Seizures and type 1 diabetes mellitus: current state of knowledge. *European Journal of Endocrinology*. 2012;167(6):749-58.

[21] Khanam J J, Foo S Y. A comparison of machine learning algorithms for diabetes prediction. *ICT Express*. 2021;7(4):432-9.

[22] O'gara P T, Kushner F G, Ascheim D D, Casey Jr D E, Chung M K, De Lemos J A, Ettinger S M, Fang J C, Fesmire F M, Franklin B A, Granger C B. 2013 ACCF/AHA guideline for the management of ST-elevation myocardial infarction: executive summary: a report of the American College of Cardiology Foundation/American Heart Association Task Force on Practice Guidelines. *Circulation*. 2013;127(4): 529-55.

[23] Papatheodorou K, Banach M, Edmonds M, Papanas N, Papazoglou D. Complications of diabetes. *Journal of Diabetes Research*. 2015.

[24] Ajani R A, Oboh G, Adefegha S A, Akindahunsi A A. Free polyphenol contents, antioxidant activity and inhibition of enzymes linked with type-2-diabetes of bread produced from cocoa powder flavoured improved variety cassava-wheat composite flours: *Tropical Journal of Natural Product Research*. 2022;6(2):227-35.

[25] Heuch L, Gomersall JS. Effectiveness of offloading methods in preventing primary diabetic foot ulcers in adults with diabetes: a systematic review. *JBI Evidence Synthesis*. 2016;14(7):236-65.

[26] Rivetti G, Hursh B E, Miraglia del Giudice E, Marzuillo P. Acute and chronic kidney complications in children with type 1 diabetes mellitus. *Pediatric Nephrology*. 2022:1-0.

[27] Davies M J, Aroda V R, Collins B S, Gabbay R A, Green J, Maruthur N M, Rosas S E, Del Prato S, Mathieu C, Mingrone G, Rossing P. Management of hyperglycemia in type 2 diabetes, 2022. A consensus report by the American Diabetes Association (ADA) and the European Association for the Study of Diabetes (EASD). *Diabetes Care*. 2022;45(11): 2753-86.

[28] Winifred U, Alexander M. Biochemical Studies of the Ameliorating Effects of Bitter Leaf and Scent Leaf Extracts on Diabetes Mellitus in Humans. *International Journal of Chemistry and Chemical Processes*. 2018;4(1):29-46.

[29] Vyshnavi P, Venkatesh P. Review on diabetes mellitus. *Journal of Innovations in Applied Pharmaceutical Sciences*. 2022:24-7.

[30] Butler A E, Misselbrook D. Distinguishing between type 1 and type 2 diabetes. *British Medical Journal*. 2020;370.

[31] Al Khafaji M M, Al-Taee H A, Al-Shaikh S F. Assessment of anti-Mullerian hormone level in reproductive age group women with diabetes mellitus type one. *Middle East Fertility Society Journal*. 2017;22(4):269-72.

[32] Repaske D R. Medication-induced diabetes mellitus. *Pediatric diabetes*. 2016;17(6):392-7.

[33] Care D. 6. Glycemic targets: standards of medical care in diabetes—2019. *Diabetes Care*. 2019;42(Supplement 1):S61-70.

[34] Delli A J, Lernmark Å. Type 1 (insulin-dependent) diabetes mellitus: etiology, pathogenesis, prediction, and prevention. *Endocrinology Adult and Pediatric: Diabetes Mellitus and Obesity E-Book*. 2013:202.

[35] Fueyo-Díaz R, Magallón-Botaya R, Masluk B, Palacios-Navarro G, Asensio-Martínez A, Gascón-Santos S, Olivan-Blázquez B, Sebastián-Domingo J J. Prevalence of celiac disease in primary care: the need for its own code. *BMC Health Services Research*. 2019;19(1):1-9.

[36] Héroux P. *Principles of Toxicology*. Lulu.com; 2014.

[37] Katsarou A, Gudbjörnsdottir S, Rawshani A, Dabelea D, Bonifacio E, Anderson B J, Jacobsen L M, Schatz D A, Lernmark Å. Type 1 diabetes mellitus. *Nature Reviews Disease Primers*. 2017;3(1):1-7.

[38] Meglio A D, Molina B E, Oram R A. Type 1 diabetes. *The Lancet*. 2018;391(10138):2449-62.

[39] Repaske D R. Medication-induced diabetes mellitus. *Pediatric diabetes*. 2016;17(6): 392-7.

[40] Bellary S, Kyrou I, Brown J E, Bailey C J. Type 2 diabetes mellitus in older adults: clinical considerations and management. *Nature Reviews Endocrinology*. 2021;17(9): 534-48.

[41] Galicia-Garcia U, Benito-Vicente A, Jebari S, Larrea-Sebal A, Siddiqi H, Uribe K B, Ostolaza H, Martín C. Pathophysiology of type 2 diabetes mellitus. *International Journal of Molecular Sciences*. 2020;21(17):6275.

[42] Gardner D G, Shoback D. Chapter 18, *Pancreatic hormones and diabetes mellitus*. Greenspan's basic & clinical endocrinology (9th ed.). New York: McGraw-Hill Medical.

[43] Vos T, Allen C, Arora M, Barber R M, Bhutta Z A, Brown A, Carter A, Casey D C, Charlson F J, Chen A Z, Coggeshall M. Global, regional, and national incidence, prevalence, and years lived with disability for 310 diseases and injuries, 1990–2015: a systematic analysis for the Global Burden of Disease Study 2015. *The Lancet*. 2016; 388(10053):1545-602.

[44] Khan M M. Factors responsible for delay in initiation of insulin treatment in type-2 diabetes mellitus patients with secondary failure of oral hypoglycemic agents. *Journal of Rawalpindi Medical College*. 2016;20(4):244-50.

[45] Ma X, Jing Z, Chang P, Liu X, Montuoro R, Small R J, Bryan F O, Greatbatch R J, Brandt P, Wu D, Lin X. Western boundary currents regulated by interaction between ocean eddies and the atmosphere. *Nature*. 2016;535(7613):533-7.

[46] Maid R, Sureshkumar T. A Study to Evaluate the Reaction Time According to the Duration of Diabetes. Website: www. ijpot. com. 2019;13(3):101.

[47] Nandan S, Rao M M, Obulesu G. The study of diabetic complications in patients of newly diagnosed type 2 diabetes mellitus. *International Archives of Integrated Medicine*. 2017;4(1):38-43.

[48] Ta S. Diagnosis and classification of diabetes mellitus. *Diabetes care*. 2014;37(1): 81-90.

[49] Singh N, Kesherwani R, Tiwari A K, Patel D K. A review on diabetes mellitus. *The Pharma Innovation*. 2016;5(7, Part A):36.

[50] Siddiqui A A, Siddiqui S A, Ahmad S, Siddiqui S, Ahsan I, Sahu K. Diabetes: Mechanism, pathophysiology and management-A review. *International Journal of Drug Development and Research*. 2013;5(2).

[51] Ozougwu J C, Obimba K C, Belonwu C D, Unakalamba C B. The pathogenesis and pathophysiology of type 1 and type 2 diabetes mellitus. *Journal of Physiology and Pathophysiology*. 2013;4(4):46-57.

[52] Laugesen E, Østergaard J A, Leslie R D, Danish Diabetes Academy Workshop and Workshop Speakers. Latent autoimmune diabetes of the adult: current knowledge and uncertainty. *Diabetic Medicine*. 2015;32(7):843-52.

[53] Deepthi B, Sowjanya K, Lidiya B, Bhargavi R S, Babu P S. A modern review of diabetes mellitus: an annihilatory metabolic disorder. *Journal of In Silico & In Vitro Pharmacology* 2017;3(1).

[54] Di Iorgi N, Napoli F, Allegri A E, Olivieri I, Bertelli E, Gallizia A, Rossi A, Maghnie M. Diabetes insipidus–diagnosis and management. *Hormone Research in Paediatrics.* 2012;77(2):69-84.

[55] Okesene-Gafa K A, Moore A E, Jordan V, McCowan L, Crowther C A. Probiotic treatment for women with gestational diabetes to improve maternal and infant health and well-being. *Cochrane Database of Systematic Reviews*. 2020(6).

[56] Sheik R. Assessment of Major Complications in Pregnancy: A Single Center Study. *Asian Journal of Pharmaceutical Research and Development*. 2017:1-6.

[57] Egan A M, Dinneen S F. What is diabetes?. *Medicine*. 2019;47(1):1-4.

[58] Hirsch I B, Gaudiani L M. A new look at brittle diabetes. *Journal of Diabetes and its Complications*. 2021;35(1):107646.

[59] Refardt J, Winzeler B, Christ-Crain M. Diabetes insipidus: an update. *Endocrinology and Metabolism Clinics*. 2020;49(3):517-31.

Chapter 2

The Pathophysiology of Diabetes Mellitus

Yachana Mishra*
Aditi Chattaraj
and Kajal
School of Bioengineering and Biosciences, Lovely Professional University, Phagwara (Punjab), India

Abstract

Diabetes mellitus is a metabolic disease. The strategy for therapy and prevention of this disease may evolve due to increased knowledge of its pathophysiology. The present chapter discusses the details of the pathogenesis of T1DM.

Keywords: diabetes mellitus, pathophysiology, T1DM, blood sugar level

1. Introduction

A genetically predisposed person with Type 1 diabetes mellitus (T1DM) will experience a specific loss of insulin-producing cells in their pancreatic islets throughout a long, quiet period before symptoms manifest clinically. Early development through early childhood may see the effects of environmental influences at play. At least two years before diagnosis, the C-peptide activity is decreased [1].

---

* Corresponding Author's Email: yachanamishra@gmail.com.

In: Management of Diabetes Mellitus Based on Natural Products
Editors: Yachana Mishra and Vijay Mishra
ISBN: 979-8-88697-853-7

2. Etiopathogenesis of Type 1 Diabetes Mellitus

There is proof that T1DM is an autoimmune condition that is organ-specific and hereditary, with strong associations to certain HLA haplotypes. It is also recognized that the beginning of T1DM is caused by inappropriate activation of the innate and adaptive immune systems, which sets off a chain of events that destroys pancreatic islets.

Eisenbarth's descriptions of the successive stages are depicted as- Genetic susceptibility is a component of stage I. In stage II, the immune system is triggered by an external stimulus. Beta-cell antibodies and role of self are both present in stage III. Metabolic problems start to show up in stage IV, which causes the symptoms to appear in stage V. In stage VI, insulin dependence manifests itself. The lower half of the illustration demonstrates how CD4+, CD8+, and NKT cells contributed to the development of T1DM [1].

2.1. Genetic Factors

The epidemiology studies' observations of family histories have continued the hunt for genetic origins of T1D. Clinical, immunological, and genetic medicine can be connected through the major histocompatibility complex (MHC), and several disorders, including T1DM, have been linked to genes in the MHC. The group of WBC antigens is coded for by the most significant genes (HLA). The wide variety of HLA genes has resulted in a wide range of immune responses and disease vulnerability. A key factor in the pathophysiology of type 1 diabetes is the overexpression of HLA molecules. The short arm of chromosome 6p21 codes for the class II HLA molecules linked to type 1 diabetes (T1D) (IDDM1) [2, 3]; They have a direct role in the antigen presentation to T CD4+ cells and are in charge of selecting T cells from the T cell repertoire in the thymus. Alleles DP, DQ, and DR make up the genetic area of class II HLA, which is further broken down into subregions. There are two HLA gene combinations. Compared to the general population, those with the HLADR3-DQ2/DR4-DQ8 gene are 20 times more likely to acquire T1DM, and 90% of children with the disease carry it. 20% of the general population and less than 1% of children with T1DM have the third protective haplotype, DR15-DQ6. More common in young patients who appear in pediatrics [4-6].

On the other hand, the World Health Organization's (WHO) Diamond Project investigated whether differences in the Expression of a subset of T1DM risk genes affected the condition's occurrence in different countries [7-10]. These findings imply that HLA DQ molecules have a larger role in diabetes susceptibility [11, 12]. Additionally, as these molecules are involved in the trimolecular complex that includes a peptide and the T cell receptor of autoreactive cells that escape from the thymus, evidence of the involvement of class II HLA in pathophysiology has been seen in the murine model. I-Ag-7, a known peptide, is one of them (part of the insulin B chain) [13]. The HLA alleles are not completely penetrating, which means that not everyone who inherits them has the illness. Nevertheless, even when the connection of HLA alleles and haplotypes is substantial, these loci constitute less than 50% of the genetic contribution to disease susceptibility. This has expanded the genetic and immunological frontiers of T1DM study. Non-HLA genes account for the remaining 50% of T1BM risk.

About 40 non-HLA polymorphisms and additional potential sites have been found through genomic association analyses in population research. A polymorphism near the insulin promotor gene on chromosome 11p15.5 is among the most significant (locus IDDM2, polymorphism that consists in the number of tandem repetitions: VNTR) [14–17].

Insulin tolerance controls glucose metabolism by translating and transcribing the insulin gene in the thymus. Following genome scanning, several more susceptibility loci have been proposed (IDDM3-15). The protein tyrosine phosphatase, nonreceptor type 22 gene, which is found on chromosome 1p13, is another non-HLA gene that has been linked to T1DM. (PTPN22). The variant that substitutes arginine for a tryptophan in position 620 alters the B and T cell response and is accompanied by a reduction in T cell inhibition, promoting multi-organic autoimmunity, but the precise genes responsible have not yet been identified [18–20]. PTPN22 codes for a specific lymphocyte phosphatase that inhibits T-cell activity. Thompson et al. used flow cytometry to measure the genetic evidence for the involvement of the peripheral B cell compartment and the production of cytokines (IL-10). They did not discover any evidence of changes in IL-10 production after in vitro stimulation with IL-21, indicating that the pathogenetic role of the B cells is restricted to the early stages of the disease in the isles of Langerhans and the draining pancreatic lymph nodes [21]. One of the confirmed susceptibility loci for T1DM is IDDM12 on chromosome 2q33 [22]. At least three genes may be found in this 300-kilobase area, including CD28, CTLA-4 (cytotoxic T-lymphocyte associated protein A), and inducible gene costimulatory molecule

(ICOS). The polymorphism A49G has been linked to a decrease in the activation and proliferation of T cells because CTLA-4 codes for a molecule that is expressed on the surface of activated T cells. According to genetic mapping, the CTLA-4 gene or a gene that is closely linked to it may have a role in T1DM susceptibility [23]. Interleukin 2 receptor alpha chain (IL2RA) and induced interferon with dominion 1 helicase C (IFIH1) are additional non-HLA risk genes [24, 25]. However, it was recently shown that there was a strong correlation between the presence of autoimmune antibodies and the non-HLA risk genes. For instance, PTPN22 and anti-GAD autoantibody are associated, but ERBB3 and anti-IA-2 antibody are associated ($p = 0.042$). Likewise, anti-insulin antibodies are associated with IL2RA and INS-VNTR [26]. Other non-HLA genes include TFPR3, which regulates intracellular calcium release, BACH2, which orchestrates the activation and repression of MAFK, and UBASH3A, which encourages the accumulation of target receptors, including T cell receptors, but is not yet connected to specific antibody positivity [27].

2.2. Immunological Factors

Regarding the immunological components of T1DM, very little is categorically demonstrated. However, "an absence of evidence should not be misconstrued with proof of absence", as stated by Mannering et al. [28]. Currently, there is evidence for the autoimmune component's engagement in diverse forms. Insulitis is characterized as an inflammation of the islets of Langerhans that kills beta cells that produce insulin. The immune response is handled by cells, and Th1 cells (CD4+) work with specialized in situ Tc cells (CD8+, associated with Th2) to activate them and guide them against the beta cell, causing primary damage. Thus, the clinical manifestation of a persistent autoimmune response is the loss of 60 to 80% of the insulin-producing cells in the pancreas [29].

Dendritic cells, B and T lymphocytes, and macrophages make up the majority of the insulitis seen in the islets and its surrounds [30]. Numerous studies have demonstrated that inflammation starts to occur before tissue damage manifests, and that the loss of beta cells stimulates dendritic cells, which in turn activate T cells in the pancreas [31]. At least three islets must have at least 15 CD45+ cells each for insulinitis to be identified. Long regarded as the pathologic hallmark of type 1 diabetes, it is typically but not always seen in conjunction with beta cells that are insulin-positive [32].

Although it has been said that younger patients are typically connected with it, this relationship may perhaps be overstated. However, the majority of people with T1DM who have recently developed the disease have been shown to have insulitis [33]. However, it has been demonstrated that the occurrence of insulitis does not correlate with age at the beginning of diabetes but rather with the duration of diabetes [32]. Even after a year of insulin therapy, insulinitis is likely the primary source of T cell loss, which may help to explain some of the disease's progression [34].

Recently, it was shown that islet-invading T cells are distinct from allogeneic T cells. Patients with T1DM and those who have experienced allograft rejection have distinct characteristics. Low levels of cytokines and chemokines are found in diabetic patients [33]. To induce an antiviral state in cells, interferon induces the upregulation of interferon-stimulated genes (ISGs). GBP1, TLR3, OAS1, EIF2AK2, HLA-E, IFI6, and STAT1 are a few of them. These genes are more prevalent in type 1 diabetes and/or insulitis. It has been discovered that insulitis can boost the levels of ISGs in the peri-islet region by a factor of five. The precise contribution of this overexpression to the development of T1DM, however, is still unclear [35]. However, the development of T1D in children and adults differs. Young people have a rapid loss of beta cells (75–85%), but they also have a great capacity for regenerating new beta cells. Most of the autoantibodies found are insulin-specific. In contrast, the loss of beta cells in T1D with adult onset is more progressive (60–75%) and has a lesser chance of regeneration. More anti-GAD antibodies are present. The causes for the wide variations in the loss of C-peptide production are yet unknown [36]. The presence of T lymphocytes that produce interferon-gamma (IFN-γ) in the islet infiltrates is directly correlated with this [37–41].

In fact, Gomez-Tourino et al. suggest that CD4 T cells can be distinguished from healthy persons' CD4 T cells by the release of either IFN- or IL-17 as opposed to IL-10. They affirm that T1 (IFN-) and T17 (IL-17) play a significant role in the development of T1DM [42]. However, Mannering et al. also reported that clones of these T cells were able to detect epitopes from the proinsulin C-peptide, demonstrating that CD4+ T cells are related with HLA risk genotypes for T1D [28, 43]. The production of specific autoantibodies against pancreatic islet autoantigens is a subsequent consequence. The measurement of antibodies against autoantigens has helped to classify and forecast the clinical condition of patients, as well as to understand the activity of the illness and the degree of its development. Antibodies against glutamic acid decarboxylase (anti-GAD) are prevalent in

60–80% of newly diagnosed patients; antibodies against zinc cation transporter (ZnT8) tyrosine (anti-IA2) are present in 60–70% of patients; and anti-insulin antibodies are detectable in only 30–50% of patients [44–46]. However, the sensitivity and specificity of these autoantibodies vary with follow-up time and ethnicity.

Velluzzi et al. research demonstrate that while the hazard ratio for positivity for one of these antibodies is 55.3, it decreases to 14.5 for two positive antibodies and 3.0 for three [47]. This suggests that CD8+ T lymphocytes are the ultimate cause of beta-cell demise. The existence of antigen-specific (GAD65) and HLA-restricted versions have confirmed this. In addition to being harmful to beta cells, CD8+ T lymphocytes can be specific for a number of epitopes, including insulin, insulinoma antigen 2 (IA 2), and GAD-65 [43]. Another study has demonstrated that autoantigens such GAD65, ZnT8, and IA-2 can cause CD8+ T cells to become autoreactive [28, 34].

2.3. Environmental Factors

The rapid rise in the prevalence of T1DM in our nation and around the world cannot be solely attributed to genetics (in individuals with risk HLA haplotypes), with epigenetic modifications being those that may be crucial in relation to environmental risk factors and which are likely in line with the hygiene hypothesis, which claims that early exposure to microbes and other pathogens, as well as their byproducts, induce immunological tolerance [48]. IFIH1, also known as MDA5, or the gene linked to the development of melanoma 5 or the detection of intracellular RNA of the picornavirus, virus family that includes enterovirus, may be one connection between the genetic and environmental factors. IFIH1 and the interferon pathway are activated in response to the detection of intracellular RNA. According to a theory, enterovirus causes IFIH1 to become active in pancreatic beta cells, raise interferon levels, and enhance the Expression of MHC class I, which in turn activates CD8 T lymphocytes and kills pancreatic beta cells. The variations that arise from IFIH1 having decreased function are T1DM protective [28]. Coxsackie B, parotitis [49], and rubella [50] are a few more viruses that have been linked to the illness as potential initiators, accelerators, or precipitators [48]. The virus that has been most clearly linked to T1DM is congenital rubella syndrome, which affects children who contract the infection while still in the womb. This syndrome carries a 30% risk of developing the disease between 5 and 30 years later, but this only accounts for a small portion of cases. Numerous viruses employ a variety of strategies that eventually result in beta-cell death. When the rubella virus is present, it triggers two-way interactions between the antigens and GAD, causing T lymphocyte activity to be stimulated and resulting in beta-cell infection. The cytomegalovirus also infects beta cells, but it does so via inducing the migration of macrophages to the pancreas through clonal activation of T cells. While rotavirus infects cells by molecular mimicry, the mumps causes increased Expression of class I and II HLA in beta cells. Instead of infecting beta cells, the parvovirus employs macrophages to stimulate a Th1 immune response while also boosting Th2 responses [51]. It has been proposed that beta cells, but not alpha cells, undergo apoptosis during the onset and progression of T1DM may be partially explained by the inability to promptly treat viral infections [52].

According to the "bystander theory," pancreatic cell infection produces pro-inflammatory cytokines, which might account for the aforementioned cell death [53, 54]. Due to inconsistent experimental data, the "molecular mimicry" process attributed to rotavirus, among other things, is still debatable [53, 55]. In reality, there are several ways that infection can prevent or postpone the onset of T1DM. There is a reciprocal adaptation over time. Infections that cause the release of immunoregulatory cytokines, such IL-10, aid in regulating inflammation, support regulatory T cell activity and stimulate NKT cell activity. On the other hand, Th1 responses are inhibited by activated macrophages and "tolerogenic" dendritic cells by a number of methods, including redirecting the response to Th2, activating T cells, and releasing enzymes that break down amino acids. Tissue pathology is restricted by this action [56]. However, because of improvements in methods to identify it, the Enterovirus genus has received considerable attention in relation to T1DM. The majority of viruses that cause illness in people, including foot-and-mouth disease and poliomyelitis, are enteroviruses. Since the majority are highly resistant to medicines and the chlorine that is often added to treated water, they can spread through soil, food, and water. The Coxsackie family, most notably Coxsackie B, belongs to this genus. In a pancreatic biopsy from a patient with T1DM, one investigation discovered enteroviral genomes in the islets [57]. In the Diabetes Virus Detection Study (DiViD), enterovirus was discovered in every sample of insulin-containing pancreatic islets from individuals with recently developed T1DM (within 10 weeks) [58]. This lends credence to the theory that viral infection occurs before diabetes manifests. The same findings have been found by a number of other pediatric investigations, including VirDiab [59] and the research by Laitinen et al. [60], both of which compared type 1 diabetic children to controls who appeared to be in good condition. With the mounting body of data, it has been hypothesised that the enterovirus infection, and perhaps other viral infections as well, may be the tipping point and cause a major loss of beta cells by tipping an already imbalanced metabolism over the edge [61]. On the other hand, nutrition, particularly during the lactation period, is one of the environmental risk factors that has been researched. Diet can affect intestinal microbiota, which is one of the processes that affect T1DM. Early exposure to cow's milk and highly hydrolyzed casein formula has been linked in several studies [62–65] to the development of autoimmunity in some genetically vulnerable people. Studies on the relationship between vitamin D, yet another hypothesised component, and the onset of T1DM are still debatable [66, 67]. The C-reactive protein and a number of cytokines, such as IFN-, TNF-, IL-6, IL-1, IL-4, and IL-10, were found to significantly correlate inversely with vitamin D in a recent research [68].

2.4. Microbiota

Numerous variables, such as nutrition, way of life, usage of antibiotics, type of delivery (natural or caesarean), and breastfeeding, impact the development of intestinal microbiota. It is well recognized that a healthy balance of the gut microbiota is crucial for many physiological processes, including the operation of the immune system. It has been proposed that the development of T1DM is associated with dysbiosis, an imbalance in the gut microbiota. Nutrition changes impact gut microbiota development, as shown by the strong connection between T1D and celiac disease. As diets alter and become more "westernized," these facts may aid in explaining why T1D is on the rise worldwide [69]. In light of these findings, a number of recent investigations have compared the microbiome profiles of healthy and T1DM people. Spanish research of this kind discovered considerable variations in Bifidobacterium, Lactobacillus, and Clostridium. Compared to controls, patients showed greater amounts of Clostridium and lower levels of Bifidobacterium, which may be related to glycemic level. Additionally, they discovered that children with T1DM had lower-quality bacteria than healthy controls [70]. Another investigation of Mexican toddlers in Sonora revealed that whereas healthy kids had high levels of Prevotella, newly diagnosed T1DM sufferers had high levels of Bacteroides. However, the levels of both bacteria had recovered to that of the healthy children after 2 years of therapy, showing that dietary modifications were likely involved and the potential for employing microbiota treatments to lower the risk of acquiring diabetes [71]. However, children with obesity had higher levels of Lactobacillus and lower levels of Bacteroidetes than children with T1D, indicating a significant difference between the two situations [71, 72]. However, in addition to the gut microbiota makeup, this difference could also be influenced by other elements, including hereditary risk. Probiotic supplementation was linked to a lower incidence of islet autoimmunity in a section of the TEDDY trial that included American and European children, but only in those with the high-risk genotype (DR3/4). The lack of any advantage in other genotypes might point to a treatment plan for people at high risk [73]. Before using this type of therapy, further study will be required, including that on genetics, the impact of infections, and the many other variables that alter microbiota profiles.

2.5. Role of NKT Cells

The involvement of acquired autoimmunity in T1DM, which corresponds to the increase and/or function of the population of regulatory T cells, is also caused by a change in the regulatory systems of acquired autoimmunity. In the development of the illness, the interplay of the immune systems, innate and adaptive is undeniable. Complex immune system reactions have developed to defend multicellular creatures against invaders; but, due to selective pressure from evolution, some of these responses may also cause tissue damage to the organisms.

The immune system is divided into two distinct parts: an innate arm that may mount nonspecific responses fast and an adaptive arm that can support more sustained, targeted responses. To perform these tasks, specialized cells have arisen due to evolution. Some cells possess both intrinsic and adaptive skills or mixed abilities. Acknowledging the physiopathology of several autoimmune illnesses, including T1DM, may depend on this cellular group. Additionally, they have just been connected to type 2 diabetes [74]. Both arms' cellular surface markers and functions are shared. Additionally, they play a key role in the homeostatic control of the immune system due to their evolutionary persistence across species. T lymphocytes CD4+CD25+ and natural killer lymphocyte type (NKT) cells are two options, albeit the regulatory cell population has not yet been precisely determined. NKT were first discovered in mice in 1987 [75]; subsequently, its human homologue was discovered. They are a group of lymphocytes that exhibit the T lymphocyte antigen (TCR) receptor as well as the universal NK cell signature (NK 1.1 for mice and CD161 in humans). These individuals exhibit a repertoire of conserved TCRs [76], which are composed of variable regions V24 and V11 in humans. The aforementioned heterogeneous population can be CD4+, CD4CD8 (double negatives), or even CD8+. NKT distinguish lipids in the presence of CD1d molecules, in contrast to most T cells. They react to antigens presented in the context of CD1d molecules, and their crucial regulatory function is carried out by releasing cytokines like INF- or IL-4 [77, 78].

At the location of inflammation, NKT cells are present in large numbers and may be a marker of diabetes risk. The relative frequency of particular tolerogenic dendritic cell subsets correlates with the number of NKT cells. According to Naumov et al. research's using non-obese diabetic mice models (NOD) [79], it appears that NKT cells regulate diabetes by altering the frequency and perhaps the function of dendritic cell subsets. They play a crucial part in the body's defense against bacteria, viruses, and parasites in addition to playing a function in immunological modulation and tumor protection. The key findings in autoimmune and inflammation came from NOD mice that did not develop diabetes [80]. The sickness may be lessened with the transfection of populations high in NKT cells because several studies demonstrate a deficiency in the amount and functionality of NKT cells in these animals [81–84]. The pathogenesis of T1DM is mediated by the numerical and functional deficit of NKT cells, which was discovered in the thyroid and spleen of NOD mice at 3 weeks of age. However, the stage of T cell development at which this deficit develops is still unclear.

According to Wagner et al. hypothesis's [85], the formation of the thymus in NOD mice has a deficiency in this lineage, which is shared by conventional T cells and doubly negative NKT. According to some data, the risk alleles IDD9 and IDD6 (locus Idd9.1, Idd6, Nkt1, and NKt2) for the condition may code for a lack of NKT cells [86–88]. In the past ten years, some investigations in humans have shown a decrease in the frequencies of NKT cells and their capacity to produce IL-4 in patients with T1D [89], while others have shown an increase in these cells' frequency [90–92]. On the other hand, during T1DM, both the frequency of NKT and the production of IL-4 are maintained. There were no differences between the T1DM group and the healthy control group in a recent study of Colombian patients with T2DM and autoimmune thyroid abnormalities, however, the numbers of NKT cells were higher in T2DM patients [93]. Since it has recently been hypothesized that the subset of CD4+ NKT cells may be activated in the prevention of autoimmune disease while the subset of double negative NKT (CD4- CD8-) may be pathogenic, the discrepancy in the data appears to be caused by the type of population chosen for the study, as well as the status of the patient in relation to the natural history of the disease, or the subpopulation of NKT cells quantified in those studies. To prove this hypothesis, In individuals at risk, the findings revealed an expansion and rise of double-negative NKT cells (CD4CD8) [94]. Our research team discovered a decrease in NKT cells in addition to identifying two populations within these cells: a majority population that expressed high levels of invariant TCR (V24/V11) and a minority population that expressed low levels of invariant TCR in children with T1DM and their first-degree relatives [95–97]. The activation marker CRTAM (class I-restricted T cell-associated molecule) was shown to be expressed in this subgroup [95]. Additionally expressed on CD4+ and CD8+ T cells, CRTAM is linked to inflammation. In NKT cells with low invariant TCR, CRTAM and CD69 are both expressed, indicating an activated state [96]. Further evidence that CRTAM may be utilised as a marker to identify the NKT cells comes from the observation of a strong correlation between the Expression of CRTAM and the production of IFN- in NKT cells in both healthy and type 1 diabetic person [98]. On the other hand, class II MHC molecules include cathepsinL lysosomal protease (CTSL), which significantly impacts the Expression of antigen-presenting cells and broad influence on the immune system. It has been demonstrated in CTSL nkt/nkt mice that the CTSL gene's activity affects the positive selection of CD4+ thymocytes and controls the expression level of different extracellular matrix components in lymphoid organs, affecting the number and makeup of central and peripheral T lymphoids [99]. However, the function of NKT cells and CTSL gene expression in humans as a biomarker in the physiopathology of T1DM has not yet been fully demonstrated. It was recently demonstrated that low levels of CTSL gene expression in T1D in humans correlate with both the percentage and absolute numbers of NKT cells, supporting the theory that CTSL is involved in the enhancement of cytotoxic T lymphocyte survival [100].

Conclusion

The whole etiology of T1DM is still a mystery. What is understood is that a wide range of variables contributes to the development of this disease. Genetically, PTPN22, CTLA-4, and IFIH1 are examples of non-HLA genes related to 50% of T1D susceptibility and HLA genes connected with the remaining 50%. New candidates for the latter are continually being found via research. The alleles associated with risk or protection against the onset of T1DM differ by nation and racial group. Furthermore, two or more autoantigen antibodies are a significant risk indication. The involved environmental variables probably have a substantial role in the sharp rise in the prevalence of T1DM. Genetic overexpression in response insulitis has been identified thanks to technological advancements. Dysbiosis has been connected to the etiology of T1D and is implicated in immune system changes. This crucial component of the disease's epigenetics is the subject of current research. Finally, NKT cells, which may be a marker of diabetes risk, are present in considerable quantities near the site of inflammation. They have drawn attention because they are involved in both innate and adaptive autoimmunity. The clinical use of this is still being researched.

References

[1] Atkinson MA, Eisenbarth GS, Michels AW. Type 1 diabetes. *Lancet.* 2014;383(9911):69–82.

[2] Todd JA, Bell JI, McDevitt HO. HLA-DQ gene contributes to susceptibility and resistance to IDDM. *Nature*. 1987;329:599–604.

[3] Undlien DE, Lie BA, Thorsby E. HLA complex genes in type 1 diabetes and other autoimmune diseases. Which genes are involved? *Trends Genet*. 2001;17:93–100.

[4] Caillat-Zucman S, Garchon HJ, Timsit J, Assan, R., Boitard, C., Djilali-Saiah, I., & Bach, J. F. Age-dependent HLA genetic heterogeneity of type 1 insulin-dependent diabetes mellitus. *J Clin Invest.* 1992;90:2242–50.

[5] Knip M, Siljander H. Autoimmune mechanisms in type 1 diabetes. *Autoimmun Rev*. 2008;7:550–7.

[6] Lambert AP, Gillespie KM, Thomson G, Cordell, HJ, Todd, JA, Gale, EAM, Bingleyet, PJ. Absolute risk of childhood-onset type 1 diabetes defined by human leukocyte antigen class II genotype: a population-based study in the United Kingdom. *J Clin Endocrinol Metab*. 2004;89:4037–43.

[7] Dorman JS, McCarthy B, McCanlies E, Kramer MK, Vergona RJ, Stone R, Steenkiste AR, Kocova M, Trucco M. Molecular IDDM epidemiology: international studies. WHO DiaMond Molecular Epidemiology Sub-Project Group. *Diabetes Res Clin Pract*. 1996;34 Suppl:S107–16.

[8] Notkins AL. Immunologic and genetic factors in type 1 diabetes. *J Biol Chem.* 2002;277:43545–8.

[9] Erlich HA, Zeidler A, Chang J, Shaw S, Raffel LJ, Klitz W, Beshkov Y, Costin G, Pressman S, Bugawan T, Rotter JI. HLA class II alleles and susceptibility and resistance to insulin dependent diabetes mellitus in Mexican-American families. *Nat Genet*. 1993;3:358–64.

[10] Godoresky C, Olivares A, Debezo H, Rodriguez L, Altamirano N, Robles C. MHC-dependent molecular mechanisms of susceptibility and protection in type 1 diabetes in Mexicans. *Gac Med Mex*. 1995;131:395–402.

[11] Thorsby E, Gjertsen HA, Lundin KE, Rønningen KS. Insulin dependent diabetes mellitus susceptibility or protection may be determined by certain HLA-DQ molecules. *Bailliere Clin Endocrinol Metab.* 1991;5:361–73.

[12] Vicario JL, Martinez-Laso J, Corell A, Martin-Villa JM, Morales P, Lledo G, Segurado OG, De Juan D, Arnaiz-Villena A. Comparison between HLA-DRB and DQ DNA sequences and classic serological markers as type 1 (insulin-dependent) diabetes mellitus predictive risk markers in the Spanish population. *Diabetologia.* 1992;35:475–81.

[13] Eisenbarth GS. Banting lecture 2009: an unfinished journey: molecular pathogenesis to prevention of type 1A diabetes. *Diabetes*. 2010;59:759–74.

[14] Thomson G, Robinson W, Kuhner M, Joe S, Klitz W. HLA and insulin gene associations with IDDM. *Genet Epidemiol.* 1989;6:155–60.

[15] Bennett ST, Lucassen AM, Gough SCL, Powell EE, Undlien DE, Pritchard LE, Merriman ME, Kawaguchi Y, Dronsfield MJ, Pociot F, Nerup J. susceptibility to human type 1 diabetes at IDDM2 is determined by tandem repeat variation at the insulin gene minisatellite locus. *Nat Genet.* 1995;9:284–92.

[16] Bell GI, Horita S, Karam JH. A polymorphic locus near the human insulin gene is associated with insulin-dependent diabetes mellitus. *Diabetes*. 1984;33:176–83.

[17] Todd JA, Farrall M. Panning for gold: genome-wide scanning for linkage in type 1 diabetes. *Hum Mol Genet*. 1995;5:1443–8.

[18] Pugliese A, Miceli D. The insulin gene in diabetes. *Diabetes Metab Res Rev.* 2002;18:13–25.

[19] Davies JL, Kawaguchi Y, Bennett ST, Copeman JB, Cordell HJ, Pritchard LE, Reed PW, Gough SC, Jenkins SC, Palmer SM, Balfour KM. A genome-wide search for human type 1 diabetes susceptibility genes. *Nature*. 1994;371:130–6.

[20] Bottini N, Musumeci L, Alonso A, Rahmouni S, Nika K, Rostamkhani M, MacMurray J, Meloni GF, Lucarelli P, Pellecchia M, Eisenbarth GS. A functional variant of lymphoid tyrosine phosphatase is associated with type I diabetes. *Nat Genet*. 2004;36:337–8.

[21] Thompson WS, Pekalski ML, Simons HZ, Smyth DJ, Castro-Dopico X, Guo H, Guy C, Dunger DB, Arif S, Peakman M, Wallace C. Multi-parametric flow cytometric and genetic investigation of the peripheral B cell compartment in human type 1 diabetes. *Clin Exp Immunol*. 2014;177:571–85.

[22] Marron MP, Zeidler A, Raffel LJ, Eckenrode SE, Yang JJ, Hopkins DI, Garchon HJ, Jacob CO, Serrano-Rios M, Martinez Larrad MT, Park Y. Genetic and physical mapping of a type 1 diabetes susceptibility gene (IDDM12) to a 100-kb phagemid artificial chromosome clone containing D2S72-CTLA4-D2S105 on chromosome 2q33. *Diabetes*. 2000;49:492–9.

[23] Ueda H, Howson JMM, Esposito L, Heward J, Chamberlain G, Rainbow DB, Hunter KM, Smith AN, Di Genova G, Herr MH, Dahlman I. Association of the T cell regulatory gene CTLA4 with susceptibility to autoimmune disease. *Nature.* 2003;423:506–11.

[24] Tang W, Cui D, Jiang L, Zhao L, Qian W, Long SA, Xu K. Association of common polymorphisms in the IL2RA gene with type 1 diabetes: evidence of 32,646 individuals from 10 independent studies. *J Cell Mol Med*. 2015;19:2481–8.

[25] Liu S, Wang H, Jin Y, Podolsky R, Reddy MP, Pedersen J, Bode B, Reed J, Steed D, Anderson S, Yang P. IFIH1 polymorphisms are significantly associated with type 1 diabetes and IFIH1 gene expression in peripheral blood mononuclear cells. *Hum Mol Genet.* 2009;18:358–65.

[26] Maziarz M, Hagopian W, Palmer JP, Sanjeevi CB, Kockum I, Breslow N, Lernmark Å. Diabetes incidence in Sweden study group; type 1 diabetes genetics consortium. Non-HLA type 1 diabetes genes modulate disease risk together with HLA-DQ and islet autoantibodies. *Genes Immun*. 2015;16:541–51.

[27] http://www.t1base.org/page/Welcome/display.

[28] Mannering SI, Pathiraja V, Kay TW. The case for an autoimmune aetiology of type 1 diabetes. *Clin Exp Immunol.* 2016;183:8–15.

[29] Foulis AK, Liddle CN, Farquharson MA, Richmond JA, Weir RS. The histopathology of the pancreas in type 1 (insulin-dependent) diabetes mellitus: a 25 years review of deaths in patients under 20 years of age in the United Kingdom. *Diabetologia.* 1986;29:267–74.

[30] Willcox A, Richardson SJ, Bone AJ, Foulis AK, Morgan NG. Analysis of islet inflammation in human type 1 diabetes. *Clin Exp Immunol.* 2009;155:173–81.

[31] Barcala Tabarrozzi AE, Castro CN, Dewey RA, Sogayar MC, Labriola L, Perone MJ. Cell-based interventions to halt autoimmunity in type 1 diabetes mellitus. *Clin Exp Immunol*. 2013;171:135–46.

[32] Pugliese A. Insulitis in the pathogenesis of type 1 diabetes. *Pediatr Diabetes*. 2016;17(Suppl 22):31–6.

[33] Krogvold L, Wiberg A, Edwin B, Buanes T, Jahnsen FL, Hanssen KF, Larsson E, Korsgren O, Skog O, Dahl-Jørgensen K. Insulitis and characterisation of infiltrating T cells in surgical pancreatic tail resections from patients at onset of type 1 diabetes. *Diabetologia.* 2016;59:492–501.

[34] Zubkiewicz-Kucharska A, Noczyńska A. Abnormal distribution of gamma-delta T lymphocytes and their subsets in type 1 diabetes. *Adv Clin Exp Med.* 2016;25:665–71.

[35] Lundberg M, Krogvold L, Kuric E, Dahl-Jørgensen K, Skog O. Expression of interferonstimulated genes in insulitic pancreatic islets of patients recently diagnosed with type 1 diabetes. *Diabetes.* 2016;65:3104–10.

[36] von Herrath MG, Korsgren O, Atkinson MA. Factors impeding the discovery of an intervention-based treatment for type 1 diabetes. *Clin Exp Immunol.* 2016;183(1):1–7.

[37] Hannirn A, Jalkanen S, Salmi M, Toikkanen S, Nikolakaros G, Simell O. Macrophages, T cell receptor usage, and endothelial cell activation in the pancreas at the onset of insulin-dependent diabetes mellitus. *J Clin Invest*. 1992;90:1901–10.

[38] Imagawa A, Hanafusa T, Tamura S, Moriwaki M, Itoh N, Yamamoto K, Iwahashi H, Yamagata K, Waguri M, Nanmo T, Uno S. Pancreatic biopsy as a procedure for detecting in situ autoimmune phenomena in type 1 diabetes. Close correlation

between serological markers and a histological evidence of cellular autoimmunity. *Diabetes*. 2001;50:1269–73.

[39] Rabinovitch A, Suares-Pinzon WL, Sorensen O, Bleackley RC, Power RF. INF-γ gene expression in pancreatic islet-infiltrating mononuclear cells correlates with autoimmune diabetes in nonobese diabetic mice. *J Immunol*. 1995;154:4878–82.

[40] Foulis AK, McGill M, Farquharson MA. Insulitis in type 1 (insulin- dependent) diabetes mellitus in ma-macrophages, lymphocytes, and interferon-gamma containing cells. *J Pathol*. 1991;165:97–103.

[41] Fowlkes BJ, Kruisbeek AM, Ton-That H, Fowlkes BJ, Kruisbeek AM, Ton-That H, Weston MA, Coligan JE, Schwartz RH, Pardoll DM. A novel population of T-cell receptor alpha beta-bearing thymocytes which predominantly expresses a single V beta gene family. *Nature*. 1987;329:251–4.

[42] Gomez-Tourino I, Arif S, Eichmann M, Peakman M. T cells in type 1 diabetes: instructors, regulators and effectors: a comprehensive review. *J Autoimmun*. 2016;66:7–16.

[43] Pathiraja V, Kuehlich JP, Campbell PD, Krishnamurthy B, Loudovaris T, Coates PT, Brodnicki TC, O'Connell PJ, Kedzierska K, Rodda C, Bergman P. Proinsulin-specific, HLA-DQ8, and HLA-DQ8-transdimer-restricted CD4+ T cells infiltrate islets in type 1 diabetes. *Diabetes*. 2015;64:172–82.

[44] Verge CF, Gianani R, Kawasaki E, Yu L, Pietropaolo M, Chase HP, Eisenbarth GS, Jackson RA. Prediction of type I diabetes in first-degree relatives using a combination of insulin, GAD, and ICA512bdc/IA-2 autoantibodies. *Diabetes*. 1996;45:926–33.

[45] Leslie D, Lipsky P, Notkins AL. Autoantibodies as predictors of disease. *J Clin Invest*. 2001;108:1417–22.

[46] Wenzlau JM, Juhl K, Yu L, Moua O, Sarkar SA, Gottlieb P, Rewers M, Eisenbarth GS, Jensen J, Davidson HW, Hutton JC. The cation efflux transporter ZnT8 (Slc30A8) is a major autoantigen in human type 1 diabetes. *Proc Natl Acad Sci USA*. 2007;104:17040–5.

[47] Velluzzi F, Secci G, Sepe V, Sardinian Autoimmunity Study Group, Klersy C, Shattock M, Foxon R, Songini M, Mariotti S, Locatelli M, Bottazzo GF, Loviselli A. Prediction of type 1 diabetes in Sardinian schoolchildren using islet cell autoantibodies: 10-year follow-up of the Sardinian schoolchildren type 1 diabetes prediction study. *Acta Diabetol*. 2016;53(1):73–9.

[48] Von Herrath MG, Holz A, Homann D, Oldstone MB. Role of viruses in type I diabetes. Role of viruses in type I diabetes. *Semin Immunol*. 1998;10:87–100.

[49] Hyoty H, Hiltunen M, Reuranen A, Leinikki P, Vesikari T, Lounamaa R, Tuomilehto J, Åkerblom HK, Childhoood Diabetes in Finland Study Group, Toivanen L, Kaprio EA. Decline of mumps antibodies in type 1(insulin-dependent) diabetic children with a plateau in the rising incidence of type 1 diabetes after introduction of the mumps-measles-rubella vaccine in Finland. *Diabetologia*. 1993;36:1303–8

[50] McIntosh EDG, Menser M. A fifty-year follow-up of congenital rubella. *Lancet*. 1992;340:414–5.

[51] Tavares RG, Trevisol RB, Comerlato J, Dalzochio T, Feksa LR, Spilki FR, Berlese DB. Enterovirus infections and type 1 diabetes mellitus: is there any relationship? *J Venom Anim Toxins Incl Trop Dis*. 2012;18:3–15.

[52] de Beeck AO, Eizirik DL. Viral infections in type 1 diabetes mellitus – why the β cells? *Nat Rev Endocrinol*. 2016;12:263–73.

[53] Petzold A, Solimena M, Knoch KP. Mechanisms of Beta cell dysfunction associated with viral infection. *Curr Diab Rep*. 2015;15:73.

[54] Seewaldt S, Thomas HE, Ejrnaes M, Christen U, Wolfe T, Rodrigo E, Coon B, Michelsen B, Kay TW, von Herrath MG. Virus-induced autoimmune diabetes: most beta-cells die through inflammatory cytokines and not perforin from autoreactive (anti-viral) cytotoxic T-lymphocytes. *Diabetes*. 2000;49:1801–9.

[55] Honeyman MC, Stone NL, Falk BA, Nepom G, Harrison LC. Evidence for molecular mimicry between human T cell epitopes in rotavirus and pancreatic islet autoantigens. *J Immunol*. 2010;15(184):2204–10.

[56] Cooke A. Review series on helminths, immune modulation and the hygiene hypothesis: how might infection modulate the onset of type 1 diabetes? *Immunology*. 2009;126:12–7.

[57] Ylipaasto P, Klingel K, Lindberg AM, Otonkoski T, Kandolf R, Hovi T, Roivainen M. Enterovirus infection in human pancreatic islet cells, islet tropism in vivo and receptor involvement in cultured islet beta cells. *Diabetologia*. 2004;47:225–39.

[58] Krogvold L, Edwin B, Buanes T, Ludvigsson J, Korsgren O, Hyöty H, Frisk G, Hanssen KF, Dahl-Jørgensen K. Pancreatic biopsy by minimal tail resection in live adult patients at the onset of type 1 diabetes: experiences from the DiViD study. *Diabetologia*. 2014;57:841–3.

[59] Oikarinen S, Tauriainen S, Hober D, Lucas B, Vazeou A, Sioofy-Khojine A, Bozas E, Muir P, Honkanen H, Ilonen J, Knip M. Virus antibody survey in different European populations indicates risk association between coxsackie virus B1 and type 1 diabetes. *Diabetes*. 2014;63:655–62.

[60] Laitinen OH, Honkanen H, Pakkanen O, Oikarinen S, Hankaniemi MM, Huhtala H, Ruokoranta T, Lecouturier V, André P, Harju R, Virtanen SM. Coxsackievirus B1 is associated with induction of β-cell autoimmunity that portends type 1 diabetes. *Diabetes*. 2014;63:446–55.

[61] Rodriguez-Calvo T, von Herrath MG. Enterovirus infection and type 1 diabetes: closing in on a link? *Diabetes*. 2015;64:1503–5.

[62] Nucci AM, Virtanen SM, Becker DJ. Infant feeding and timing of complementary foods in the development of type 1 diabetes. *Curr Diab Rep*. 2015;15:62.

[63] Griebler U, Bruckmüller MU, Kien C, Dieminger B, Meidlinger B, Seper K, Hitthaller A, Emprechtinger R, Wolf A, Gartlehner G. Health effects of cow's milk consumption in infants up to 3 years of age: a systematic review and meta-analysis. *Public Health Nutr*. 2016;19:293–307.

[64] Krishna CS, Srikanta S. Type 1 diabetes pathogenesis – prevention??? *Indian J Endocrinol Metab*. 2015;19(Suppl 1):S58–63.

[65] Lamb MM, Miller M, Seifert JA, Frederiksen B, Kroehl M, Rewers M, Norris JM. The effect of childhood cow's milk intake and HLA-DR genotype on risk of islet

autoimmunity and type 1 diabetes: the diabetes autoimmunity study in the young. *Pediatr Diabetes*. 2015;16:31–8.

[66] Liu C, Lu M, Xia X, Wang J, Wan Y, He L, Li M. Correlation of serum vitamin D level with type 1 diabetes mellitus in children: a meta-analysis. *Nutr Hosp.* 2015;32:1591–4.

[67] Mäkinen M, Mykkänen J, Koskinen M, Simell V, Veijola R, Hyöty H, Ilonen J, Knip M, Simell O, Toppari J. Serum 25-hydroxyvitamin D concentrations in children progressing to autoimmunity and clinical type 1 diabetes. *J Clin Endocrinol Metab.* 2016;101:723–9.

[68] Talaat IM, Nasr A, Alsulaimani AA, Alghamdi H, Alswat KA, Almalki DM, Abushouk A, Saleh AM, Allam G. Association between type 1, type 2 cytokines, diabetic autoantibodies and 25-hydroxyvitamin D in children with type 1 diabetes. *J Endocrinol Investig*. 2016;39(12):1425–34.

[69] Gianchecchi E, Fierabracci A. On the pathogenesis of insulindependent diabetes mellitus: the role of microbiota. *Immunol Res.* 2017;65(1):242–56.

[70] Murri M, Leiva I, Gomez-Zumaquero JM, Tinahones FJ, Cardona F, Soriguer F, Queipo-Ortuño MI. Gut microbiota inchildren with type 1 diabetes differs from that in healthy children: a case-control study. *BMC Med*. 2013;11:46.

[71] Mejía-León ME, Petrosino JF, Ajami NJ, Domínguez-Bello MG, de la Barca AM. Fecal microbiota imbalance in Mexican children with type 1 diabetes. *Sci Rep.* 2014;4:3814.

[72] Armougom F, Henry M, Vialettes B, Raccah D, Raoult D. Monitoring bacterial community of human gut microbiota reveals an increase in lactobacillus in obese patients and methanogens in anorexic patients. *PLoS One*. 2009;4(9):e7125.

[73] Uusitalo U, Liu X, Yang J, Aronsson CA, Hummel S, Butterworth M, Lernmark Å, Rewers M, Hagopian W, She JX, Simell O. Association of early exposure of probiotics and islet autoimmunity in the TEDDY study. *JAMA Pediatr.* 2016;170(1):20–8.

[74] Tard C, Rouxel O, Lehuen A. Regulatory role of natural killer T cells in diabetes. *Biom J.* 2015;38:484–95.

[75] Porcelli S, Yockey CE, Brenner MB, Balk SP. Analysis of T cell antigen receptor (TCR) expression by human peripheral blood CD4-8- alpha/beta T cells demonstrates preferential use of several Vß genes and an invariant TCR alpha chain. *J Exp Med.* 1993;178:1–16.

[76] Baxter AG, Hammond KJ, Scollay R, Godfrey DI. Association between alphabeta TCR+CD-CD- T-cell deficiency and IDMM in NOD/Lt mice. *Diabetes.* 1997;46:572–82.

[77] Lantz O, Bendelac A. An invariant T cell receptor alpha chain is used by a unique subset of MHC class I-specific CD4+ and CD4- 8- T cells in mice and humans. *J Exp Med*. 1994;180:1097–106.

[78] Kronenberg M, Gapin L. The unconventional lifestyle of NKT cells. *Nat Rev Immunol*. 2002;2:557–8.

[79] Naumov YN, Bahjat KS, Gausling R, Abraham R, Exley MA, Koezuka Y, Balk SB, Strominger JL, Clare-Salzer M, Wilson SB. Activation of CD1drestricted T cells

protects NOD mice from developing diabetes by regulating dendritic cell subsets. *Proc Natl Acad Sci USA*. 2001;98:13838–43.

[80] Hammond KJ, Pellicci DG, Poulton LD, Naidenko OV, Scalzo AA, Baxter AG, Godfrey DI. CD1drestricted NKT cells: an interstrain comparison. *J Immunol.* 2001;167:1164–73.

[81] Lehuen A, Lantz O, Beaudoin L, Laloux V, Carnaud C, Bendelac A, Bach JF, Monteiro RC. Overexpression of natural killer T cells protects Va14-Ja281 transgenic nonobese mice against diabetes. *J Exp Med.* 1998;188:1831–9.

[82] Falcone M, Brian Y, Tucker L, Rodriguez E, Sarvetnick N. A defect in interleukin 12-induced activation and interferon-gamma secretion of peripheral natural killer T cells in nonobese diabetic mice suggests new pathogenic mechanism for insulin-dependent diabetes mellitus. *J Exp Med.* 1999;190:963–72.

[83] Poulon LD, Smyth MJ, Hawke CG, Silveira P, Shepherd D, Naidenko OV, Godfrey DI, Baxter AG. Cytometric and functional analysis of NK- and NKT cell deficiencies in NOD mice. *Int Immunol.* 2001;13:887–96.

[84] Berzins SP, Kyparissoudis K, Pellicci DG, Hammond KJ, Sidobre S, Baxter A, Smyth MJ, Kronenberg M, Godfrey DI. Systemic NKT cell deficiency in NOD mice is not detected in peripheral blood: implications for human studies. *Immunol Cell Biol*. 2004;82:247–52.

[85] Wagner MJD, Hussain S, Mehan M, Verdi JM, Delovitch TL. A defect in lineage fate decision during fetal thymic invariant NKT cell development may regulate susceptibility to type 1 diabetes. *J Immunol.* 2005;174:6764–71.

[86] Carnaud C, Gombert J, Donnars O, Garchon HJ, Herbelin A. Protection against diabetes and improved NK/NKT cell performance in NOD.NK1.1 mice congenic at the NK complex. *J Immunol.* 2001;166:2404–11.

[87] Esteban LM, Tsoutsman T, Jordan MA, Roach D, Poulton LD, Brooks A, Naidenko OV, Sidobre S, Godfrey DI, Baxter AG. Genetic control of NKT cell numbers maps to major diabetes and lupus loci. *J Immunol*. 2003;171:2873–8.

[88] Rocha-Campos AC, Melki R, Zhu R, Deruytter N, Damotte D, Dy M, Herbelin A, Garchon HJ. Genetic and functional analysis of the Nkt1 locus using congenic NOD mice: improved Vα14-NKT cell performance but failure to protect against type 1 diabetes. *Diabetes.* 2006;55:1163–70.

[89] Kent S, Chen Y, Clemmings SM, Viglietta V, Kenyon NS, Ricordi C, Hering B, Hafler DA. Loss of IL-4 secretion from human type 1a diabetic pancreatic draining lymph node NKT cells. *J Immunol*. 2005;175:4458–64.

[90] Kukreja A, Cost G, Marker J, Zhang C, Sun Z, Lin-Su K, Ten S, Sanz M, Exley M, Wilson B, Porcelli S. Multiple immuno-regulatory defects in type 1 diabetes. *J Clin Invest*. 2002;109:131–40.

[91] Rodacki M, Svoren B, Butty V, Besse W, Laffel L, Benoist C, Mathis D. Altered natural killer cells in type 1 diabetic patients. *Diabetes.* 2007;56:177–85.

[92] Janos K, Engelmann P, Farkas K, Richman G, Eck S, Lolley J, Jalahej H, Borowiec M, Kent SC, Treszl A, Orban T. Reduced CD4- subset and Th1 bias of the human iNKT cells in type 1 diabetes mellitus. *J Leukoc Biol*. 2006;81:654–62.

[93] Roman-Gonzalez A, Moreno ME, Alfaro JM, Uribe F, Latorre-Sierra G, Rugeles MT, Montoya CJ. Frequency and function of circulating invariant NKT cells in

autoimmune diabetes mellitus and thyroid diseases in Colombian patients. *Human Immunol.* 2009;70:262–8.

[94] Montoya CJ, Pollard D, Martinson J, Kumari K, Wasserfall C, Mulder CB, Rugeles MT, Atkinson MA, Landay AL, Wilson SB. Characterization of human invariant natural killer T subsets in health and disease using a novel invariant natural killer T cell-clonotypic monoclonal antibody, 6B11. *Immunology*. 2007;122:1–14.

[95] Ortiz-Navarrete V, Canche-Pool E, Gómez-Díaz R, Medina-Contreras O, Valle-Rios R, Patiño-Lopez G. CRTAM molecule is expressed at the cell surface of NKT cells from patients with type 1 diabetes mellitus. *Clin Immunol.* 2009;131:S145.

[96] Beristain-Covarrubias N, Canche-Pool E, Gomez-Diaz R, Sanchez-Torres LE, Ortiz-Navarrete V. Reduced iNKT cells numbers in type 1 diabetes patients and their first-degree relatives. *Immun Inflamm Dis.* 2015;3:411–9.

[97] Gómez-Díaz RA, Aguilar MV, Meguro EN, Marquez RH, Magana EG, Carmen Martinez-Garcia M, Rodarte NW, Aguilar-Salinas CA, Canché-Pool E, Ortiz-Navarrete V. The role of natural killer T (NKT) cells in the pathogenesis of type 1 diabetes. *Curr Diabetes Rev*. 2011;7:278–83.

[98] Beristain-Covarrubias N, Canche-Pool EB, Ramirez-Velazquez C, Barragan-Galvez JC, Gomez-Diaz RA, Ortiz-Navarrete V. Class I-restricted T cell-associated molecule is a Marker for IFN-γ-producing iNKT cells in healthy subjects and patients with type 1 diabetes. *J Interf Cytokine Res*. 2017;37(1):39–49.

[99] Lombardi G, Burzyn D, Mundiñiano J, Berguer P, Bekinschtein P, Costa H, Castillo LF, Goldman A, Meiss R, Piazzon I, Nepomnaschy I. Cathepsin-L influences the Expression of extracellular matrix in lymphoid organs and plays a role in the regulation of thymic output and of peripheral T cell number. *J Immunol.* 2005;174:7022–32.

[100] Gómez-Díaz RA, Medina-Santillán R, Castro Magdonel BE, Association of NKT cells with Expression of the CTSL gene in Mexican pediatric population with recently-diagnosed type 1 diabetes. *Gac Med Mex.* 2016;152:14–21.

Chapter 3

The Social Determinants of Diabetes

Yachana Mishra*
Kajal
and Aditi Chattaraj
School of Bioengineering and Biosciences, Lovely Professional University, Phagwara (Punjab), India

Abstract

This chapter aims to introduce the idea of "social determinants of diabetes" and to explain how important it is for conversations about public policy to address the social problem that diabetes poses. The evidence available on how diabetes is spread in society and how it affects people is briefly reviewed. The detrimental effects of social stigma on diabetes patients, which may prevent them from practicing good self-care and diabetes-aware behavior, are also discussed. The chapter finishes with some policy and research ideas on the social causes of diabetes. It also explores how the social determinants of diabetes may be converted into policy involvements to address the inequality in the problem of diabetes among communities.

Keywords: diabetes, social determinants, communities

* Corresponding Author's Email: yachanamishra@gmail.com.

In: Management of Diabetes Mellitus Based on Natural Products
Editors: Yachana Mishra and Vijay Mishra
ISBN: 979-8-88697-853-7

1. Introduction

Diabetes poses a serious threat to global health [1, 2]. In recent years, research of the biological reasons for diabetes, such as insulin sensitivity and beta cell malfunction, has advanced significantly [3]. As a result, novel pharmacological treatments, such as DPP-4 inhibitors, have been created to more effectively treat the condition. Despite advancements in science and technology, diabetes continues to be a social problem since the causes and effects of the illness are intrinsically linked to human behavior and life experiences. In fact, accumulating data have shown that the disease's impact is unevenly spread between peoples and nations [4].

The majority of the attention in this chapter is given to type 2 diabetes mellitus (T2DM), although various effects on type 1 diabetes mellitus (T1DM) have also been studied in regards to mortality, morbidity, and contact with or loyalty to high-quality diabetes care among individuals with various socioeconomic conditions that are imitated in career class, educational achievement, and income levels [5]. There is ongoing academic and clinical discussion over the mechanism by which T1DM affects those in lower socioeconomic positions more severely, and it is unclear if this process differs from that of T2DM. The "break budgets" of effectively guiding self-care groups, in terms of internal, economic (including time), and social charges, may be higher for those with lower socioeconomic sites, and this likely prevents them from effectively defending their own health, according to some, even though access to high-quality healthcare is suspected of playing a role.

2. Community Difference in the Diabetes Load

The prevalence, comorbidity, and humanity of T2DM among individuals, tentatively based on pay close, occupational class, educational attainment, sex, race/origin, and the financial development stage of the nation where they reside [4]. The situation in low- and medium-income nations [6]. The relationship, nevertheless, could be gender specific. In contrast to women, there was a significant and negative correlation between these variables among men in a study using data from a European cross-country panel survey of the elderly population [7]. This correlation persisted even after adjusting for body mass index and lifestyle factors like physical activity [8]. Research that used data from the Canadian Public Health Examination similarly discovered a body mass indicator increase in the prevalence of diabetes, which was more pronounced in women than in men and may be partially explained by education [9]. Incidence of diabetes and education had a more difficult correlation among women than males, according to a nationally representative study employing the US National Health and Nutrition Examination Examination Survey [10]. In contrast to women, males had a negative connection between diabetics and education, according to this study [11]. Regarding diabetes death, a US study found that increased diabetes-related mortality was linked to lower income and education levels [12–15]. Turning to the prevalence of the disease or the percentage of people who now have the disease in the general public, [16, 17] studies from high-income nations generally demonstrate that those with lower socioeconomic position have a greater incidence of diabetes [7, 18, 19]. Within urban and rural areas of Ghana, different relationships between diabetes prevalence and socioeconomic status have been discovered [20, 21]. The relationships between socioeconomic position and diabetes incidence and mortality that differ among regions and nations by level of economic development might be used to explain the inconsistent results for diabetes prevalence by socioeconomic position. Recent research has centred on the socioeconomic circumstances of children. Although the connection varied by gender and conditional adult risk factors (such as obesity), a review of 10 prior research found a link between early life poor socioeconomic status and present diabetes illness [21]. Low childhood socioeconomic level has a protective effect on adult diabetes status [22-24]. Contrary skill in youth had a substantial influence on diabetes risk, despite the previous researchers' generally greater and comparable educational attainment [25].

3. Hypothetical Device of Common Difference in Diabetes

Different diabetes risk factors are connected to lifestyle choices, and healthy alteration of these choices is necessary for diabetes control [6, 26]. This does not, however, yet explain why or how socioeconomic status and gender variations in lifestyle choices result in inequalities in the diabetes burden. In order to better understand the intricate process of disease development within a social setting, Brown et al., devised a model, which further supported the inclusion of literacy levels, psychological stress, and demands conflicting with self-care activities [27]. However, the most current study on type 2 diabetes and environmental factors [28] and other relevant review studies on diet and obesity [29-31]. Several research studies have shown that socioeconomic factors impact both the availability and efficacy of diabetes management [13, 15, 26]. The distribution of obesity in society is strongly influenced by social ties within the community and family [32, 33]. Recent research has focused on the social impact of the stigma that diabetic patients experience [27, 34-38]. The hypothesis that people who suffer inadequate nutrition during infancy have increased risks of fat, insulin sensitivity, and diabetes is supported by several epidemiological studies [39-41]. More recent epigenetic studies have looked at the "metabolic memory"—a mark that the early environment leaves on the epigenome—which manifests later on as metabolic malfunction [42]. According to a UK-based longitudinal investigation, lifestyle factors account for around 50% of the elevated risk of T2DM incidence linked with poor socioeconomic status [43, 44]. The molecular process by which poor socioeconomic status-related social stress is translated into a pathological course leading to insulin sensitivity and beta cell malfunctioning may be shown by chronic irritation. Each stage has a distinct window with particular vulnerabilities to chronic illness's biological, behavioural, and psychological risk factors. The effects of one stage will reverberate across following stages [45]. According to this idea, health is influenced by healthcare systems andjust by medical systems but also by circumstances in which individuals are born, raised, educated, and employed [46]. Diabetes can benefit from the socioeconomic determinants of health theory. According to the analysis above, [47] equality in diabetes outcomes must be achieved. Macroeconomic policy appears to be a significant social structural driver of health. The government and international institutions must collaborate across the health, financial, labour and industrial, educational, civil works, and other sectors to address the socioeconomic determinants of health [46].

4. Community Factors Interferences in Diabetes Outcomes

One of the top priorities for decreasing the gap is the implementation of universal health care [1, 2]. This is insufficient, though; while access to high-quality care may help decrease the diabetes humanities gap, it will do nothing to stop a gap in diabetic mortality and, especially, incidence [48]. However, the variation that was first experienced between the treatment and control groups significantly decreased with time, according to a longer join of the same randomized clinical study [49]. The current evidence is conflicting, and more research on the impact of environment and situation and other intervention strategies on the social determinants of diabetes is needed [28, 29, 31], according to existing studies on the impact of policy interventions like the creation of walkable cities and enhancing community access to healthier food. Sugar taxes have started to emerge as potential strategic interferences [50]. The consumption of sugar-sweetened beverages has decreased as a result, and as was predicted, the impact was greater among low-income families than among high-income families [51, 52]. The effect of this plan on lowering consumption would likely result in a substantial decrease in obesity and the prevalence of linked diseases like diabetes, according to more recent research that used simulation models [53]. Taxes for the purpose of promoting health are not always efficient or politically viable [54-56]. As we established previously, people who have diabetes are susceptible to societal stigma and high-risk practises that recognize those with elevated chances of developing diabetes.

Conclusion

Because the incidence, mortality, and sickness of diabetes are impacted by the socioeconomic and environmental aspects of diabetes, epidemiological and clinical research have persuasively demonstrated that the illness load of diabetes is disproportionately affecting distribution across society. Diet and exercise are important lifestyle choices that can help control diabetes. These choices are influenced not only by an individual's capacity but also by the social environment in which they occur. The effectiveness of interventions to regain diabetes control by lifestyle adjustment in specific high-risk groups has been demonstrated. However, this selective strategy may increase societal stigma toward those with a high risk of developing diabetes, which might substantially impede good self-care. Although it will need more research and policy analysis to effectively put the concept into practise and assist people in overcoming the social challenges of diabetes, the balanced breadth approach is a promising alternative that targets structural external interference to change the social environmental determinants of diabetes.

References

[1] Bommer C, Heesemann E, Sagalova V, Manne-Goehler J, Atun R, Barnighausen T, Vollmer S. The global economic burden of diabetes in adults aged 20–79 years: a cost-of-illness study. *Lancet Diabetes Endocrinol*. 2017;5:423–30.

[2] World Health Organization. *Global report on diabetes* 2021.

[3] Kahn S E, Cooper M E, Del Prato S. Pathophysiology and treatment of type 2 diabetes: perspectives on the past, present, and future. *Lancet*. 2014;383:1068–83.

[4] World Health Organization. *Equity, social determinants and public health programmes 2010*. http://www.who.int/iris/ handle/10665/44289.

[5] Scott A, Chambers D, Goyder E, O'Cathain A. Socioeconomic inequalities in mortality, morbidity and diabetes management for adults with type 1 diabetes: a systematic review. *PLoS One*. 2017;12:e0177210. .

[6] Agardh E, Allebeck P, Hallqvist J, Moradi T, Sidorchuk A. Type 2 diabetes incidence and socio-economic position: a systematic review and meta-analysis. *Int. J. Epidemiol. 2011*;40:804–18.

[7] Espelt A, Arriola L, Borrell C, Larranaga I, Sandin M, EscolarPujolar A. Socioeconomic position and type 2 diabetes mellitus in Europe 1999–2009: a panorama of inequalities. *Curr. Diabetes Rev*. 2011;7:148–58.

[8] Sacerdote C, Ricceri F, Rolandsson O, Baldi I, Chirlaque M D, Feskens E, Bendinelli B, Ardanaz E, Arriola L, Balkau B, Bergmann M. Lower educational level is a predictor of incident type 2 diabetes in European countries: the EPIC–InterAct study. *Int. J. Epidemiol.* 2012;41:1162–73.

[9] Smith P M, Smith B T, Mustard C A, Lu H, Glazier RH. Estimating the direct and indirect pathways between education and diabetes incidence among Canadian men and women: a mediation analysis. *Ann. Epidemiol.* 2013;23:143–9.

[10] Robbins JM, Vaccarino V, Zhang H, Kasl SV. Socioeconomic status and diagnosed diabetes incidence. Diabetes Res Clin Pract. 2005;68:230–6.

[11] Shang X, Li J, Tao Q, Li J, Li X, Zhang L, Liu X, Wang Q, Shi X, Zhao Y, Hu S. Educational level, obesity and incidence of diabetes among Chinese adult men and women aged 18–59 years old: an 11-year follow-up study. *PLoS One.* 2013;8:e66479.

[12] Saydah S, Lochner K. Socioeconomic status and risk of diabetes related mortality in the U.S. *Public Health Rep.* 2010;125:377–88.

[13] Funakoshi M, Azami Y, Matsumoto H, Ikota A, Ito K, Okimoto H, Shimizu N, Tsujimura F, Fukuda H, Miyagi C, Osawa S. Socioeconomic status and type 2 diabetes complications among young adult patients in Japan. *PLoS One.* 2017;12:e0176087. .

[14] Grintsova O, Maier W, Mielck A. Inequalities in health care among patients with type 2 diabetes by individual socioeconomic status (SES) and regional deprivation: a systematic literature review. *Int. J. Equity Health.* 2014;13:43.

[15] Lamy S, Ducros D, Dimeglio C, Colineaux H, Fantin R, Berger E, Grosclaude P, Delpierre C, Bouhanick B. Disentangling the influence of living place and socioeconomic position on health services use among diabetes patients: a population-based study. *PLoS One*. 2017;12:e0188295.

[16] Corsi D J, Subramanian S V. Association between socioeconomic status and self-reported diabetes in India: a cross-sectional multilevel analysis. *BMJ Open.* 2012;2:e000895.

[17] Tareque MI, Koshio A, Tiedt AD, Hasegawa T. Are the rates of hypertension and diabetes higher in people from lower socioeconomic status in Bangladesh? Results from a nationally representative survey. *PLoS One*. 2015;10:e0127954.

[18] Jaffiol C, Thomas F, Bean K, Jego B, Danchin N. Impact of socioeconomic status on diabetes and cardiovascular risk factors: results of a large French survey. *Diabetes Metab*. 2013;39:56–62.

[19] Wikstrom K, Lindstrom J, Tuomilehto J, Saaristo TE, KorpiHyovalti E, Vanhala M, Niskanen L, Keinänen-Kiukaanniemi S, Uusitupa M, Peltonen M. Socio-economic differences in dysglycemia and lifestyle-related risk factors in the Finnish middleaged population. *Eur. J. Pub. Health.* 2011;21:768–74.

[20] Addo J, Agyemang C, de-Graft Aikins A, Beune E, Schulze MB, Danquah I, Galbete C, Nicolaou M, Meeks K, Klipstein-Grobusch K, Bahendaka S. Association between socioeconomic position and the prevalence of type 2 diabetes in Ghanaians in different geographic locations: the RODAM study. *J. Epidemiol. Community Health.* 2017;71:633–9.

[21] Tamayo T, Christian H, Rathmann W. Impact of early psychosocial factors (childhood socioeconomic factors and adversities) on future risk of type 2 diabetes, metabolic disturbances and obesity: a systematic review. *BMC Public Health.* 2010;10:525.

[22] Tsenkova V, Pudrovska T, Karlamangla A. Childhood socioeconomic disadvantage and prediabetes and diabetes in later life: a study of biopsychosocial pathways. *Psychosom. Med.* 2014;76:622–8.

[23] Derks I P, Koster A, Schram M T, Stehouwer C D, Dagnelie P C, Groffen D A, Bosma H. The association of early life socioeconomic conditions with prediabetes and type 2 diabetes: results from the Maastricht study. *Int. J. Equity Health.* 2017;16:61.

[24] Shields M E, Hovdestad W E, Pelletier C, Dykxhoorn J L, O'Donnell SC, Tonmyr L. Childhood maltreatment as a risk factor for diabetes: findings from a population-based survey of Canadian adults. *BMC Public Health.* 2016;16:879.

[25] Rich-Edwards J W, Spiegelman D, Lividoti Hibert E N, Jun H J, Todd T J, Kawachi I, Wright RJ. Abuse in childhood and adolescence as a predictor of type 2 diabetes in adult women. *Am. J. Prev. Med.* 2010;39:529–36.

[26] Chaturvedi N, Jarrett J, Shipley M J, Fuller J H. Socioeconomic gradient in morbidity and mortality in people with diabetes: cohort study findings from the Whitehall Study and the WHO Multinational Study of Vascular Disease in Diabetes. *BMJ.* 1998;316:100–5.

[27] Brown A F, Ettner S L, Piette J, Weinberger M, Gregg E, Shapiro M, Karter A J, Safford M, Waitzfelder B, Prata P A, Beckles G L. Socioeconomic position and health among persons with diabetes mellitus: a conceptual framework and review of the literature. *Epidemiol. Rev.* 2004;26:63–77.

[28] Dendup T, Feng X, Clingan S, Astell-Burt T. Environmental risk factors for developing type 2 diabetes mellitus: a systematic review. *Int. J. Environ. Res. Public Health.* 2018;15.

[29] Feng J, Glass T A, Curriero F C, Stewart WF, Schwartz BS. The built environment and obesity: a systematic review of the epidemiologic evidence. *Health Place.* 2010;16:175–90.

[30] Black C, Moon G, Baird J. Dietary inequalities: what is the evidence for the effect of the neighbourhood food environment? *Health Place*. 2014;27:229–42.

[31] Gary-Webb TL, Suglia SF, Tehranifar P. Social epidemiology of diabetes and associated conditions. *Curr. Diab. Rep*. 2013;13:850–9.

[32] Christakis NA, Fowler JH. The spread of obesity in a large social network over 32 years. *N. Engl. J. Med.* 2007;357:370–9.

[33] Powell K, Wilcox J, Clonan A, Bissell P, Preston L, Peacock M, Holdsworth M. The role of social networks in the development of overweight and obesity among adults: a scoping review. *BMC Public Health.* 2015;15.

[34] Browne J L, Ventura A, Mosely K, Speight J. 'I call it the blame and shame disease': a qualitative study about perceptions of social stigma surrounding type 2 diabetes. *BMJ Open.* 2013;3:e003384. .

[35] Browne J L, Ventura A, Mosely K, Speight J. 'I'm not a druggie, I'm just a diabetic': a qualitative study of stigma from the perspective of adults with type 1 diabetes. *BMJ Open*. 2014;4:e005625.

[36] Kato A, Fujimaki Y, Fujimori S, Isogawa A, Onishi Y, Suzuki R, Yamauchi T, Ueki K, Kadowaki T, Hashimoto H. Psychological and behavioural patterns of stigma among patients with type 2 diabetes: a cross-sectional study. *BMJ Open.* 2017;7:e013425

[37] Kato A, Fujimaki Y, Fujimori S, Izumida Y, Suzuki R, Ueki K, Kadowaki T, Hashimoto H. A qualitative study on the impact of internalized stigma on type 2 diabetes self-management. *Patient Educ. Couns.* 2016;99:1233–9.

[38] Hales C N, Barker D J. Type 2 (non-insulin-dependent) diabetes mellitus: the thrifty phenotype hypothesis. *Diabetologia*. 1992;35:595–601.

[39] Painter RC, Roseboom TJ, Bleker OP. Prenatal exposure to the Dutch famine and disease in later life: an overview. *Reprod. Toxicol.* 2005;20:345–52.

[40] Singhal A, Fewtrell M, Cole T J, Lucas A. Low nutrient intake and early growth for later insulin resistance in adolescents born preterm. *Lancet.* 2003;361:1089–97.

[41] Symonds ME, Sebert SP, Hyatt MA, Budge H. Nutritional programming of the metabolic syndrome. *Nat. Rev. Endocrinol.* 2009;5:604–10.

[42] Waki H, Yamauchi T, Kadowaki T. The epigenome and its role in diabetes. *Curr. Diab. Rep.* 2012;12:673–85.

[43] Stringhini S, Zaninotto P, Kumari M, Kivimaki M, Batty G D. Lifecourse, socioeconomic status and type 2 diabetes: the role of chronic inflammation in the English Longitudinal Study of Ageing. *Sci. Rep.* 2016;6:24780. .

[44] Stringhini S, Batty G D, Bovet P, Shipley M J, Marmot M G, Kumari M, Tabak A G, Kivimäki M. Association of lifecourse socioeconomic status with chronic inflammation and type 2 diabetes risk: the Whitehall II prospective cohort study. *PLoS Med*. 2013;10:e1001479.

[45] Kuh D, Ben-Shlomo Y. A life-course approach to chronic disease epidemiology. Oxford: Oxford University Press; 1997.

[46] World Health Organization. *A Conceptual Framework for Action on the Social Determinants of Health 2010*. http://www.who.int/ sdhconference/resources/ ConceptualframeworkforactiononSDH_ eng.pdf.

[47] Read S H, Kerssens J J, McAllister D A, Colhoun H M, Fischbacher C M, Lindsay RS, for Scottish Diabetes Research Network Epidemiology Group. Trends in type 2 diabetes incidence and mortality in Scotland between 2004 and 2013. *Diabetologia.* 2016;59: 2106–13.

[48] Knowler W C, Barrett-Connor E, Fowler S E, Hamman R F, Lachin J M, Walker, E A, Nathan D M, Watson P G, Mendoza J T, Smith K A, Caro J. Reduction in the incidence of type 2 diabetes with lifestyle intervention or metformin. *N. Engl. J. Med.* 2002;346:393–403.

[49] Knowler W C, Fowler S E, Hamman R F, Christophi C A, Hoffman H J, Nathan D M. 10-year follow-up of diabetes incidence and weight loss in the Diabetes Prevention Program Outcomes Study. *Lancet.* 2009;374:1677–86.

[50] Backholer K, Sarink D, Beauchamp A, Keating C, Loh V, Ball K, Martin J, Peeters A. The impact of a tax on sugar-sweetened beverages according to socio-economic position: a systematic review of the evidence. *Public Health Nutr.* 2016;19:3070–84.

[51] Colchero M A, Guerrero-Lopez C M, Molina M, Rivera JA. Beverages sales in Mexico before and after implementation of a sugar sweetened beverage tax. *PLoS One.* 2016;11:e0163463. .

[52] Colchero M A, Popkin B M, Rivera J A, Ng S W. Beverage purchases from stores in Mexico under the excise tax on sugar sweetened beverages: observational study. *BMJ.* 2016;352:h6704.

[53] Barrientos-Gutierrez T, Zepeda-Tello R, Rodrigues E R, Colchero M A, Rojas-Martinez R, Lazcano-Ponce E, Hernández-Ávila M, Rivera-Dommarco J, Meza R. Expected population weight and diabetes impact of the 1-peso-per-litre tax to sugar sweetened beverages in Mexico. *PLoS One*. 2017;12:e0176336. .

[54] Bodker M, Pisinger C, Toft U, Jorgensen T. The rise and fall of the world's first fat tax. *Health Policy*. 2015;119:737–42.

[55] Wright A, Smith K E, Hellowell M. Policy lessons from health taxes: a systematic review of empirical studies. *BMC Public Health.* 2017;17:583.

[56] Carey G, Crammond B, De Leeuw E. Towards health equity: a framework for the application of proportionate universalism. *Int. J. Equity Health.* 2015;14:81.

Chapter 4

Diabetes Mellitus in Pregnancy

Yachana Mishra*
School of Bioengineering and Biosciences,
Lovely Professional University, Phagwara (Punjab), India

Abstract

Medical practitioners who care for pregnant patients must be knowledgeable on diabetes mellitus in pregnancy to reduce maternal and fetal morbidity in pregnant diabetic women. Adopting strategies, including preconception and nutritional counseling, supporting active lifestyle modifications, and rapid medical management utilizing the variety of alternatives available are critical, as is the identification of patients with risk factors at the initial stage of therapy.

Keywords: diabetes mellitus, pregnancy, therapy

1. Introduction

Improper dietary patterns and a sedentary lifestyle are the major causes of the rising rate of obesity, which is a global issue. Pregnancy obesity increases the chance of diabetes, which increases the risk to the mother and fetus as well as the likelihood of hypertensive diseases. Obesity affects people of reproductive age in general and women in particular [1, 2]. As a result, diabetes during pregnancy is becoming increasingly common depending on the demographic investigated; it is estimated that it considerably complicates 1–16% of all

* Corresponding Author's Email: yachanamishra@gmail.com.

In: Management of Diabetes Mellitus Based on Natural Products
Editors: Yachana Mishra and Vijay Mishra
ISBN: 979-8-88697-853-7

births globally. Depending on the community, the incidence of gestational diabetes (GD) varies in direct proportion to the prevalence of type 1 diabetes mellitus (T1DM) and type 2 diabetes mellitus (T2DM). According to some estimates, this illness complicates 6-7% of pregnancies, and women with T1DM and T2DM account for 90% of the cases. Additionally, it has been proven that Afro-Americans, Hispanics, and natives of Asia, America, and the Pacific islands had the highest incidence [3, 4].

In comparison to a healthy pregnancy, suffering from GD significantly increases the risk of undesirable pregnancy outcomes: congenital malformations occur in 5% of cases versus 2% in the general population, perinatal mortality occurs in 2.7% of cases versus 0.72%, premature birth occurs in 25% of cases versus 6%, and fetal macrosomia occurs in 54% of cases versus 10% in the general population [5]. There is the possibility that increased total abdominal obesity is related to fetal overnutrition after maternal exposure to GD [6]. The higher risk of metabolic changes, obesity, and diabetes among the children of women who had a pregnancy linked with diabetes may be explained by intrauterine programming related to hyperglycemia during pregnancy [7]. To minimize maternal and fetal morbidity in diabetic pregnant women, knowledge of this topic is essential for medical professionals caring for pregnant women. Identifying patients with risk factors at the initial level of treatment is crucial, as is the implementation of measures such as preconception and nutritional counseling, encouraging active lifestyle changes, and prompt medical management using the range of available options [8]. Fortunately, the situation for those who are pregnant now has drastically changed; in the past, a diabetic pregnant woman was unthinkable. The University of Toronto researchers Banting, MacLeod, and Bets discovered insulin in 1921, completely altering the outlook for diabetic patients and pregnant women with the disease. Similarly, the recent acceptance of glyburide and metformin during pregnancy adds another therapy option for pregestational and gestational diabetes. However, diabetes has not stopped being a health issue since pregnant diabetic women still face significant obstetric risk and heightened perinatal morbidity.

2. Classification and Diagnosis of Diabetes

Four broad kinds of diabetes are outlined in the classification [9, 10].

1. Type 1 diabetes (T1DM), which results from the pancreatic beta cells being destroyed and, in most cases, causes a complete lack of insulin;
2. Type 2 diabetes (T2DM) is brought on by an ever-declining level of insulin secretion;
3. Gestational diabetes (GD), which is discovered in the second or third trimester of pregnancy; and
4. Specific diabetes, caused by various factors such as chemically induced diabetes (treatment for HIV/AIDS or use of glucocorticoids after transplant). The possibility that both T1DM and T2DM may be present or have already developed during pregnancy is acknowledged in this category.

The World Health Organization's (WHO) general criteria for plasma glucose, the glucose tolerance test following oral administration of 75 g of glucose, or the criteria for glycosylated hemoglobin are used to diagnose GD. The definition of fasting is the absence of food consumption for eight hours. Concerning the determination of A1c, it is essential to note that it requires defined procedures and certification. When the patient's risk of developing GD is stratified during the first prenatal appointment, the American Diabetes Association (ADA) advises selective screening. The following list of risk factors: older than 25 years, overweight, and first-degree relatives with diabetes. High-risk patients should consent to an oral glucose tolerance test. The test should be repeated between 24 and 28 weeks of pregnancy if the results do not support the diagnosis. According to the Hyperglycemia and Adverse Pregnancy Outcomes (HAPO) study, even a one-standard-deviation increase in fasting glucose and 2-hour postprandial levels are linked to a higher risk of premature birth before 37 weeks, shoulder dystocia or other congenital disabilities requiring intensive neonatal care, hyperbilirubinemia, and preeclampsia [11]. It should be noted that the ADA and the American College of Obstetricians and Gynecologists (ACOG) support the two-step approach recommended by the National Institutes of Health (NIH), which entails performing a first glucose tolerance test with 50 g and in positive cases, a second test with 100 g of oral glucose. It is obvious that there are distinctions amongst diagnosis methods when it comes to glucose levels, but they all enable us to reach a diabetes diagnosis [12]. Similar relationships are seen in both systems when comparing diagnostic criteria in meta-analysis studies.

3. Recommendations for Diabetes Diagnosis in Pregnant Woman

1. Determine the fasting blood sugar of every pregnant woman during her initial prenatal checkup following the accepted diagnostic criteria, especially for pregnancies with risk factors in which T2DM has not yet been diagnosed [13].
2. In pregnant women who have never been diagnosed with diabetes before, a diabetes diagnosis should be made between weeks 24 and 28 of pregnancy.
3. Between weeks 6 and 12 postpartum, all women with GD should be screened with a glucose tolerance test to look for the development of T2DM and the persistence of hyperglycemia.
4. Since it is believed that a significant portion of women with GD acquire T2DM within a time frame of no longer than 10 years, women with a history of GD should have a permanent follow-up for developing diabetes or prediabetes at least every 3 years [14].
5. Metformin usage or lifestyle changes should be implemented for all women with a proven history of gestational diabetes or a prediabetic condition to prevent or postpone the onset of diabetes.

4. Carbohydrate Metabolism in Pregnant Woman

Development of the fetal placental unit during a normal pregnancy raises growth hormone, cortisol, estrogens, prolactin, human placental lactogens, and progesterone levels directly or indirectly. The pancreatic beta cells hyperplasia that results from the rise in estrogen and progesterone synthesis during the first week of pregnancy is followed by an increase in insulin production. The increased synthesis of human placental chorionic gonadotropin, tumor necrosis factor, prolactin, cortisol, and glucagon during the second half of pregnancy (especially weeks 24-28) affect glucose metabolism [15]. Improved glucose tolerance, higher insulin resistance, decreased hepatic glycogen stores, and enhanced hepatic glycogenesis are all effects of these alterations. Lipogenesis, macrosomia, polyhydramnios, organomegaly, etc., are all connected with diabetes-related pregnancies because of enhanced fetal insulin, which promotes the development of the fetus along with increased fatty tissue and increased hepatic glycogen stores

[16, 17]. Its function is connected to mitogenic and angiogenic activities, immune response control, and nutrition transport, all crucial processes during placentation and embryonic development [18].

5. Treatment of Diabetes in Pregnant Woman

Information on sexual and reproductive health, a method of family planning, and ways to prevent STDs, as well as information on the risk that pregnancy poses for developing overweight and obesity, nutritional guidance during pregnancy, and encouragement of breastfeeding because quitting this practice increases the risk of developing maternal overweight and obesity. Pregnancy weight increase should be negatively correlated with pre-pregnancy body mass index (BMI). Pregnancies in people with pregestational diabetes must occur in euglycemic conditions to prevent fetal problems associated with preconception hyperglycemia, congenital abnormalities, and recurrent miscarriages. Education on self-monitoring of glucose and the prevalence of ketonuria in patients who develop diabetes during pregnancy is essential, as is training families to recognize signs of hypoglycemia. Appropriate management of GD will significantly reduce perinatal complications like fetal death, congenital malformations, fetal macrosomia, shoulder dystocia, bone fractures resulting from obstetric trauma, nerve lesions, and newborns with delayed intrauterine growth [15]. It will even play a role in the future decline in the risk of juvenile obesity in the offspring of diabetic mothers. Patients with pre-existing diabetes (T1DM or T2DM) who are likely to become pregnant are given prompt referrals to second or third-level care for managing their pregnancy, with the primary goal of therapy being the rigorous control of blood glucose levels.

ADA suggested the following general guidelines for the care of diabetic patients [15]:

1. A1c should ideally be fasting glucose levels 90 mg/dL (5.0 mmol/L), in the first postprandial hour 130 to 140 mg/dL (7.2-7.8 mmol/L), and at 2-hours postprandial 120 mg/dL (6.7 mmol/L). Provide preconception information on the need for glycemia regulation as naturally and securely as feasible.
2. Family planning is a necessary topic that recommends a secure, effective contraceptive strategy till the woman is ready and able to get pregnant.

3. Pregnant or planning to become pregnant women with T1DM or T2DM should be informed about the possibility of developing and/or progressing diabetic retinopathy. Vision tests before becoming pregnant or during the first trimester of pregnancy, followed by tests every trimester, a year after the baby is born, and as recommended by the doctor, depending on the severity of the retinopathy.
4. A lifestyle change is a crucial part of managing GD and may be the primary course of therapy.
5. If additional medication is required, it should be administered to achieve glycemic goals. Compared to insulin or metformin, glyburide has a greater likelihood of neonatal hypoglycemia and macrosomia, making it less commonly used as a medication for GD.
6. The adjustment in lifestyle entails minimizing sedentary behavior and maintaining a healthy diet. Since dietary advice can typically be sufficient to provide optimal management of glucose levels, it is crucial for patients with pre-existing diabetes or diabetes that manifests during pregnancy. Since the doctor or prenatal nurse may guide the pregnant woman, whether or not she has diabetes, from the first office visit, nutritional advice is not just available from nutritionists.

5.1. Insulin

The Food and Drug Administration (FDA), the ADA, and the ACOG all support it as the cornerstone of treatment for glycemic control in pregnant women. The immediate and rapid (INPH and IR) insulins that have been approved for use during pregnancy may be difficult for patients to understand. The success of their administration depends on several variables, including the patient's capacity and the level of training provided before application. If the patient is slender, 0.1–0.3 IU/Kg of weight/day is taken into account, and if the patient is obese, 0.4–0.7 IU/Kg of weight/day. The total dose may vary from patient to patient. One typical dosage method involves splitting the total amount into two administrations, with two-thirds being administered in the morning before breakfast and one-third before supper. If so, the morning dose would consist of one-third rapid action and two-thirds INPH, while the evening dose would consist of half rapid action and half INPH. The dose for this scheme can be changed up to 1.5 IU/Kg of weight/day [19].

5.2. Oral Hypoglycemic Drugs

The FDA has not expressly authorized any oral hypoglycemic medications to treat GD. But over the past 10 years, there has been mounting scientific evidence in favor of oral hypoglycemic drugs, which, in comparison to insulin, have the benefit of requiring fewer injections, leading to fewer hypoglycemia incidents, and being less expensive. Their usage during pregnancy is rising, particularly in overweight women and women with GD and pre-existing T2DM. Although they have been licensed for use during pregnancy, there is no research in this area. One should remember that oral hypoglycemic drugs pass the fetal placental barrier before prescribing them. Two oral hypoglycemic drugs, i.e., glyburide and metformin, have been discussed below:

5.2.1. Glyburide

Glyburide, commonly known as glibenclamide, is a strong anti-diabetic drug (Figure 1). The activation of beta cells in the pancreatic islets, which increases insulin release, gives the drug its hypoglycemic effects. Orally, it is absorbed. Sulfonylureas bind to the receptors in ATP-dependent potassium channels, decreasing potassium flow and resulting in membrane depolarization. By stimulating calcium entry through calcium channels and raising intracellular calcium concentrations, this depolarization increases insulin secretion and/or exocytosis. There must be a certain minimum quantity of viable beta cells for this medication to work. Glyburide is most effective in people of normal weight and lowers blood glucose by 20%. It was the first oral hypoglycemic medication to be prospectively evaluated and used to control GD, and its efficacy is comparable to insulin's. The most frequent gastrointestinal adverse effects are mild nausea and burning in the epigastrium. Currently, a daily dose of 2.5–5 mg, or twice daily, is advised, with a maximum dose of 20 mg. Its usage is not recommended if the patient is nursing, yet this is not a reason to stop lactation, as breastfeeding has several advantages for both the mother and the fetus [20].

5.2.2. Metformin

Metformin (Figure 2) reduces postprandial and fasting glucose levels. It works in three different ways: (1) by lowering hepatic glucose production by blocking gluconeogenesis and glycogenolysis; (2) by improving insulin sensitivity in muscle and enhancing the uptake and use of peripheral glucose; and (3) by delaying intestinal glucose absorption. It does not cause hypoglycemia since it does not increase insulin secretion. It can be taken either by itself or with glibenclamide or insulin. The dosage ranges from 1000 to 2000 mg daily, split into two doses with or after meals. Increased bowel movement, nausea, and vomiting are the most often reported adverse effects. The pattern for its use in pregnant patients with diabetes was set by the prevalence of its use in women with pregestational diabetes, polycystic ovary syndrome, and poor fertility. No adverse effects on either the mother or the fetus were noticed when metformin therapy persisted through the third trimester. Metformin is an effective medication for achieving optimal glycemic control, according to recent trials that compared its effectiveness to insulin in treating GD in women [21]. In terms of neonatal hypoglycemia, the prevalence of products with higher weight for gestational age, infant admission into phototherapy, respiratory stress syndrome, and perinatal mortality, meta-analysis studies have determined that metformin has equivalent efficacy and safety to insulin [22].

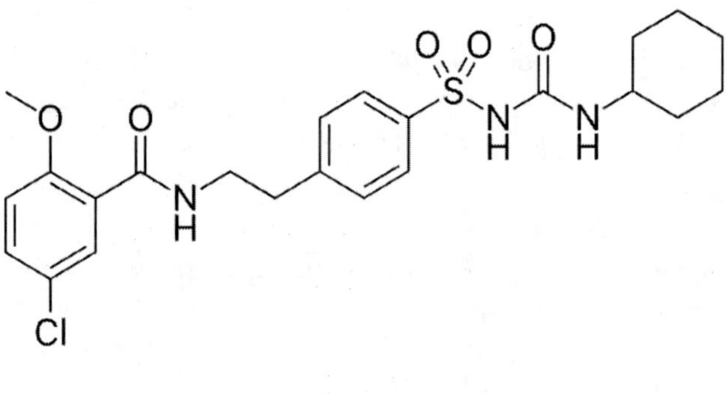

Figure 1. Glyburide, commonly known as glibenclamide.

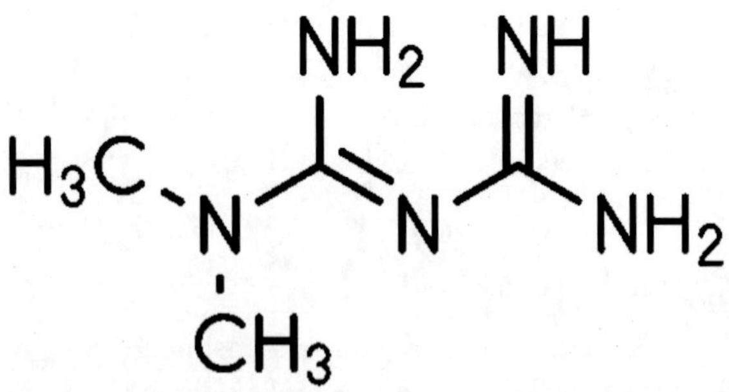

Figure 2. Metformin.

Regarding the frequency of hypoglycemia peaks, metformin is safe. Human milk contains metformin secreted by the body. Newborns and breastfed infants have not had any negative consequences [23]. However, breastfeeding is not advised when using metformin since adequate data is lacking.

6. Pregnancy Management in Gestational Diabetic Patients

Every patient with GD should be referred, as soon as the diagnosis is made, to a second- or third-level hospital with a multidisciplinary team that offers obstetrics, endocrinology, perinatology, nutrition and diet services, social work, psychology, etc., for the control and treatment of the condition. Between weeks 18 and 22, a structural ultrasound should be done to rule out fetal abnormalities, and a series of ultrasounds every four weeks with measurement of the fetal abdominal perimeter at the beginning of the third trimester should be done to identify babies at higher risk of macrosomia. Cardiotocographic examinations should begin without stress at week 32 of pregnancy and expand to twice-weekly examinations by week 36. The amount of amniotic fluid, the estimated weight, and the fetal abdominal circumference should all be assessed using ultrasound technology. Any data do not support whether to induce labor or wait, but the obstetrician is concerned about it since these patients have a greater incidence of intrauterine fetal mortality. Compared to straightforward pregnancies, induced labor at term may have an 80% success rate, but cesarean sections are far more common. For women whose blood sugar levels are managed with insulin or oral hypoglycemic medications, studies advise inducing labor at 39 weeks of gestation [24, 25].

As recommended by ACOG and the American College of Endocrinology (ACE), glucose levels during labor in patients with pre-existing or gestational diabetes should be monitored and kept within the range of 70 and 110 mg/dL (3.6-6.1 mm/L). High glucose levels during labor have been linked to an increased risk of neonatal hypoglycemia [26]. To achieve this goal, take intravenous glucose solutions, continuous insulin infusions, or fast-acting insulin before capillary glucose treatment. To maintain sufficient blood levels and prevent ketoacidosis, women with T1DM need glucose supplementation. Women with T2DM and GD may have enough glycogen in their bodies to keep their blood sugar levels around 70 mg/dL during the latent phase of labor without the need for additional glucose. However, glucose needs to rise during active labor, the expulsion phase, and prolonged labor induction. Monitoring for hypoglycemia, hypocalcemia, and hyperbilirubinemia in the neonate is necessary. Women should be able to resume their usual diet throughout the postpartum period. After delivery, placental hormones' hyperglycemic effects immediately subside, and plasma glucose levels revert to normal. However, measuring glucose concentrations using capillary glucose during the first 24-72 hours is advised to rule out chronic hyperglycemia in the postpartum period. Given that there is a 70% chance that these women may acquire T2DM up to 10 years after giving a child, women with a history of GD should be monitored for the next 6 to 12 weeks postpartum with a glucose tolerance test to rule out diabetes or carbohydrate intolerance [27]. To reduce the consequences of an intrauterine hyperglycemic environment on neonates and babies of mothers with obesity or T2DM, women should breastfeed exclusively for the first six months and then supplementally for the next two years [28, 29].

Conclusion

For the welfare of the fetus and the mother, women with GD should get dietary treatment and, if required, medication. Both insulin and oral hypoglycemic drugs are equally effective and can be used as a first-line treatment for GD. All pregnant women should have GD screening in the first trimester of their pregnancies, whether based on the patient's medical history, clinical risk factors, or the findings of laboratory screening tests that measure blood glucose levels. When the expected fetal weight is 4500 g or above, women with GD should get advice on planned cesarean birth. Expectant management is an option for women with GD who have satisfactory glycemic control and no additional problems. Most of the time, medically treated pregnant women with adequate glycemic control don't need to deliver their babies before 39 weeks. For all women who have GD, postpartum screening between 6 and 12 weeks after delivery is advised to detect women who have T2DM, impaired fasting glucose, or glucose tolerance. Repeat testing at least every three years.

References

[1] Liat S, Cabrero L, Hod M, Yogev Y. Obesity in obstetrics. *Best Pract. Res. Clin. Obstet. and Gynaecol.* 2015;29: 79–90.

[2] Aviram A, Hod M, Yogev Y. Maternal obesity: implications for pregnancy outcome and long-term risks—a link to maternal nutrition. *Int. J. Gynecol. Obstet.* 2011; 115(Suppl 1):S6–S10.

[3] Albrecht S S, Barquera S, Popkin B M. Exploring secular changes in the association between BMI and waist circumference in MexicanOrigin and White women: a comparison of Mexico and the United States. *Am. J. of Hum. Biol.* 2014;26:627–34.

[4] ACOG. Committee on Practice Bulletins-Obstetrics. Practice Bulletin No. 137: Gestational diabetes mellitus. *Obstet. Gynecol*. 2013;122(2 Pt 1):406–16.

[5] McCance D R. Diabetes in pregnancy. *Best Pract. Res. Clin. Obstet. Gynaecol.* 2015;29:685–99.

[6] Lawrence J M. Women with diabetes in pregnancy: different perceptions and expectations. *Best Pract. Res. Clin. Obstet. Gynaecol.* 2011;25:15–24.

[7] Crume T L, Ogden L, West N A, Vehik K S, Scherzinger A, Daniels S, McDuffie R, Bischoff K, Hamman R F, Norris J M, Dabelea D. Association of exposure to diabetes in utero with adiposity and fat distribution in a multiethnic population of youth: The Exploring Perinatal Outcomes among Children (EPOCH) Study. *Diabetologia*. 2011;54:87–92.

[8] Hadar E, Ashwal E, Hod M. The preconceptional period as an opportunity for prediction and prevention of non-communicable disease. *Best Pract. Res. Clin. Obstet. Gynaecol.* 2015;29:54–62.

[9] American Diabetes Association. Classification and diagnosis of diabetes. Sec. 2. In standards of medical care in diabetes 2016. *Diabetes Care*. 2016;39(Suppl. 1):S13–22.

[10] Sacks D A, Metzger B E. Classification of diabetes in pregnancy. Time to reassess the alphabet. *Obstet. Gynecol.* 2013;121(2):345–8.

[11] The HAPO Study Cooperative Research Group. Hyperglycemia and adverse pregnancy outcomes. *N. Engl. J. Med*. 2008;358(19):1991–2002.

[12] Ogunyemi D A, Fong A, Rad S, Fong S, Kjos S L. Attitudes and practices of health care providers regarding gestational diabetes: results of a survey conducted at the 2010 meeting of the International Association of Diabetes in Pregnancy Study Group (IADPSG). *Diabet. Med.* 2011;28(8):976–86.

[13] Wendland E M, Torloni M R, Falavigna M, Trujillo J, Dode M A, Campos M A, Duncan B B, Schmidt M I. Gestational diabetes and pregnancy outcomes – a systematic review of the World Health Organization (WHO) and the International Association of Diabetes in Pregnancy Study Groups (IADPSG) diagnostic criteria. *BMC Pregnancy Childbirth*. 2012;12:23.

[14] McIntyre H D, Metzger B E, Coustan D R, Dyer A R, Hadden D R, Hod M, Lowe L P, Oats J J, Persson B. Counterpoint: establishing consensus in the diagnosis of GDM following the HAPO study. *Curr. Diab. Rep*. 2014;14:497.

[15] American Diabetes Association. Management of diabetes in pregnancy. Sec. 12. In standards of medical care in diabetes. *Diabetes Care*. 2016;39(Suppl 1):S94–8.

[16] Buchanan T A. *Intermediary metabolism durin pregnancy: implication for diabtes mellitus*. En: Le Roith D, Olefsky J M, Tyalor S I. Diabetes mellitus: a fundamental and clinical text (3). Philadelphia: Wolters Kluwer Health; 2003. Pro Quest Library. pp. 1237–50.

[17] Buchanan T A. *Effects of maternal diabetes mellitus on intrauterine development.* En: Le Roith D, Olefsky J M, Tyalor S I. Diabetes mellitus: a fundamental and clinical text (3). Philadelphia: Wolters Kluwer Health; 2003. Pro Qeust ebrary. pp. 1251–64.
[18] Tessier D R, Ferraro Z M, Gruslin A. Role of leptin in pregnancy: consequences of maternal obesity. *Placenta*. 2013;34: 205–11.
[19] Guía de Práctica Clínica. Diagnóstico y Tratamiento de la Diabetes en el Embarazo. México: Secretaria de Salud; 2009.
[20] Berggren E K, Boggess K A. *Oral agents for the management of gestational diabetes.* Clinical Obstet Gynecol Lippincott Williams and Wilkins. 2013;56(4):827–36.
[21] Spaulonci C P, Bernardes L S, Trindade T C, Zugaib M, Francisco R P. Randomized trial of metformin vs insulin in the management of gestational diabetes. *Am. J. Obstet. Gynecol.* 2013;209:34. e1–7.
[22] Zhao L P, Sheng X Y, Zhou S, Yang T, Ma L Y, Zhou Y, Cui Y M. Metformin versus insulin for gestational diabetes mellitus: a meta-analysis. *Br. J. Clin. Pharmacol.* 2015;80(5): 1224–34.
[23] Singh A K, Singh R. Metformin in gestational diabetes: an emerging contender. *Indian J. Endocrinol. Metab.* 2015;19(2): 236–44.
[24] Korkmazer E, Solak N, Tokgöz V Y. Gestational diabetes: screening, management, timing of delivery. *Curr. Obstet. Gynecol. Rep.* 2015;4:132–8.
[25] Benhalima K, Devlieger R, Van Assche A. Screening and management of gestational diabetes. *Best Pract. Res. Clin. Obstet. Gynaecol.* 2015;29:339–49.
[26] Garrison E A, Jagasia S. Inpatient management of women with gestational and pregestational diabetes in pregnancy. *Curr. Diab. Rep.* 2014;14:457.
[27] Theodoraki A, Baldeweg S E. Symposium on diabetes. Gestational diabetes mellitus. *Br. J. Hosp. Med.* 2008;69(10):562–7.
[28] Gunderson E P. Breastfeeding after gestational diabetes pregnancy. *Diabetes Care ProQuest.* 2007;30(S2):S161–8.
[29] Trout K K, Averbuch T, Barowski M. Promoting breastfeeding among obese women and women with gestational diabetes mellitus. *Curr. Diab. Rep.* 2011;11(7): 7–12.

Chapter 5

Current Treatment Methods for Diabetes Mellitus

Vijay Mishra*
and Abhigyan Ranjan
School of Pharmaceutical Sciences, Lovely Professional University, Phagwara, (Punjab), India

Abstract

Diabetes mellitus, a metabolic disease, is characterized by hyperglycemia. In recent years, the number of glucose-lowering drugs increased. The present chapter discusses the currently available diabetes treatment strategies incorporating various antidiabetic agents.

Keywords: diabetes mellitus, hyperglycemia, blood sugar, insulin

1. Introduction

A lack of insulin causes a severe catabolic condition that impacts protein, glucose, and fat reserves. Insulin is a strong anabolic hormone. If left untreated, absolute insulin shortage, such as that caused by type 1 diabetes (T1DM), can cause mortality. The study of diabetic patients in the pre-insulin era informs us that diabetes may be managed without insulin for an incredibly long time. Leonard Thompson was the first patient to get successful insulin therapy. When he received his first insulin injection at 11 a.m. on January 22,

* Corresponding Author's Email: vijaymishra2@gmail.com.

In: Management of Diabetes Mellitus Based on Natural Products
Editors: Yachana Mishra and Vijay Mishra
ISBN: 979-8-88697-853-7

1922, he had been living with diabetes for more than 2 years and was 12 years old when he was diagnosed with it in 1919. Despite this, life without insulin was unpleasant. Aside from the weight loss, ongoing fatigue, thirst, frequent urination, and infections, there was also the assurance that one had been sentenced to death and that it would be a painful and drawn-out procedure. Severe dietary restriction, possibly most popularized by Allen of the Rockefeller Institute in New York, appeared to be the most successful treatment [1]. However, this was a challenging diet that did not seem to increase life expectancy appreciably. When death did occur, it was unclear if it was due to malnutrition or diabetes.

1.1. Historical Background of Insulin

The story of insulin may be regarded as having begun in the fall of 1920, when Frederick Grant Banting while preparing a lecture on carbohydrate metabolism, considered a way to isolate the internal secretion of the pancreas. However, there had been prior attempts to identify a pancreatic agent that could control blood sugar, most notably by the Romanian physiologist Nicolas Paulesco. By the summer of the following year, he had made arrangements with John Macleod, a professor of physiology at the University of Toronto, to use lab space and Charles Best's assistance to begin his experiments. They demonstrated that blocking the pancreatic ducts caused the exocrine glands of the pancreas to atrophy, enabling the separation of the "internal" secretions. By administering this internal secretion to dogs that had had pancreatectomy to make them diabetic, they examined how it affected blood sugar levels. James Collip, a scientist, assisted them in properly purifying this abstract for the initial patient studies. Banting and Macleod shared the 1923 Nobel Prize in Medicine for this accomplishment. This discovery was by no means simple, and one especially critical writer claimed that "the creation of insulin... started in badly conceived, incorrectly conducted, and improperly understood set of studies" [2].

Nevertheless, the discovery of insulin was a turning point in the history of diabetes. The molecule has since undergone extensive research, leading to three additional Nobel Prizes: Frederick Sanger in 1958 for determining the primary amino acid sequence, Dorothy Hodgkin in 1964 for X-ray crystallographic studies, and Rosalyn Yalow et al. in 1977 for their work on the development of radioimmuno assays.

Initially, pancreatic tissue from pigs and cows was used to create the commercially available insulin. To stop the enzymatic breakdown of the insulin protein, the organs would be newly removed from the slaughterhouses and instantly frozen. To solubilize insulin, the tissue would be treated with acid and ethanol. The insulin would then be salted out with sodium chloride, precipitated, and finally crystallized [3]. The process produced insulin with approximately 80–90% purity; the main impurities were pancreatic polypeptides and glucagon. Although this insulin was successful, immune-mediated side effects, particularly lipoatrophy and antibody-mediated insulin resistance, which may both significantly affect the kinetics of insulin action, frequently hindered its use. These contaminants also had a role in an allergic reaction, which occasionally caused discomfort and swelling at the injection site [4].

1.2. Animal and Human Insulins

Animal insulin is still generated from pigs and cows. Bovine insulin varies from human insulin in its amino acid structure by three amino acids (position 30 of the B chain and positions 8 and 10 of the A chain), while pig insulin differs from human insulin in its amino acid structure by just one amino acid (position 30 of the B chain) [5, 6]. Despite these variations, the purity of the insulin preparation seemed to have an impact on how immunogenic it was.

In the 1970s, further purification procedures, including gel filtration and ion exchange chromatography, produced mono-component or single-component insulin that was better accepted and had fewer side effects. As these purer insulins were more widely accessible, the incidence of lipoatrophy and allergy was reduced. Moving on to therapy with human insulin was, therefore a reasonable next step to further minimize immune-mediated problems and enhance glucose management.

Three methods have been used to obtain human insulin. The initial efforts were directly isolating and purifying it from human cadaveric pancreata. However, there has never been a significant supply of human tissue to make this procedure feasible. Through the substitution of the one amino acid variation in the main sequence, the "semi-synthesis" method chemically changes swine insulin to the human sequence. Human insulin treatment wasn't generally available until the invention of recombinant DNA technology in 1980. In order for the host cell to produce insulin, generally baker's yeast or the bacterium Escherichia coli, the human DNA sequence must be inserted into it [7]. The protein would next be refined to a 99.5–99.9% purity, often using chromatography columns. As with pure porcine insulin, the quality of the human insulin formulation made possible by this method has essentially removed issues related to immune-mediated adverse effects.

Recombinant human insulin has been widely adopted, and fewer than 7% of all insulin sales worldwide are currently made from animal sources. The phase-out of animal insulins by the top insulin producers is likely responsible for this trend, at least in part. This alternative supply is still offered by a number of businesses, and both porcine- and bovine-derived insulin are still accessible. Animal insulins are priced similarly to recombinant human insulin in the UK, despite being less expensive to produce. The cost of animal insulin is around half that of recombinant human insulin in the poor world, for instance, which may affect the choice of insulin production. This pricing approach is not the same everywhere [8].

1.3. Long-Acting Insulin

Since soluble insulin's biologic effect doesn't last more than 5 to 6 hours, the early preparations were frequently accompanied by discomfort and edema at the injection site. Therefore, efforts to meet patients' daily insulin needs with a single injection were attempted in the 1920s and 1930s. Lecithin, oil, and cholesterol were utilized as modifying agents to achieve this, but their duration of action varied greatly from injection to injection, making clinical application highly challenging [9].

Insulin incorporation into a poorly soluble complex was first described in 1936, reducing the absorption of the drug [10]. Protamine, a highly basic protein produced from salmon or trout sperm, was used in this method. Protamine-zinc insulin was created by further stabilizing the combination with a modest quantity of zinc, which persisted for around 24 hours. Making uniform batches was challenging, and absorption was once more inconsistent. Protamine and zinc were added in stoichiometric amounts (such that there was no free protamine or zinc) in 1946, which further improved the procedure and produced a preparation that was absorbed more steadily and lasted for 12 to 24 hours. This insulin was called isophane or neutral protamine Hagedorn (NPH) and became available clinically in 1940.

It was discovered in 1951 that adding sufficient zinc to an acetate buffer might extend the action of insulin without the requirement for protamine, creating crystals of somewhat insoluble zinc-insulin complexes known as

Lente insulins [11]. By altering the pH, it was possible to make both smaller (semilente) and bigger (ultralente) crystals, depending on how quickly the crystals were absorbed. The most frequently used version of the zinc insulins was Lente insulin, which was utilized extensively in clinical practice. Lente insulin was a formulation that had a 70:30 ratio of ultralente and semilente insulins.

1.4. Rapid and Long-Acting Insulin Analogs

Approximately 109 mol/L of insulin circulates in the blood as a single molecule. Insulin molecules often form non-covalent associations into dimers, tetramers, and hexamers at larger concentrations, such as those in commercial preparations [12]. The zinc presence further stabilizes the hexamer interaction. After injection, fluid is attracted by osmosis into the insulin depot. Before insulin can pass the capillary walls as monomers into the blood circulation, it must first undergo a spontaneous but slow process known as dilution and dissociation of the insulin molecules [13, 14]. Therefore, patients should provide their soluble insulin 15 to 20 minutes before eating to ensure optimal circulation insulin levels at meal absorption. Due to the preparation needed to implement this guidance, many patients struggle. Even then, the predicted dosages could be off, especially if the patient does not influence how the food is prepared.

Specific modifications to the amino acid sequence of insulin can be made to lessen the interaction between insulin molecules [15]. Because of these modifications, insulin is absorbed more quickly into circulation, enabling it to be administered shortly before or after eating [16]. Currently, three such rapid-acting analogs (RAIs) are commercially available: insulin glulisine (Apidra ®, Sanofi-Aventis), insulin aspart (Novorapid ®, Novo Nordisk), and insulin lispro (Humalog ®, Lilly). These analogs have a shorter duration of action (3 to 5 hours) and a quicker onset of action (10 to 20 minutes) than soluble insulin (30 to 60 minutes and 6 to 8 hours, respectively). Several studies have now shown that RAIs are safe for people with type 1 and type 2 diabetes (T1DM and T2DM) when used in continuous subcutaneous insulin infusion (CSII) and as part of a "basal-bolus" insulin injection regimen with intermediate-acting insulins. RAIs likely regulate post-prandial hyperglycemia more efficiently than soluble insulin because their time-action profile is best adapted to imitating the need during mealtimes. Patients can therefore obtain better glycemic control with RAIs than with soluble insulin while experiencing fewer hypoglycemic episodes. Studies including individuals with T1DM as opposed to T2DM, and employing CSII as opposed to repeated dosage injections seem to make the advantages of RAI over soluble insulin more obvious [17].

Even though delayed-action insulins like insulin Lente and isophane can last for 12 to 24 hours, their absorption from subcutaneous tissue might vary greatly [18]. As a result, efforts to maintain strict glucose control may lead to a higher risk of hypoglycemia. The isoelectric point of the insulin molecule may change towards neutrality due to altering its core amino acid sequence (the isoelectric point is that at which the molecule is least soluble). As a result, after injecting insulin into the subcutaneous tissue (which has a neutral pH), the isoelectric point change causes insulin to precipitate, which causes absorption to be slower and, more significantly, more repeatable [19]. Early research on long-acting analog insulins, intended to prove equivalence rather than superiority over isophane NPH insulins, has not been able to clearly demonstrate an advantage in glycemic control [20]. The findings do, however, indicate that using long-acting insulin analogs to achieve glycemic control is related to reduced symptoms and nocturnal hypoglycemia [21].

1.5. Route of Insulin Administration

1.5.1 Subcutaneous

The most common method of administering insulin is subcutaneously, and the belly, thigh, and deltoid are recommended injection locations. Although there are few scientific trials on this topic, the current advice is to squeeze the skin to lessen the chance of injecting into muscle and to inject at right angles to the skin. The fold should then be kept for 5 to 10 seconds before removing the needle [22]. There has been a move to using insulin pens instead of the conventional needle and syringe since they are more widely available and simpler to use. The needle lengths that are currently available are 12.7, 8, 6, and 5 mm. Shorter needles are connected with a decreased risk of intramuscular injection and may be seen as less traumatic. There are few, if any, justifications for prescribing the 12.7 mm needle. However, some data suggest that shorter needles are linked to a higher risk of insulin back-leakage unless the injection technique is good. The 6 to 8 mm needle is often best for non-obese patients who employ the pinch method on the belly, arm, or legs.

When kept below 25 °C, standard insulin formulations have a shelf life of 4 to 6 weeks. They must be kept in a refrigerator (4 °C) for extended lengths to be kept until their expiration date. Patients who want to alter their therapy surreptitiously may use the method of rendering insulin inactive by exposing it to high temperatures or microwaves. Some delayed-action insulin formulations come in a two-phase solution that requires thorough mixing to achieve total suspension. To ensure that consistent doses of insulin are drawn up each time, it is crucial that patients are informed of the significance of this [23].

The long-acting insulin analogs do not require mixing. Insulin at or above 40 U/mL, mostly monomers, dimers, or hexamers, makes up insulin preparations. Following injection, fluid is pulled into the injection depot by osmosis, which causes the oligomers to split into single molecules that may pass through the capillary membrane and enter the bloodstream. Circulating insulin attaches to the target cell's insulin receptor, internalizes the cell, and starts various intracellular processes. Less than 1% of insulin is excreted by the kidney, most of which is internalized and degraded [24]. The liver, kidney, skeletal muscle, and adipose tissue all break down between 60 and 80 percent of insulin [25]. Therefore, persistent insulin in the bloodstream can increase the risk of hypoglycemia when the liver or renal function is impaired.

Numerous methods, including utilizing a gamma counter to measure the rate of loss of ^{125}I-labeled insulin from the injection site, have been utilized in studies evaluating the absorption of subcutaneously injected insulin [26]. The pace might vary dramatically across persons and from one injection to another within a single individual, according to studies [27]. While there do not seem to be any apparent changes in the absorption rate between the various injection sites, absorption rates in obese patients are slower than in non-obese patients. The upper abdomen appears to absorb soluble insulin from the body more quickly than the lower abdomen in the non-obese patient compared to the arm or leg [28].

1.5.2. Intramuscular

Although intramuscular injection is more painful and has a quicker absorption rate than the subcutaneous injection, it is still effective in emergencies where intravenous access is problematic. The thin diabetic patient who complains of discomfort after insulin injections and who may have irregular glucose control and hypoglycemia should be evaluated for accidental intramuscular delivery. This issue can be solved with the appropriate selection of insulin needles [29].

1.5.3. Intraperitoneal

Recently, interest has grown in using implanted insulin pump treatment with intraperitoneal insulin injection since it absorbs insulin more rapidly than the subcutaneous approach [30]. The fact that most of the absorbed insulin goes into the portal circulation [31] is a benefit, as it lowers the possibility of high levels of peripheral insulin contributing to the development of obesity and vascular problems associated with diabetes [32, 33]. Compared to the subcutaneous method, implanted intraperitoneal pumps appear to provide better glucose management and less hypoglycemia in early investigations. In patients requiring renal replacement treatment utilizing continuous ambulatory peritoneal dialysis, where the insulin is provided simultaneously with the dialysis fluid, a long experience of intraperitoneal insulin administration has been attained. There are some claims that this route is linked to more reliable absorption and lower levels of peripheral insulin, but there are no conclusive studies to support this [34, 35].

1.5.4. Oral

Frederick Banting's early tests rapidly demonstrated that the oral way of administering insulin was unreliable and those gut peptides later functionally destroyed the insulin molecule. Because of its relatively predictable absorption kinetics and relative simplicity of administration, subcutaneous injection of insulin has grown to be the most preferred method of delivering the hormone. However, it is still worthwhile to explore some of the other delivery methods.

In order to avoid excessive levels of peripheral insulin, this medication can reach the portal circulation through oral administration. Reports suggest that such a strategy would be feasible. Early-phase clinical trials have shown that methods like insulin modification to create resistance to degradation efficiently boost circulating insulin concentrations and lower blood glucose [36, 37].

1.6. Insulin Pumps

When Dr. Arnold Kadish of Los Angeles, California, first conceived of a closed-loop system that supplied the components of blood glucose monitoring paired with insulin infusion, it was the 1960s and insulin pump or continuous subcutaneous insulin infusion (CSII) technology was in its infancy. It was designed to be worn on the back to make intravenous access easier. Although it was undoubtedly portable, its size and weight also proved to be a significant disadvantage. This insulin pump prototype had a glucose autoanalyzer to detect blood sugar and an on/off switch to operate an insulin pump. When the autoanalyzer identified glucose levels beyond the usual range, insulin was automatically switched off—the computer-controlled glucose sensing and insulin delivery system. Biostater was a newly released and highly praised gadget in the next decade. The Biostater had a number of parts, including a pump that withdrew blood for analysis, a glucose analyzer for continuous glucose readings, computerized algorithms for calculating the amount of insulin or dextrose to be infused based on glucose blood levels, a computer-driven infusion pump for insulin or dextrose delivery, and a printout of blood readings based on per minute determinations. However, these drawbacks caused it to be abandoned. Although it was also utilized in obstetrical settings, this device was mostly employed in research [38].

To address the portability limitations of earlier designs, the insulin pump's next generation was created to be worn as a shoulder bag. Slama et al. reported on an insulin delivery system that delivered insulin over a period of 1 to 5 days at a consistent rate for the basal insulin and a fixed 15-fold greater rate for the prandial insulin boluses [39]. Unfortunately, the intravenous nature of insulin administration and the associated hazards of infection, thrombosis, and phlebitis prevented further development of this model. A portable concept was advanced even further at the National Institute for Medical Research in England. The Mill Hill Infuser was designed to give insulin at two different rates: a basal rate and a prandial rate that was eightfold higher. It was initially used for studies that involved injecting hormones into animals.

A battery-powered syringe pump that weighed only 5.6 ounces, or approximately a third of a pound, was available for delivery at the touch of a button [40]. The first commercial pump, known as the "Big Blue Brick" because of its look, debuted in 1978 under Auto-Syringe as a sign of how far technology had come. When initial sales of 600 pumps per month exceeded estimates, numerous device firms in the early 1980s became interested in developing commercial pumps [41]. Initially, there were several setbacks due to issues with the safety of insulin administration, inflexible insulin doses, metal needles that regularly came loose, and constantly draining batteries.

Technology underwent a significant metamorphosis in the 1990s, making insulin pumps considerably safer and more dependable. User safety was increased by reducing insulin leakage, more reliable warnings for these possible failures, and more constant insulin administration. Alarms boosted users' perception of confidence in relying on insulin pump therapy for low battery or low insulin levels in the pump reservoir. It is obvious that more dependable pump devices have increased doctors' confidence in prescribing them for more diabetic patients rather than only those with the most complex needs. Pumps now work even more efficiently by saving numerous pre-programmed basal insulin rates in their memory. The carbohydrate composition of an approaching meal, a glucose goal range, and a correction factor for both pre-meal and post-meal glucose adjustments may all be entered to estimate the appropriate bolus dosages. The idea of insulin on board based on the pharmacodynamics of fast analogue insulin enables the pump to calculate a corrective insulin dose with greater accuracy—typically, a dose that is more advantageous than would be obvious to the pump user, who might be tempted to wing it! These so-called "smart pumps" are also capable of delivering insulin boluses to extend the duration of the insulin's activity [42].

1.7. Inhaled Insulin

According to surveys, many patients with T2DM find it challenging to utilize insulin due to their fear of needles, pain from insulin injections, and other factors. Therefore, there may be advantages to an efficient alternate insulin delivery method. Because insulin is a peptide hormone, it cannot be administered orally because the digestive enzymes in the stomach would quickly break it down. The administration of insulin via transdermal, transbuccal, and transpulmonary (inhaled) routes are other options that have been studied [43, 44].

Due to its substantial area for drug absorption and accessibility, the lung is a desirable route for systemic medication delivery. The first insulin to be inhaled was Exubera® (Pfizer), and the FDA gave its usage the go-ahead in January 2006. However, smoking can significantly alter the pharmacokinetics of inhaled insulin [45, 46] and even passive smoke exposure in non-smokers can affect bioavailability [47]. Clinical studies have shown that pre-meal inhaled insulin achieves comparable glycemic control to subcutaneous regular insulin administration [48, 49].

Concerns regarding the possible long-term toxicity of insulin administered through the pulmonary route have been raised by the follow-up of the patients who had taken Exubera in clinical trials. As of April 2008, just one of the 4292 patients in the placebo group got lung cancer, as opposed to six of the 4740 individuals who received Exubera in clinical trials. The six lung cancer patients were all former smokers (Exubera label, FDA clearance September 29, 2008), although due to the limited sample size, this connection was not statistically significant. However, because of these safety worries and Exubera's inability to win over patients and medical professionals, Pfizer pulled the drug off the market, and Eli Lilly and Novo Nordisk also abandoned their efforts to develop their insulin inhalation systems.

Technosphere® insulin, an inhaled form of insulin, is currently being developed by one firm, MannKind Corporation [50]. A new drug application was submitted to the FDA in March 2009 to sell this insulin. Technosphere insulin is made of insulin particles with a diameter of 2.5 m designed for inhalation and dissolving quickly (pH-sensitive carrier particles). Pharmacokinetic studies have shown that this formulation has a very quick systemic insulin uptake (insulin T_{max} is approximately 12–14 minutes), a quick onset of action (maximum activity is approximately 20–30 minutes), and a quick duration of action (approximately 2–3 hours) [51], which may provide better postprandial control than insulin administered subcutaneously.

1.8. Closed-Loop/Artificial Pancreas

In its current form, insulin pump therapy is regarded as an "open-loop system," in which the patient must make executive choices on how often to check their blood glucose and what to do with the results. There is undoubtedly room for human error in this method, and either overdosing or underdosing based on a minor error in computation might lead to a series of hypoglycemia or hyperglycemic episodes. The patient would be removed from the decision-making process in a "closed-loop system" that incorporates an insulin pump, continuous glucose monitor, and an automated algorithm to govern insulin delivery. The device would effectively act as an artificial pancreas.

The development of a fail-safe algorithm that can "interpret" a person's metabolic state based on data from the continuous glucose monitor and then relay this information to the pump for automatic insulin delivery of the proper dose of insulin may currently be one of the major challenges for the fully automated closed-loop system. Model predictive control and proportional integral derivative control are two methods that are now being tested in both in vivo and in silico situations [52]. The development of a closed-loop system also faces several technical challenges, such as the need for accurate and dependable glucose sensors (e.g., minimal calibration drift, limited potential mechanisms for sensor failure), as well as physiologic lag, which can be particularly troublesome during periods of rapid blood glucose change (e.g., during meals or exercise) [53]. Thus, building a sensor with minimal lag time would also be crucial. Currently being tested are the first closed-loop prototype devices that can give glucagon to avoid hypoglycemia [54].

Many studies have previously shown that glycemic control can be achieved using an automated closed-loop device in exploratory and controlled hospital settings, and the first generations of an artificial pancreas are now being developed. In order to mimic the physiologic properties of the - cell, Medtronic MiniMed has created an external physiologic insulin delivery system that incorporates an external insulin pump, a continuous glucose sensor, and a variable insulin infusion rate algorithm. Other businesses, such as Abbott Laboratories, are also creating and testing similar devices [55, 56].

2. Oral Hypoglycemic Drugs

The attempts to maintain near-normal blood glucose levels in people with T2DM (also known as non-insulin-dependent diabetes mellitus) have not been successful despite extensive management efforts. The fact that this condition is becoming more common worldwide is a significant issue for medical professionals. Insulin insufficiency, insulin resistance, and increased hepatic glucose production are the hallmarks of T2DM. One or more of these metabolic abnormalities are intended to be corrected by medications used to treat T2DM.

There are five groups of hypoglycemic drugs, each with pharmacologic characteristics. These classes include alpha-glucosidase inhibitors, sulfonylureas, meglitinides, biguanides, and thiazolidinediones. Therapy with a single oral medication can be considered in people for whom diet and exercise do not produce appropriate glucose control. When selecting an agent, it is advisable to consider both patient- and drug-specific factors. If optimal blood glucose control cannot be achieved with a single oral medication, a combination of drugs with various modes of action may have therapeutic benefits that add up and improve glycemic control.

2.1. Sulfonylureas

Sulfonylureas are secretagogues that induce pancreatic -cells to secrete natural insulin. It works best when there are still some remaining pancreatic beta cells and primarily targets the ATP-sensitive potassium channels on β-cells [57].

Sulfonylureas may hasten -cell failure and have no sustained protective impact on -cell activities [58]. It has been demonstrated that HbA1c concentrations rise after the first decline in glucose levels. Sulfonylureas have been shown to often lead to hypoglycemia, especially in patients on older medications. HbA1c levels can decrease by 1 to 2%, but blood glucose levels can be reduced by over 20%. Weight gain is a side effect of sulfonylureas [59].

2.2. Biguanides

Metformin is the most popular anti-diabetic drug, used mainly in obese and overweight people. Still, this is the top option for monotherapy. It improves glucose uptake by phosphorylating GLUT enhancer factors, suppresses hepatic gluconeogenesis, and increases insulin sensitivity [60]. In addition to reducing blood LDL cholesterol and triglycerides, metformin can help people lose weight [61]. Along with blocking mitochondrial complex 1 and the enzyme glycerophosphate dehydrogenase in the mitochondria, metformin also works by activating AMP-activated protein kinase, one of the enzymes implicated in the expression of hepatic gluconeogenic genes. All of these result in reduced glucose and HbA1c readings. Metformin does not affect beta cells, and if weight gain persists, insulin sensitivity in muscles does not improve, with HbA1c levels progressively returning to their initial level [62].

2.3. Thiazolidinediones

Thiazolidinediones (TZDs), which improve insulin sensitivity in adipocytes, cardiac muscles, and the liver, are peroxisome proliferator-activated receptor (PPAR) activators [63]. To maintain insulin secretion, they operate on cells. As a result, it is applied as a therapy strategy for T2DM patients who are insulin resistant, with results that extend for up to 5 years [64]. TZD often causes weight gain as a side effect. However, HbA1c decreases and improvement in β-cell functioning and insulin sensitivity are better the more weight gained [65]. TZD has the potential to reduce carotid artery thickness in T2DM patients. Due to the significant number of cardiovascular-related incidents, the FDA initially prohibited rosiglitazone; however, the prohibition has since been overturned. Patients with class III to IV cardiac failure should not use pioglitazone. Due to the increased risk of female fractures, it is recommended not to be suggested in senior congestive heart failure patients, despite being well-tolerated even in older renal-impaired individuals [66].

2.4. Dipeptidyl Peptidase-4 (DPP4) Inhibitors

Gliptins, commonly known as dipeptidyl peptidase 4 (DPP4) inhibitors, are a class of relatively recent medications that prevent the DPP4 enzyme from doing its job. A gastric inhibitory polypeptide (GIP) and glucagon-like peptide 1 (GLP-1) are incretin hormones that play a role in physically maintaining glucose homeostasis. Inhibition of this enzyme delays the inactivation of these hormones [67]. The production of insulin by pancreatic β-cells is stimulated by GLP-1 and GIP [68]. Additionally, pancreatic -cells' release of glucagon is reduced by GLP-1. Individuals with T2DM get improved glycemic control due to these benefits taken together. These medications have fewer side effects that have been documented, reduced risk of hypoglycemia, and weight neutrality [69].

2.5. Glucagon-Like Peptide 1 (GLP-1) Analogues

GLP-1 analogues are primarily used as incretin-based medicines that restrict the synthesis of hepatic glucose by decreasing glucagon secretion, increasing insulin secretion in a glucose-dependent manner, and increasing insulin secretion via a glucose-dependent manner [70]. Up to three years' worth of HbA1c reduction has been seen. Although these medications are not as well tolerated as DPP4 inhibitors, they result in greater HbA1c level reductions and promote weight loss [71]. They enhance lipid profiles, lengthen stomach emptying time, correct endothelial dysfunctions, and reduce blood pressure [72]. According to some evidence, incretin-based medicines are beneficial for the central nervous system, hepatic and cardiovascular health, inflammation (by lowering reactive protein levels), sleep, and inflammation [73].

2.6. Sodium-Glucose Co-Transporter-2 (SGLT2) Inhibitors

By blocking glucose absorption in the proximal renal tubules, SGLT2 inhibitors, often referred to as Gliflozins, reduce plasma blood glucose levels and increase glucose excretion via the kidneys [74]. This family of pharmaceuticals includes the drugs canagliflozin, dapagliflozin, and empagliflozin. Because they operate independently of insulin, they can be utilized in people with diabetes at any stage. These medications can boost insulin sensitivity, promote beta-cell functionality, and lessen the effects of glucosuria-related glucotoxicity. They can lower blood pressure, lose weight, and cut HbA1c levels by 0.5 to 1% [75]. Urinary tract infections, vaginal mycotic infections, particularly in women, and symptoms associated with volume depletion have all been reported as side effects. Patients who are old or on diuretics should be prescribed this medication with extra caution [76].

3. Combination Drug Therapy

Combination treatment is initiated for quicker, more efficient blood glucose management and dose reductions for individual drugs. It is often started after monotherapy is ineffective at controlling blood glucose levels. Exogenous insulin can be used in conjunction with various oral diabetes medications to reduce insulin doses. Glycemic control is improved when metformin or TZD are combined with insulin. HbA1c levels fall along with weight loss when basal insulin and GLP-1 receptor agonists are used together. SGLT2 inhibitors are typically used in conjunction with metformin or other medications [77]. Without increasing the risk of hypoglycemia, it can also be administered with DPP4 inhibitors to enhance glycemic control and reduce weight [78]. Pioglitazone and rosiglitazone, medications from the TZD family, as well as low-dosage metformin, have demonstrated efficacy in reducing the development of diabetes in prediabetic people [79].

4. Islet Transplantation

The development of insulin significantly improved the prognosis for people with T1DM, allowing for the proper management of the disease's most severe and deadly consequences, such as diabetic ketoacidosis. However, the increased longevity allowed for the emergence of diabetes secondary problems [80]. Over time, retinopathy, nephropathy, neuropathy, or vascular disease are frequently developed in T1DM patients. It wasn't until 1993 that the need of having effective glycemic control was shown without a doubt. Good glycemic control, which requires rigorous insulin therapy, might postpone or prevent the microvascular consequences of diabetes, according to the landmark Diabetes Control and Complications Trial (DCCT) trial [81].

Hemoglobin A1c (HbA1c) levels linked with such treatment were 1% (11 mmol/mol) lower than those of the control group. It should be highlighted that the HbA1c did not normalize and remained at least 1% (11 mmol/mol) beyond the upper limit of normal in the intensively treated group. Similar data were presented by the UK Prospective Diabetes Study (UKPDS), which demonstrated a substantial improvement for a drop of 1% (11 mmol/mol) in the HbA1c in T2DM with microvascular illness [82]. In order to prevent the microvascular consequences of diabetes, glycemic management is crucial. Glycemia control with exogenous insulin is still difficult. Even with extensive therapy, normoglycemia is challenging because of the unpredictability and delay in absorption introduced by the more recent insulin analogs. Continuous subcutaneous insulin treatment furthers the beneficial effects, although neither earlier nor more recent investigations have been successful in bringing glucose levels back to normal. Counting carbohydrates and paying attention to nutrition help in the quest for normoglycemia, but they are not a panacea. The most extensive trial that utilized every method available to enhance treatment was still linked to an elevated risk of hypoglycemia [81]. In the DCCT, there was a threefold increase in the probability of severe hypoglycemia, defined as requiring outside intervention. The obstacle to achieving ideal glycemic control continues to worry about hypoglycemia.

There have been several attempts to develop a closed-loop system for glucose regulation. The first successful attempts used the Biostator®, which used a computer-derived algorithm to continuously check blood glucose levels before administering insulin. It was unwieldy, had flow issues with the twin lumen catheter being used to sense the glucose level, and although successful for a brief amount of time. Although helpful, insulin infusion pumps that use insulin analogs, such as lispro or insulin aspart, are not closed-loop devices and frequently need glucose monitoring. As a result, normal glycemia is seldom achieved without severe hypoglycemia. Any closed-loop system's objective is to continuously link accurate glucose detection to optimal insulin administration. Mechanical closed-loop systems may eventually do this, but they have proved rife with issues despite early promise. The islets of Langerhans or the whole pancreas can now be transplanted to create a physiologic closed-loop system [83].

Although prolonged storage before islet isolation hindered viable islets' recovery, the University of Wisconsin solution (UW) proved beneficial in pancreatic preservation [84]. To save ischemically injured pancreas, the two-layer approach utilizing perfluorodecalin (PFC) and UW for entire pancreatic preservation was recommended. This was made possible by the capacity to maintain enough oxygenation to the pancreas during preservation and by encouraging the formation of adenosine triphosphate, which lessens the effects of cold ischemia damage [85]. Additionally, it was shown that preservation in PFC caused anti-apoptotic genes to be upregulated and pro-apoptotic genes to be downregulated [86].

Once sufficient pure islets have been produced, the patient is sent to radiology, where percutaneous access is made while they are sedated with midazolam and fentanyl. After local anesthetic infiltration under fluoroscopic guidance, a 22-gauge Cheba needle is inserted into the portal vein. Others have employed computer tomography (CT) guidance, and access can also be obtained via laparoscopy or the transjugular route [87]. The primary portal vein is then punctured with a guidewire, and a catheter is positioned with a portal venogram. Then, after regular portal pressure monitoring, purified islets are injected. The danger of liver hemorrhage from this percutaneous technique exists, as was noted in the original study. The catheter tract was then sealed with Gelfoam® pledgets and coils, and no further bleeding was observed in the following 28 cases. However, in 2003, there was a spate of post-procedural bleeding, defined as an acute fall in hemoglobin of 20% or more, coupled with free fluid on ultrasound, the requirement for blood transfusion, or the need for surgical intervention for the control of bleeding. Since then, the tract was ablated using tissue glue (Tisseel®), and the portal tributary cannulation site was sealed with coils, with no subsequent bleeding occurring in the next 35 surgeries. To seal the catheter tract Avitene® paste mixed in radiologic contrast and saline has been employed more recently. This has the benefit of being visibly apparent during deployment on fluoroscopy and has eliminated bleeding hazards when deployed properly [88, 89].

After receiving a minimum of 9000 IE/kg in transplants, 11 of the first 12 patients were no longer dependent on insulin. All patients had lower HbA1c levels, which were attained without hypoglycemia and were accompanied by better stability of glucose management [90]. Unfortunately, the majority of patients were unable to maintain insulin independence over time. Only 10% of patients were still without insulin after five years, according to a survival analysis, even though the majority of patients (80%) still had C-peptide in their bodies. Patients who continued to be insulin-free fared the best in terms of overall blood glucose management (median HbA1c of 6.2%, 44 mmol/mol), along with those who were put back on insulin but still had C peptide (median HbA1c of 6.7%, 50 mmol/mol). The glycemic management of patients who had completely lost graft function was rather poor (median HbA1c of 9.0%, 75 mmol/mol), and they needed more insulin than they did in the pre-transplantation period [88].

5. Gene Therapy

The transport of the insulin gene into several tissues, including the pancreas, liver, adipocytes, and muscle, has been done using viral and nonviral methods, including lentivirus, adenovirus, and AAV as well as liposomes and bare DNA [91]. Intriguingly, intestinal cells like enteroendocrine K-cells, which generate glucose-dependent insulinotropic polypeptide (GIP) and include prohormone convertases essential for digesting proinsulin, exhibited numerous similarities with pancreatic β-cells [92]. As a result, several scientists tried to modify K-cells in vitro so that they would make and release insulin, but the implantation of these cells did not successfully correct diabetes in a safe manner. Surprisingly, after utilizing streptozotocin (STZ) to induce diabetes, transgenic mice engineered to produce insulin under the GIP promoter had normal glucose levels. This proved that K cells generated insulin in sufficient amounts to maintain glucose homeostasis [93].

Adeno-associated viral (AAV) vectors have recently been used in managing diabetes mellitus (DM) to co-express the genes for insulin and glucokinase in skeletal muscles. The long-term effectiveness of diabetic gene therapy without the administration of exogenous insulin might lead to normoglycemia [94]. AAV vectors infect both dividing and quiescent cells without integrating into the host cell's DNA and trigger a moderate immune response. AAV vectors are the ideal choice for gene therapy because of these characteristics. In the study, STZ-induced diabetes mice and dogs had their skeletal muscles implanted with AAV vectors encoding the genes for insulin and glucokinase. The translocation of the GLUT4 and glucokinase enzyme is accelerated by the co-expression of two genes, facilitating glucose absorption into modified muscle cells. Additionally, it serves as a glucose sensor, measuring blood sugar levels and indicating how much insulin must be generated to achieve normoglycemia [95].

On the other side, a humanized liver mouse model is used in gene therapy to treat diabetes. In order to transfect the pancreatic and duodenal homeobox 1 (pdx-1) gene, also known as the insulin promoter factor 1 for the formation and maturation of the pancreatic β-cells, Li et al. employed AAV serotype 2 (AAV2) as a medium [96]. In order to maintain glycemic control, the PDX1 gene in the liver will release insulin ectopically, as seen by the presence of green fluorescent protein expression. According to the study, the AAV-pdx-1 gene injection lowered the elevated glucose content in STZ-induced diabetic mice. Neurogenin 3 (Ngn3) is another gene that determines the pancreas' endocrine destiny [4].

Insulin production and oval cell population transdifferentiation result after the transfection of hepatic cells with an adenovirus that carried Ngn3 [97]. The elevation of downstream and upstream pancreatic transcription factors, such as Pax4, Pax6, Ngn3, Nkx6.1, and Nkx2.2, was caused by the injection of NeuroD1 into the liver of STZ-induced diabetic mice, without appreciable hepatitis or hepatotoxicity [98, 99]. Additionally, when compared to Ngn3, pdx-1, and Pax4 in primary duct cells, NeuroD1 had the largest effect on triggering insulin expression [100]. Targeting promoters in other cells, such as liver-type pyruvate kinase (L-PK), glucose 6-phosphatase (G6Pase), phosphoenolpyruvate carboxykinase (PEPCK), S-14, albumin, and insulin-like growth factor binding protein-1, would be the ideal DNA construct (IGFBP-1). Although insulin secretion was demonstrated when these genes were promoted in the liver as part of a hepatic insulin gene therapy, the secretion was weak due to their modest promoting activity compared to powerful constitutive promoters like CMV [101]. For instance, L-PK was modified to increase insulin expression in the liver, which improved glucose sensitivity and allowed for the restoration of normoglycemia for up to one month. The suppression of this promoter by insulin is the only restriction. S14 and albumin may be utilized to prevent this feedback [102].

Intravenous injection of insulin fragments with plasmid DNA allows for the non-viral introduction. The liver and muscles of STZ-induced diabetic rats who received injections of this plasmid exhibited normoglycemia for 1 week and 30 weeks, respectively. The brief duration of expression in liver injection was resolved by introducing the gene into the host chromosome via a DNA transposon technique. However, the co-injection of plasmid DNA carrying insulin and furin resulted in a significant amount of active insulin in the muscle [103].

Pigs' insulin production, hyperglycemia, and diabetes sequelae significantly improved for more than 47 weeks after ex vivo transfection and autologous transplant of human insulin into pancreatic or liver cells [104]. Gene silencing occurred; however, the mechanism of this silencing is unknown, therefore this improvement stopped. Another effective strategy involves injecting a lentivirus vector—carrying human-modified insulin gene—into the portal system of the liver of diabetic rats. Unexpectedly, this technique enables liver cells to detect glucose and, in reaction, produce, release, and store human insulin [105].

6. Stem Cells

Studies into alternate β-cell sources, such as embryonic stem cells, have been conducted due to the limitations of pancreatic progenitor cells (ESCs). The pancreatic epithelium, which contains multipotent progenitors, will evolve during embryonic development into different pancreatic cell types, including ductal, endocrine, and exocrine lineages [106]. The use of human stem cells at the embryonic stage is the biggest drawback of this approach. This creates a constraint by raising the ethical question. In order to get over this restriction, somatic cell nucleus reprogramming was used to create induced pluripotent stem cells (iPSCs) [107]. iPSCs and ESCs share several characteristics. Small chemicals and ribonucleic acids are both capable of producing iPSCs. Since most patients' iPSCs share the same genetic makeup, immunological responses are avoided.

A small variation between iPSCs and ESCs raises the potential for patient-specific cell replacement treatment [108]. These alternate sources have an infinite capacity for growth and differentiation into various germ-layer cells. HiPSCs are created by combining multiple factors, including Klf4, lenti-Oct3/4, Sox2, and c-Myc, into human pancreatic duct cells [109]. These hiPSCs had equivalent amounts of specific ESCs markers, which instantly differentiate into three germ layers where hiPSCs form an embryoid body [110]. Recent investigations revealed procedures that produced -cells with considerably comparable expression to -cells obtained from humans [111]. Within two weeks of being transplanted into diabetic mice, the new stem cell-derived -cells began to produce insulin in response to high glucose levels and kept the normoglycemic level. This result increases the likelihood that ESC or iPSC replacement therapy for diabetic patients may be used in the future [112]. However, the differentiation of ESCs and iPSCs imposes numerous phases and requires that various aspects be considered.

Additionally, undifferentiated ESCs and IPSCs have a risk of malignancy, and clinical trials of differentiation methods take time [113]. The use of ESCs and iPSCs for treating diabetes has been constrained by hurdles. Interestingly, the presence of pancreatic lineage in pancreatic progenitor cells (PPCs) allows them to circumvent the constraints imposed on ESCs and iPSCs.

Mesenchymal stem cell (MSC) treatment for diabetics has been shown to be beneficial through immunomodulatory pathways in several trials. A microenvironment is produced where destructive T-Helper1 (Th1) cells are largely inhibited and β-cells are replenished [114]. The experts concurred that the control of hyperglycemia had improved in these investigations. However, combining MSCs therapy with other forms of treatment is recommended. According to strong histologic evidence, undifferentiated MSCs are not directly responsible for the regeneration of new cells. Additionally, when administered to diabetic rats, the MSC culture medium had efficient therapeutic effects [63].

Due to the cell-free nature of this approach, it offers an effective therapy and averts the problems of autoimmunity and oncogenesis. In conclusion, if the collection methods are improved, the MSC medium may be used in conjunction with other tried-and-true treatments to lessen insulin reliance or with the transplantation of insulin-producing cells generated from different pluripotent sources [115].

In order to replace injured beta cells, bone marrow stem cells (BMSC) are employed; however, they generate little insulin. Thankfully, adipose tissue has a stronger immunomodulatory capacity, a lower immunogenicity, and the capacity to create more stem cells than bone marrow [116]. Additionally, adipose-derived stem cells (ADSCs) are characterized by their straightforward isolation process, simple accessibility, and ability to proliferate unaffected by the patient's age [117].

In research, insulin-producing cells (IPCs) were created from ADSCs, which were subsequently injected into the pancreas of STZ rats. The results of the histological investigation showed that the pancreatic regeneration process had been induced, as seen by the many dilated blood capillaries and diffusely proliferating islet cells. Intriguingly, the IPC transplanted group's blood glucose levels were not noticeably different from those of the control (diabetic-free) group, and the IPCs rats' pancreas looked to be identical to those of the control group. Overall, the appearance and performance of the islet cells in diabetic rats were enhanced by the transplantation of differentiated IPCs. More research has been done to support the efficacy of ADSCs in reducing T2DM in rats. Through the promotion of islet angiogenesis, reduction of cell death, and improvement of insulin sensitivity, ADSCs infusion might repair islet -cells and alleviate hyperglycemia [118].

Another study found that employing human eyelid adipose tissue-derived stem cells resulted in higher levels of human insulin and c-peptide in type 2 diabetic mice and lower levels of IL-6, triglycerides, and free fatty acids [119].

Adenoviral vectors encoding for mouse pdx-1 and human BM-MSCs were used in a first effort to induce BM-MSCs to differentiate into IPCs. IPCs that were created demonstrated the ability to release insulin in a glucose-dependent manner [120, 121]. Numerous investigations examined BM-MSCs with umbilical cord (UC)-MSCs, notably those produced from Wharton's jelly (WJ-MSCs), and concluded that WJ-MSCs had a higher differentiation ability toward a mature-cell phenotype than BM-MSCs [122]. Additionally, compared to BMMSCs, WJMSCs showed a higher ability for insulin and C-peptide mRNA expression. In light of this, if ADSCs' safety and efficacy are shown, they may provide patients with T1DM and T2DM with a favorable treatment approach.

Scientists were drawn to human placenta-derived MSC (PD-MSC) because of their capacity to make insulin. In a pilot trial, 10 T2DM patients received intravenous injections of PD-MSC to evaluate its effects. According to the data, all ten patients had a considerable reduction in glycosylated hemoglobin, and their levels of insulin and C-peptide were greater than they had been with earlier therapies. Additionally, the cardiac and renal functions improved, and no adverse effects such as chills, liver damage, fever, or immunological rejection appeared [123].

7. Complementary Diabetes Treatments

The usage of traditional anti-diabetic medications has significant risks. They could be harmful in some situations and harm the patient's health. Numerous studies have revealed that lifestyle treatments centered on increased physical activity and diet may aid in improved illness management to fight this condition and enhance the quality of life for diabetes patients.

7.1. Exercise

Exercise improves the overall quality of life and is known to lower the risk for several lifestyle-related disorders, including cardiovascular disease, obesity, and T2DM. The skeletal muscles enhance glucose absorption by many folds during a regular physical activity session, lowering the blood's hyperglycemic conditions [124]. The two key variables that affect the kind of fuel used during exercise are the intensity and duration of the physical activity. The energy source shifts from stored muscle glycogen to circulatory glucose, free fatty acids, and increased carbohydrate oxidation as the muscle glycogen gradually depletes. Additionally, gluconeogenesis replaces hepatic glycogenolysis as the source of circulatory glucose [125].

According to a meta-analysis of 8538 patients, organized exercise programs lasting more than 150 minutes per week—whether they involve weight training, aerobic activity, or both—lead to higher reductions in HbA1c than programs lasting just 150 minutes or less [126]. Similarly, a comprehensive analysis of 10 prospective cohort studies found that moderately vigorous exercise, such as walking, is similarly linked to a decreased risk of T2DM [127]. Various clinical studies show that aerobic, resistance, stretching, and upper and lower body activities might assist diabetes individuals lower their HbA1c levels. In addition to these clinical studies, Boule' et al. investigated the effects of various activities on body mass and HbA1C levels in 504 T2DM patients for a period of eight weeks. The results were evaluated using statistical models, which confirms the aforementioned study [128]. Additionally, research by Ishii et al. suggests that doing efficient workouts might enhance insulin sensitivity [129]. In a study by Cuff et al., 28 postmenopausal T2D patients were given aerobic resistance training for 16 weeks. Results were assessed by glucose disposal using a hyperinsulinemic-euglycemic clamp and computed tomography scans of the abdominal and mid-thigh skeletal muscles. The exercise group showed higher infusion rates and lower muscle density than the control group, which received no exercise [130].

7.2. Yoga

Yoga, a physical and spiritual exercise program, has enormous potential as a co-intervention in enhancing diabetes patients' quality of life. It involves a variety of physical postures and motions (referred to as asanas), breathing exercises, and meditation, all of which are intended to enhance physical comfort and mental stability. Research conducted in India on 123 diabetes individuals revealed that yoga significantly decreased BMI and improved glycemic control. Additionally, glutathione and vitamin C levels rose, considerably reducing the oxidative stress experienced by diabetes individuals. Diabetes and its accompanying clinical problems, including atherosclerosis, microvascular issues, and neuropathy, have all been linked to the development of oxidative stress as the primary factor [131]. In a 12-week yoga program, 23 persons at high risk for T2D showed improvements in their weight, blood pressure, insulin levels, and triglycerides compared to the control group [132]. Research showed that 20 T2DM patients who followed and practiced several asanas constantly for 40 days saw a discernible change in their lipid profiles and blood glucose levels [133].

Additionally, Nisha et al. in Kerala conducted a clinical experiment over three months with hypertensive diabetic patients taking diabetes medications and practicing yoga for an hour. Patients with diabetes who had just taken diabetic medications and did not practice yoga served as the control group in this study. After three months, blood pressure and blood sugar levels were examined between the two groups, and it was shown that patients who had been practicing yoga had relatively low blood pressure and blood sugar levels [134]. Similar research by Savita and colleagues on twenty-four T2DM cases showed metabolic and clinical evidence of improvements in blood glucose level management and cardiac functioning after 20-40 minutes of yoga with a variety of asanas every day for 40 days under the guidance of the experts [135].

7.3. Diet

One of the most critical factors affecting someone's health is their diet. Numerous studies support the importance of food for a healthy life. Low-fat vegetarian diets that include fruits, vegetables, grains, etc. have been demonstrated in studies to promote insulin sensitivity, improve glycemic control, cause weight reduction, and help manage diabetes. Diabetic patients are strongly advised to eat a diet high in dietary fiber, low in carbohydrates, and low in fat since these are proven to stop blood glucose levels from rising. High-fiber carbohydrates, sometimes referred to as slow-release carbs, assist in controlling blood sugar levels because they break down slowly, reducing the body's need for excessive insulin [136, 137].

Dietary fat is also of special importance because fatty acids affect glucose metabolism by changing the structure and activity of several enzymes involved in glucose metabolism as well as the function of cell membranes. It is also known that fatty meals slow down the action of insulin, causing high blood sugar levels to persist after the meal. Dietary control aids in controlling blood glucose levels [138]. A low-fat vegan diet significantly helps regulate glycemia and plasma lipid concentrations, according to research done on 99 T2DM patients in America [139]. Another randomized control experiment (RCT) with 99 people conducted in America further showed the benefits of a low-fat vegan diet for glycemic, plasma lipid, and weight control in individuals with T2D [140]. Dietary carbs affect the onset of T2DM, according to prospective cohort research on 35,988 older Iowa women who were previously free of diabetes [141]. A randomized, crossover research with 13 T2DM patients found that eating a diet high in soluble fiber helped them regulate their blood sugar levels, reduced hyperinsulinemia, and reduced their plasma lipid levels [142]. Therefore, there should be a stronger focus on encouraging these individuals to eat a diet high in fiber.

7.4. Vitamins

When taken as supplements, vitamins have a high potential to treat disorders like T2DM. Diabetes is thought to be a condition characterized by oxidative damage. As a result, oxidative stress and antioxidants have a strong relationship. However, several vitamins, including vitamins D, C, and E, are recognized potential antioxidants and may thus be utilized to treat diabetes by reducing oxidative stress [143, 144].

7.4.1. Vitamin D

Sunshine provides the majority of the vitamin D that the body needs, but due to lifestyle changes, sunlight exposure has dramatically decreased, which has resulted in vitamin D insufficiency, which in turn may result in several health problems. Numerous association-based studies have suggested that those with the lowest blood levels of vitamin D are more likely to acquire type 2 diabetes. According to recent research, the majority of diabetes patients are also shown to have lower vitamin D levels than non-diabetics. The presence of several vitamin D receptors and vitamin D binding proteins in pancreatic tissues suggests a potential involvement of this organ in the production and release of insulin [145].

Lower circulating vitamin D levels have been linked to insulin resistance and hyperglycemia in a meta-analysis that included 21 prospective trials [146]. Short-term vitamin D treatment enhanced pancreatic cell function in an RCT with 92 adult patients at risk of T2D. Low blood levels of 25-hydroxyvitamin D have been linked to diabetes and reduced glucose tolerance, according to cross-sectional studies [147]. The study done on 83,779 women over the course of 20 years [148] revealed that vitamin D has a role in lowering the risk of T2D. Additionally, it has been noted that glucose tolerance returns after vitamin D levels are back to normal [149].

7.4.2. Vitamin E

A fat-soluble vitamin called vitamin E serves as an antioxidant as well as other crucial biological functions. Vegetable oils, almonds, green leafy vegetables, and fortified cereals are typical dietary sources of vitamin E. When lipids in the tissues are being oxidized, it acts as an antioxidant to scavenge reactive oxygen species (ROS). The pathophysiology of T2DM and its consequences have been linked to oxidative stress caused by increased ROS generation and a drop in antioxidant levels. In five randomized placebo-controlled trials, with a sample size ranging from 15 to 57 participants, vitamin E supplementation at doses of 600 to 1,600 IU significantly decreased oxidative stress and improved glycemic control in diabetic patients over 4 to 16 weeks, according to a meta-analysis conducted among American women [150]. Contrarily, a Heart Outcomes Prevention Evaluation (HOPE) trial involving 3654 participants who were both diabetic and at risk of cardiovascular disease revealed that despite the daily administration of 400 IU of vitamin E, there was no difference in the outcomes for glycemic control and cardiovascular health in diabetic patients. Further studies are required to fully comprehend the effects of vitamin E administration in T2DM patients [151].

7.4.3. Vitamin C

Vitamin C is essential in controlling blood glucose levels as an antioxidant. Population-based prospective cohort research involving 21,831 people found that T2DM risk was lowered by greater plasma levels of vitamin C [152]. Another study that involved 10 healthy and 10 diabetic participants concluded that vitamin C infusions are crucial for improving non-oxidative glucose metabolism and controlling insulin action in diabetes patients [153].

7.5. Nutraceuticals

Various goods are supplied to enhance a person's health, including separated nutrients, dietary supplements, and herbal products. Growing evidence has surfaced in recent years that supports the therapeutic use of nutraceuticals for the management and complementary care of T2DM patients as well as those with other conditions. Berberine, garlic, and cinnamon are a few of the popular supplements among these nutraceuticals that are suggested to help enhance the health of diabetic people [154].

7.5.1. Cinnamon

Cinnamon is said to have the potential to regulate blood sugar, total cholesterol, and triglyceride levels, among other things. The active ingredient in cinnamon, cinnamaldehyde, largely aids in increasing insulin production and glucose absorption. Increasing the kinase activity of the insulin receptor and causing auto-phosphorylation of the insulin receptor, which activates the cascade of pathways and ultimately causes GLUT4 activation, improves glucose absorption. It was discovered that after 40 days, there was a significant reduction in the mean fasting serum glucose, triglyceride, low-density lipid, cholesterol, and total cholesterol levels as compared to placebo groups that did not consume cinnamon. This was the result of the first clinical trial to examine the effect of cinnamon in controlling T2DM, which was conducted in Pakistan on 60 diabetic individuals who were supplemented with different doses of cinnamon [155]. The meta-analysis of 10 RCTs with a sample size of 543 patients, which found that cinnamon consumption is associated with a statistically significant decrease in levels of fasting plasma glucose, total cholesterol, low-density lipid-cholesterol (LDL-C), and triglyceride levels, could be used to demonstrate the significant effect of cinnamon on blood glucose. As a result of many investigations, it has been suggested that including cinnamon in the diet may help to treat diabetes [156, 157].

7.5.2. Garlic

All around the world, it has been used to add taste and perfume to cuisine. In addition, its antioxidant action makes it effective for various medical conditions. Studies have revealed that the antioxidant S-allyl cysteine sulfoxide extracted from garlic may help garlic positively impact diabetes [158]. The results of a clinical investigation involving 50 T2DM patients with hyperlipidemia showed that taking 900 mg of garlic powder per day for six weeks dramatically reduced total cholesterol, LDL-C, systolic blood pressure, and increased HDL-C levels [159].

Another randomized, single-blind, placebo-controlled study that involved 70 T2DM patients with newly diagnosed dyslipidemia for 12 weeks and found that garlic exhibits a short-term benefit on lipid profile and more significant reductions in total cholesterol and LDL-C and moderate increases in HDL-C compared to that with placebo further demonstrated its anti-diabetic effects [160]. More research must be done to assess the anti-diabetic effects of garlic fully.

7.5.3. Berberine

A plant alkaloid known as berberine has a long history of usage in both Chinese and Ayurvedic medicine. It has a broad spectrum of effects, although its major antibacterial (against bacterial diarrhea, intestinal parasites, fungal infections, *Candida albicans*, yeast, and maybe methicillin-resistant *Staphylococcus aureus*) and anti-inflammatory actions are most notable. Several plants, including Hydrastiscanadensis, Coptischinensis, Berberisaquifolium, *Berberis vulgaris*, and Berberisaristata, have it in their roots, rhizomes, and stem bark (Although the exact mechanism of action of berberine's anti-diabetic effects is unclear, this property has been demonstrated. The adenosine monophosphate-activated protein kinase (AMPK), which phosphorylates key targets such as the enzymes involved in lipid metabolism, lipolysis, fatty acid oxidation, and glucose absorption, is one of the processes that suggest the health advantages of berberine. Research in rat models has demonstrated that berberine-induced activation of AMPK triggers a series of events that cause GLUT4 to go into the muscles and reduce lipid levels in adipocytes [161]. There aren't many case-control studies that show berberine has a hypoglycemic impact. Significant reductions in fasting and postprandial plasma glucose levels, as well as in HbA1c levels, were seen in an RCT done in China with 106 T2D patients who also had dyslipidemia when participants received a daily dose of 1 g berberine for 3 months [162].

Conclusion

The study of diabetic patients in the pre-insulin era informs us that diabetes may be managed without insulin for a long time. There are five groups of hypoglycemic drugs, each with pharmacologic characteristics. These classes include alpha-glucosidase inhibitors, sulfonylureas, meglitinides, biguanides, and thiazolidinediones. Therapy with a single oral medication can be considered in people whose diet and exercise do not produce appropriate glucose control. Combination treatment is initiated for quicker, more efficient blood glucose management and dose reductions for individual drugs. The development of insulin significantly improved the prognosis for people with T1DM, allowing for the proper management of the disease's most severe and deadly consequences, such as diabetic ketoacidosis. The transport of the insulin gene into several tissues, including the pancreas, liver, adipocytes, and muscle, has been done using viral and nonviral methods, including lentivirus, adenovirus, and AAV as well as liposomes and bare DNA. Studies into alternate β-cell sources, such as embryonic stem cells, have been conducted due to the limitations of pancreatic progenitor cells. The usage of traditional anti-diabetic medications has significant risks. They could be harmful in some situations and harm the patient's health. Numerous studies have revealed that lifestyle treatments centered on increased physical activity and diet may aid in improved illness management to fight this condition and enhance the quality of life for diabetes patients.

References

[1] Allen, Frederick Madison, Edgar Stillman, and Reginald Fitz. *Total dietary regulation in the treatment of diabetes*. New York, NY, USA: Rockefeller Institute for Medical Research, 1919.

[2] Bliss, Michael. *The Discovery of Insulin: Special Centenary Edition*. University of Toronto Press, 2021.

[3] Shah, Siddharth N., S. R. Joshi, and D. V. Parmar. "History of insulin." *Journal of the Association of Physicians of India* 97 (1997): 1-1.

[4] Schwitzgebel, Valérie M., David W. Scheel, Jennifer R. Conners, Julie Kalamaras, Jacqueline E. Lee, David J. Anderson, Lori Sussel, Jeffrey D. Johnson, and Michael S. German. "Expression of neurogenin3 reveals an islet cell precursor population in the pancreas." *Development* 127, no. 16 (2000): 3533-3542.

[5] Brogden, Rex N., and R. C. Heel. "Human insulin." *Drugs* 34, no. 3 (1987): 350-371.

[6] Heinemann, Lutz, and Bernd Richter. "Clinical pharmacology of human insulin." *Diabetes Care* 16, no. Supplement_3 (1993): 90-100.

[7] Chien, Yie W. "Human insulin: Basic sciences to therapeutic uses." *Drug development and industrial pharmacy* 22, no. 8 (1996): 753-789.

[8] Yadav, S., and Ankit Parakh. "Insulin therapy." *Indian pediatrics* 43, no. 10 (2006): 863-872.

[9] Bauman, Louis. "Clinical experience with globin insulin." *Proceedings of the Society for Experimental Biology and Medicine* 40, no. 2 (1939): 170-171.

[10] Hagedors, H. C., B. Norman Jensen, N. B. Krarup, and I. Wodstrup. "Protamine insulinate." *Journal of the American Medical Association* 106 (1936): 177-180.

[11] Hallas-Møller, K., K. Petersen, and J. Schlichtkrull. "Crystalline and amorphous insulin-zinc compounds with prolonged action." *Science* 116, no. 3015 (1952): 394-398.

[12] Søeborg, Tue, Christian Hove Rasmussen, Erik Mosekilde, and Morten Colding-Jørgensen. "Absorption kinetics of insulin after subcutaneous administration." *European journal of pharmaceutical sciences* 36, no. 1 (2009): 78-90.

[13] Brange, Jens, David R. Owens, Steven Kang, and Aage Vølund. "Monomeric insulins and their experimental and clinical implications." *Diabetes Care* 13, no. 9 (1990): 923-954.

[14] Kang, Steven, Jens Brange, Anna Burch, Aage Vølund, and David R. Owens. "Subcutaneous insulin absorption explained by insulin's physicochemical properties: evidence from absorption studies of soluble human insulin and insulin analogues in humans." *Diabetes care* 14, no. 11 (1991): 942-948.

[15] Heinemann, L., T. Heise, L. N. Jorgensen, and A. A. R. Starke. "Action profile of the rapid acting insulin analogue: human insulin B28Asp." *Diabetic medicine* 10, no. 6 (1993): 535-539.

[16] Howey, Daniel C., Ronald R. Bowsher, Rocco L. Brunelle, and James R. Woodworth. "[Lys (B28), Pro (B29)]-human insulin: a rapidly absorbed analogue of human insulin." *Diabetes* 43, no. 3 (1994): 396-402.

[17] Hirsch, Irl B. "Insulin analogues." *New England Journal of Medicine* 352, no. 2 (2005): 174-183.

[18] Bode, Bruce W. "Use of rapid-acting insulin analogues in the treatment of patients with type 1 and type 2 diabetes mellitus: insulin pump therapy versus multiple daily injections." *Clinical Therapeutics* 29 (2007): S135-S144.

[19] Owens, David R., Phillip A. Coates, Stephen D. Luzio, Jeroen P. Tinbergen, and Reiner Kurzhals. "Pharmacokinetics of 125I-labeled insulin glargine (HOE 901) in healthy men: comparison with NPH insulin and the influence of different subcutaneous injection sites." *Diabetes Care* 23, no. 6 (2000): 813-819.

[20] Horvath, Karl, Klaus Jeitler, Andrea Berghold, Susanne H. Ebrahim, Thomas W. Gratzer, Johannes Plank, Thomas Kaiser, Thomas R. Pieber, and Andrea Siebenhofer. "Long-acting insulin analogues versus NPH insulin (human isophane insulin) for type 2 diabetes mellitus." *Cochrane database of systematic reviews* 2 (2007).

[21] Monami, Matteo, Niccolò Marchionni, and Edoardo Mannucci. "Long-acting insulin analogues versus NPH human insulin in type 2 diabetes: a meta-analysis." *Diabetes research and clinical practice* 81, no. 2 (2008): 184-189.

[22] Strauss, Kenneth. "Insulin injection techniques. Report from the 1st International Insulin Injection Technique Workshop, Strasbourg, France—June 1997." *Practical Diabetes International* 15, no. 6 (1998): 181-184.

[23] Jehle, Peter M., Clemens Micheler, Daniela R. Jehle, Dieter Breitig, and Bernhard O. Boehm. "Inadequate suspension of neutral protamine Hagendorn (NPH) insulin in pens." *The Lancet* 354, no. 9190 (1999): 1604-1607.

[24] Rubenstein, A. H., and I. Spitz. "Role of the kidney in insulin metabolism and excretion." *Diabetes* 17, no. 3 (1968): 161-169.

[25] Duckworth, William C. "Insulin degradation: mechanisms, products, and significance." *Endocrine reviews* 9, no. 3 (1988): 319-345.

[26] Binder, Christian. "Absorption of Injected Insulin: A Clinical-Pharmacological Study." *Acta Pharmacologica et toxicologica* 27, no. S2 (1969): 1-83.

[27] Binder, Christian, Torsten Lauritzen, Ole Faber, and Stig Pramming. "Insulin pharmacokinetics." Diabetes care 7, no. 2 (1984): 188-199.

[28] Koivisto, Velkko A., and Philip Felig. "Alterations in insulin absorption and in blood glucose control associated with varying insulin injection sites in diabetic patients." *Annals of Internal Medicine* 92, no. 1 (1980): 59-61.

[29] Vaag, Allan, Aase Handberg, Mogens Lauritzen, Jan Erik Henriksen, Karen Damgaard Pedersen, and Henning Beck-Nielsen. "Variation in absorption of NPH insulin due to intramuscular injection." *Diabetes Care* 13, no. 1 (1990): 74-76.

[30] Selam, J. L. "External and implantable insulin pumps: current place in the treatment of diabetes." *Experimental and Clinical Endocrinology & Diabetes* 109, no. Suppl 2 (2001): S333-S340

[31] Duckworth, William C., Christopher D. Saudek, and Robert R. Henry. "Why intraperitoneal delivery of insulin with implantable pumps in NIDDM?." *Diabetes* 41, no. 6 (1992): 657-661.

[32] Henry, Robert R., Barry Gumbiner, Timothy Ditzler, Penny Wallace, Rachel Lyon, and Harry S. Glauber. "Intensive conventional insulin therapy for type II diabetes: metabolic effects during a 6-mo outpatient trial." *Diabetes care* 16, no. 1 (1993): 21-31.

[33] Feskens, E. J., and Daan Kromhout. "Hyperinsulinemia, risk factors, and coronary heart disease. The Zutphen Elderly Study." *Arteriosclerosis and Thrombosis: A Journal of Vascular Biology 14*, no. 10 (1994): 1641-1647.

[34] Chan, Edwina, and Patricia A. Montgomery. "Administration of insulin by continuous ambulatory peritoneal dialysis." *Pharmacotherapy: The Journal of Human Pharmacology and Drug Therapy* 13, no. 5 (1993): 455-460.

[35] Quellhorst, Eduard. "Insulin therapy during peritoneal dialysis: pros and cons of various forms of administration." *Journal of the American Society of Nephrology* 13, no. suppl 1 (2002): S92-S96.

[36] Kipnes, Mark, Paresh Dandona, Devjit Tripathy, J. Gordon Still, and Gordana Kosutic. "Control of postprandial plasma glucose by an oral insulin product (HIM2) in patients with type 2 diabetes." *Diabetes care* 26, no. 2 (2003): 421-426.

[37] Silva, Catarina M., António J. Ribeiro, Domingos Ferreira, and Francisco Veiga. "Insulin encapsulation in reinforced alginate microspheres prepared by internal gelation." *european journal of pharmaceutical sciences* 29, no. 2 (2006): 148-159.

[38] Alsaleh, F. M., Felicity J. Smith, S. Keady, and K. M. G. Taylor. "Insulin pumps: from inception to the present and toward the future." *Journal of clinical pharmacy and therapeutics* 35, no. 2 (2010): 127-138.

[39] Slama, Gerard, Michel Hautecouverture, Roger Assan, and Georges Tchobroutsky. "One to five days of continuous intravenous insulin infusion on seven diabetic patients." *Diabetes* 23, no. 9 (1974): 732-738.

[40] Pickup, J. C., H. Keen, J. A. Parsons, and K. G. Alberti. "Continuous subcutaneous insulin infusion: an approach to achieving normoglycaemia." *Br Med J* 1, no. 6107 (1978): 204-207.

[41] Hauge, C. "Insulin pumps: evolution of an industry Medtronic MiniMed Europe." *Switzerland: Business Briefing: European Pharmacology* (2003): 1-3.

[42] Hirsch, Irl B. "Insulin analogues." *New England Journal of Medicine* 352, no. 2 (2005): 174-183.

[43] Hunt, Linda M., Miguel A. Valenzuela, and Jacqueline A. Pugh. "NIDDM patients' fears and hopes about insulin therapy: the basis of patient reluctance." *Diabetes care* 20, no. 3 (1997): 292-298.

[44] Zambanini, Andrew, Roger B. Newson, Mari Maisey, and Michael D. Feher. "Injection related anxiety in insulin-treated diabetes." *Diabetes research and clinical practice* 46, no. 3 (1999): 239-246.

[45] Himmelmann, Anders, Johan Jendle, Anders Mellén, Astrid H. Petersen, Ulf L. Dahl, and Per Wollmer. "The impact of smoking on inhaled insulin." *Diabetes Care* 26, no. 3 (2003): 677-682.

[46] Becker, Reinhard HA, Sue Sha, Annke D. Frick, and Robert J. Fountaine. "The effect of smoking cessation and subsequent resumption on absorption of inhaled insulin." *Diabetes Care* 29, no. 2 (2006): 277-282.

[47] Fountaine, Robert, Ashley Milton, Tina Checchio, Greg Wei, Marilyn Stolar, John Teeter, Rudolph Jaeger, and David Fryburg. "Acute passive cigarette smoke exposure and inhaled human insulin (Exubera®) pharmacokinetics." *British journal of clinical pharmacology* 65, no. 6 (2008): 864-870.

[48] Hollander, Priscilla A., Lawrence Blonde, Richard Rowe, Adi E. Mehta, Joseph L. Milburn, Kenneth S. Hershon, Jean-Louis Chiasson, Seymour R. Levin, and Exubera Phase III Study Group. "Efficacy and safety of inhaled insulin (Exubera) compared with subcutaneous insulin therapy in patients with type 2 diabetes: results of a 6-month, randomized, comparative trial." *Diabetes care* 27, no. 10 (2004): 2356-2362.

[49] Ceglia, Lisa, Joseph Lau, and Anastassios G. Pittas. "Meta-analysis: efficacy and safety of inhaled insulin therapy in adults with diabetes mellitus." *Annals of internal medicine* 145, no. 9 (2006): 665-675.

[50] Rosenstock, Julio, Richard Bergenstal, Ralph A. DeFronzo, Irl B. Hirsch, David Klonoff, Anders H. Boss, David Kramer. "Efficacy and safety of Technosphere inhaled insulin compared with Technosphere powder placebo in insulin-naive type 2 diabetes suboptimally controlled with oral agents." *Diabetes Care* 31, no. 11 (2008): 2177-2182.

[51] Pfützner, Andreas, Alfred E. Mann, and Solomon S. Steiner. "Technosphere™/ Insulin—a new approach for effective delivery of human insulin via the pulmonary route." *Diabetes technology & therapeutics* 4, no. 5 (2002): 589-594.

[52] Hovorka, Roman. "The future of continuous glucose monitoring: closed loop." *Current Diabetes Reviews* 4, no. 3 (2008): 269-279.

[53] Hovorka, Roman. "Continuous glucose monitoring and closed-loop systems." *Diabetic medicine* 23, no. 1 (2006): 1-12.

[54] Russell, Steven J. "Continuous glucose monitoring awaits its "killer app"." *Journal of diabetes science and technology* 2, no. 3 (2008): 490-494.

[55] Steil, Garry M., Kerstin Rebrin, Christine Darwin, Farzam Hariri, and Mohammed F. Saad. "Feasibility of automating insulin delivery for the treatment of type 1 diabetes." *Diabetes* 55, no. 12 (2006): 3344-3350.

[56] Cordingley, Jeremy J., Dirk Vlasselaers, Natalie C. Dormand, Pieter J. Wouters, Stephen D. Squire, Ludovic J. Chassin, Malgorzata E. Wilinska, Clifford J. Morgan, Roman Hovorka, and Greet Van den Berghe. "Intensive insulin therapy: enhanced

Model Predictive Control algorithm versus standard care." *Intensive care medicine* 35, no. 1 (2009): 123-128.

[57] Proks, Peter, Frank Reimann, Nick Green, Fiona Gribble, and Frances Ashcroft. "Sulfonylurea stimulation of insulin secretion." *Diabetes* 51, no. suppl_3 (2002): S368-S376.

[58] Sola, Daniele, Luca Rossi, Gian Piero Carnevale Schianca, Pamela Maffioli, Marcello Bigliocca, Roberto Mella, Francesca Corlianò, Gian Paolo Fra, Ettore Bartoli, and Giuseppe Derosa. "State of the art paper sulfonylureas and their use in clinical practice." *Archives of Medical Science* 11, no. 4 (2015): 840-848.

[59] Roumie, Christianne L., Adriana M. Hung, Robert A. Greevy, Carlos G. Grijalva, Xulei Liu, Harvey J. Murff, Tom A. Elasy, and Marie R. Griffin. "Comparative effectiveness of sulfonylurea and metformin monotherapy on cardiovascular events in type 2 diabetes mellitus: a cohort study." *Annals of internal medicine* 157, no. 9 (2012): 601-610.

[60] He, Ling, Amin Sabet, Stephen Djedjos, Ryan Miller, Xiaojian Sun, Mehboob A. Hussain, Sally Radovick, and Fredric E. Wondisford. "Metformin and insulin suppress hepatic gluconeogenesis through phosphorylation of CREB binding protein." *Cell* 137, no. 4 (2009): 635-646.

[61] Lin, Szu Han, Po Chung Cheng, Shih Te Tu, Shang Ren Hsu, Yun Chung Cheng, and Yu Hsiu Liu. "Effect of metformin monotherapy on serum lipid profile in statin-naïve individuals with newly diagnosed type 2 diabetes mellitus: a cohort study." *PeerJ* 6 (2018): e4578.

[62] Rena, Graham, D. Grahame Hardie, and Ewan R. Pearson. "The mechanisms of action of metformin." *Diabetologia* 60, no. 9 (2017): 1577-1585.

[63] Eldor, Roy, Ralph A. DeFronzo, and Muhammad Abdul-Ghani. "In vivo actions of peroxisome proliferator–activated receptors: glycemic control, insulin sensitivity, and insulin secretion." *Diabetes care* 36, no. Supplement_2 (2013): S162-S174.

[64] DeFronzo, Ralph A., Devjit Tripathy, Dawn C. Schwenke, MaryAnn Banerji, George A. Bray, Thomas A. Buchanan, Stephen C. Clement SC, Gastaldelli A, Henry RR, Kitabchi AE, Mudaliar S. "Prevention of diabetes with pioglitazone in ACT NOW: physiologic correlates." *Diabetes* 62, no. 11 (2013): 3920-3926.

[65] Gastaldelli, Amalia, Ele Ferrannini, Yoshinori Miyazaki, Masafumi Matsuda, Andrea Mari, and Ralph A. DeFronzo. "Thiazolidinediones improve β-cell function in type 2 diabetic patients." *American Journal of Physiology-Endocrinology and Metabolism* 292, no. 3 (2007): E871-E883.

[66] Jearath, Vaneet, Rajan Vashisht, Vipul Rustagi, Sujeet Raina, and Rajesh Sharma. "Pioglitazone-induced congestive heart failure and pulmonary edema in a patient with preserved ejection fraction." *Journal of Pharmacology and Pharmacotherapeutics* 7, no. 1 (2016): 41-43.

[67] Singh, Awadhesh Kumar. "Dipeptidyl peptidase-4 inhibitors: Novel mechanism of actions." *Indian journal of endocrinology and metabolism* 18, no. 6 (2014): 753.

[68] Pathak, Rolee, and Mary Barna Bridgeman. "Dipeptidyl peptidase-4 (DPP-4) inhibitors in the management of diabetes." *Pharmacy and Therapeutics* 35, no. 9 (2010): 509.

[69] Brunton, S. "GLP-1 receptor agonists vs. DPP-4 inhibitors for type 2 diabetes: is one approach more successful or preferable than the other?." *International journal of clinical practice* 68, no. 5 (2014): 557-567.

[70] Bunck, Mathijs C., Anja Cornér, Bjorn Eliasson, Robert J. Heine, Rimma M. Shaginian, Marja-Riitta Taskinen, Ulf Smith, Hannele Yki-Järvinen, and Michaela Diamant. "Effects of exenatide on measures of β-cell function after 3 years in metformin-treated patients with type 2 diabetes." *Diabetes care* 34, no. 9 (2011): 2041-2047.

[71] Stonehouse, Anthony H., Tamara Darsow, and David G. Maggs. "Incretin-based therapies." *Journal of diabetes* 4, no. 1 (2012): 55-67.

[72] Klonoff, David C., John B. Buse, Loretta L. Nielsen, Xuesong Guan, Christopher L. Bowlus, John H. Holcombe, Matthew E. Wintle, and David G. Maggs. "Exenatide effects on diabetes, obesity, cardiovascular risk factors and hepatic biomarkers in patients with type 2 diabetes treated for at least 3 years." *Current medical research and opinion* 24, no. 1 (2008): 275-286.

[73] Inzucchi, Silvio E., Richard M. Bergenstal, John B. Buse, Michaela Diamant, Ele Ferrannini, Michael Nauck, Anne L. Peters, Apostolos Tsapas, Richard Wender, and David R. Matthews. "Management of hyperglycemia in type 2 diabetes: a patient-centered approach: position statement of the American Diabetes Association (ADA) and the European Association for the Study of Diabetes (EASD)." *Diabetes care* 35, no. 6 (2012): 1364-1379.

[74] Kalra, Sanjay. "Sodium glucose co-transporter-2 (SGLT2) inhibitors: a review of their basic and clinical pharmacology." *Diabetes Therapy* 5, no. 2 (2014): 355-366.

[75] Abdul-Ghani, Muhammad A., Luke Norton, and Ralph A. DeFronzo. "Role of sodium-glucose cotransporter 2 (SGLT 2) inhibitors in the treatment of type 2 diabetes." *Endocrine reviews* 32, no. 4 (2011): 515-531.

[76] Cherney, David ZI, Bruce A. Perkins, Nima Soleymanlou, Maria Maione, Vesta Lai, Alana Lee, Nora M. Fagan NM, Woerle HJ, Johansen OE, Broedl UC, von Eynatten M. "Renal hemodynamic effect of sodium-glucose cotransporter 2 inhibition in patients with type 1 diabetes mellitus." *Circulation* 129, no. 5 (2014): 587-597.

[77] Eng, Conrad, Caroline K. Kramer, Bernard Zinman, and Ravi Retnakaran. "Glucagon-like peptide-1 receptor agonist and basal insulin combination treatment for the management of type 2 diabetes: a systematic review and meta-analysis." *The Lancet* 384, no. 9961 (2014): 2228-2234.

[78] Min, Se Hee, Jeong-Hwa Yoon, Sun Joon Moon, Seokyung Hahn, and Young Min Cho. "Combination of sodium-glucose cotransporter 2 inhibitor and dipeptidyl peptidase-4 inhibitor in type 2 diabetes: a systematic review with meta-analysis." *Scientific reports* 8, no. 1 (2018): 1-8.

[79] Zinman, Bernard, Stewart B. Harris, Jan Neuman, Hertzel C. Gerstein, Ravi R. Retnakaran, Janet Raboud, Ying Qi, and Anthony JG Hanley. "Low-dose combination therapy with rosiglitazone and metformin to prevent type 2 diabetes mellitus (CANOE trial): a double-blind randomised controlled study." *The Lancet* 376, no. 9735 (2010): 103-111.

[80] Banting, F. G., C. H. Best, J. B. Collip, W. R. Campbell, and A. A. Fletcher. "Pancreatic Extracts in The Treatment of Diabetes Mellitus." *Diabetes* 5, no. 1 (1956): 69-71.

[81] Diabetes Control and Complications Trial Research Group. "The effect of intensive treatment of diabetes on the development and progression of long-term complications in insulin-dependent diabetes mellitus." *New England journal of medicine* 329, no. 14 (1993): 977-986.

[82] UK Prospective Diabetes Study (UKPDS) Group. "Intensive blood-glucose control with sulphonylureas or insulin compared with conventional treatment and risk of complications in patients with type 2 diabetes (UKPDS 33)." *The Lancet* 352, no. 9131 (1998): 837-853

[83] Ratzmann, Klaus Peter, Waldemar Bruns, Bernd Schulz, and Eckhard Zander. "Use of the artificial B-cell (Biostator) in improving insulin therapy in unstable insulin-dependent diabetes." *Diabetes care* 5, no. 1 (1982): 11-17.

[84] Lakey, J. R., Ray V. Rajotte, Garth L. Warnock, and Norman M. Kneteman. "Human pancreas preservation prior to islet isolation. Cold ischemic tolerance." *Transplantation* 59, no. 5 (1995): 689-694.

[85] Tsujimura, Toshiaki, Yoshikazu Kuroda, Tatsuya Kin, Jose G. Avila, Ray V. Rajotte, Gregory S. Korbutt, Edmond A. Ryan, AM James Shapiro, and Jonathan RT Lakey. "Human islet transplantation from pancreases with prolonged cold ischemia using additional preservation by the two-layer (UW solution/perfluorochemical) cold-storage method." *Transplantation* 74, no. 12 (2002): 1687-1691.

[86] Ramachandran, S., N. M. Desai, T. A. Goers, N. Benshoff, B. Olack, S. Shenoy, M. D. Jendrisak, W. C. Chapman, and T. Mohanakumar. "Improved islet yields from pancreas preserved in perflurocarbon is via inhibition of apoptosis mediated by mitochondrial pathway." *American Journal of Transplantation* 6, no. 7 (2006): 1696-1703.

[87] Weimar, Bernd, Klaus Rauber, Mathias D. Brendel, Reinhard G. Bretzel, and Wigbert S. Rau. "Percutaneous transhepatic catheterization of the portal vein: a combined CT-and fluoroscopy-guided technique." *Cardiovascular and interventional radiology* 22, no. 4 (1999): 342-344.

[88] Ryan, Edmond A., Breay W. Paty, Peter A. Senior, David Bigam, Eman Alfadhli, Norman M. Kneteman, Jonathan RT Lakey, and AM James Shapiro. "Five-year follow-up after clinical islet transplantation." *Diabetes* 54, no. 7 (2005): 2060-2069.

[89] Shapiro, AM James, Camillo Ricordi, Bernhard J. Hering, Hugh Auchincloss, Robert Lindblad, R. Paul Robertson, Antonio Secchi. "International trial of the Edmonton protocol for islet transplantation." *New England Journal of Medicine* 355, no. 13 (2006): 1318-1330.

[90] Shapiro, AM James, Jonathan RT Lakey, Edmond A. Ryan, Gregory S. Korbutt, Ellen Toth, Garth L. Warnock, Norman M. Kneteman, and Ray V. Rajotte. "Islet transplantation in seven patients with type 1 diabetes mellitus using a glucocorticoid-free immunosuppressive regimen." *New England Journal of Medicine* 343, no. 4 (2000): 230-238.

[91] Wong, Mary S., Wayne J. Hawthorne, and Nicholas Manolios. "Gene therapy in diabetes." *Self/nonself* 1, no. 3 (2010): 165-175.

[92] Ahmad, Zalinah, Mina Rasouli, Ahmad Zaid Fattah Azman, and Abdul Rahman Omar. "Evaluation of insulin expression and secretion in genetically engineered gut K and L-cells." *BMC biotechnology* 12, no. 1 (2012): 1-9.

[93] Tudurí, Eva, Jennifer E. Bruin, and Timothy J. Kieffer. "Restoring insulin production for type 1 diabetes." *Journal of diabetes* 4, no. 4 (2012): 319-331.

[94] Jaén ML, Vilà L, Elias I, Jimenez V, Rodó J, Maggioni L, Ruiz-de Gopegui R, Garcia M, Muñoz S, Callejas D, Ayuso E. "Long-term efficacy and safety of insulin and glucokinase gene therapy for diabetes: 8-year follow-up in dogs." Molecular therapy-methods & clinical development 6 (2017): 1-7.

[95] Romer, Anthony I., and Lori Sussel. "Pancreatic islet cell development and regeneration."*Current opinion in endocrinology, diabetes, and obesity* 22, no. 4 (2015): 255.

[96] Li, Hua, Xinyan Li, Karen SL Lam, Sidney Tam, Weidong Xiao, and Ruian Xu. "Adeno-associated virus-mediated pancreatic and duodenal homeobox gene-1 expression enhanced differentiation of hepatic oval stem cells to insulin-producing cells in diabetic rats." *Journal of biomedical science* 15, no. 4 (2008): 487-497.

[97] Abed, Arif, Charlotte Critchlow, Peter R. Flatt, Neville H. McClenaghan, and Catriona Kelly. "Directed differentiation of progenitor cells towards an islet-cell phenotype." *American journal of stem cells* 1, no. 3 (2012): 196.

[98] Zhao, Min, Stephanie A. Amiel, Sanaz Ajami, Jie Jiang, Mohamed Rela, Nigel Heaton, and Guo Cai Huang. "Amelioration of streptozotocin-induced diabetes in mice with cells derived from human marrow stromal cells." *Plos one* 3, no. 7 (2008): e2666.

[99] Dassaye, Reshmi, Strini Naidoo, and Marlon E. Cerf. "Transcription factor regulation of pancreatic organogenesis, differentiation and maturation." *Islets* 8, no. 1 (2016): 13-34.

[100] Mastracci, Teresa L., Keith R. Anderson, James B. Papizan, and Lori Sussel. "Regulation of Neurod1 contributes to the lineage potential of Neurogenin3+ endocrine precursor cells in the pancreas." *PLoS genetics* 9, no. 2 (2013): e1003278.

[101] Handorf, Andrew M., Hans W. Sollinger, and Tausif Alam. "Genetic engineering of surrogate β cells for treatment of type 1 diabetes mellitus." *Journal of Diabetes Mellitus* 5, no. 04 (2015): 295.

[102] Handorf, Andrew M., Hans W. Sollinger, and Tausif Alam. "Insulin gene therapy for type 1 diabetes mellitus." *Exp clin transplant* 13, no. Suppl 1 (2015): 37-45.

[103] Yoon, Ji-Won, and Hee-Sook Jun. "Recent advances in insulin gene therapy for type 1 diabetes." *Trends in molecular medicine* 8, no. 2 (2002): 62-68.

[104] Chen, Nelson KF, Jen San Wong, Irene HC Kee, Siang Hui Lai, Choon Hua Thng, Wai Har Ng, Robert TH Ng Tan SY, Lee SY, Tan ME, Sivalingam J. "Nonvirally modified autologous primary hepatocytes correct diabetes and prevent target organ injury in a large preclinical model." *PLoS One* 3, no. 3 (2008): e1734.

[105] Calne, Roy Y., Shu Uin Gan, and Kok Onn Lee. "Stem cell and gene therapies for diabetes mellitus." *Nature Reviews Endocrinology* 6, no. 3 (2010): 173-177.

[106] Guney, Michelle A., and Maureen Gannon. "Pancreas cell fate." *Birth Defects Research Part C: Embryo Today: Reviews* 87, no. 3 (2009): 232-248.

[107] Medvedev, S. P., A. I. Shevchenko, and S. M. Zakian. "Induced pluripotent stem cells: problems and advantages when applying them in regenerative medicine." *Acta Naturae* 2, no. 2 (5) (2010): 18-27.

[108] Liang, Gaoyang, and Yi Zhang. "Genetic and epigenetic variations in iPSCs: potential causes and implications for application." *Cell stem cell* 13, no. 2 (2013): 149-159.

[109] Schmidt, Ryan, and Kathrin Plath. "The roles of the reprogramming factors Oct4, Sox2 and Klf4 in resetting the somatic cell epigenome during induced pluripotent stem cell generation." *Genome biology* 13, no. 10 (2012): 1-11.

[110] Sheridan, Steven D., Vasudha Surampudi, and Raj R. Rao. "Analysis of embryoid bodies derived from human induced pluripotent stem cells as a means to assess pluripotency." *Stem cells international* 2012 (2012).

[111] Chen, Chunguang, Christian M. Cohrs, Julia Stertmann, Robert Bozsak, and Stephan Speier. "Human beta cell mass and function in diabetes: Recent advances in knowledge and technologies to understand disease pathogenesis." *Molecular metabolism* 6, no. 9 (2017): 943-957.

[112] Millman, Jeffrey R., Chunhui Xie, Alana Van Dervort, Mads Gürtler, Felicia W. Pagliuca, and Douglas A. Melton. "Generation of stem cell-derived β-cells from patients with type 1 diabetes." *Nature communications* 7, no. 1 (2016): 1-9.

[113] Youssef, Amr A., Elsie Gyang Ross, Roberto Bolli, Carl J. Pepine, Nicholas J. Leeper, and Phillip C. Yang. "The promise and challenge of induced pluripotent stem cells for cardiovascular applications." *JACC: Basic to Translational Science* 1, no. 6 (2016): 510-523.

[114] Xiao, Xiangwei, and George K. Gittes. "Concise review: new insights into the role of macrophages in β-cell proliferation." *Stem cells translational medicine* 4, no. 6 (2015): 655-658.

[115] Li, Haisen, Hao Zhu, Ting Ge, Zhifeng Wang, and Chao Zhang. "Mesenchymal stem cell-based therapy for diabetes mellitus: enhancement strategies and future perspectives." *Stem Cell Reviews and Reports* 17, no. 5 (2021): 1552-1569.

[116] Frese, Laura, Petra E. Dijkman, and Simon P. Hoerstrup. "Adipose tissue-derived stem cells in regenerative medicine." *Transfusion Medicine and Hemotherapy* 43, no. 4 (2016): 268-274.

[117] Amer, Mona G., Azza S. Embaby, Rehab A. Karam, and Marwa G. Amer. "Role of adipose tissue derived stem cells differentiated into insulin producing cells in the treatment of type I diabetes mellitus." *Gene* 654 (2018): 87-94.

[118] Hu, Jianxia, Zhengju Fu, Ying Chen, Nina Tang, Luan Wang, Fang Wang, Ruixia Sun, and Shengli Yan. "Effects of autologous adipose-derived stem cell infusion on type 2 diabetic rats." *Endocrine Journal* (2015): EJ14-0584.

[119] Nam, Ji Sun, Hyun Mi Kang, Jiyoung Kim, Seah Park, Haekwon Kim, Chul Woo Ahn, Jin Oh Park, and Kyung Rae Kim. "Transplantation of insulin-secreting cells differentiated from human adipose tissue-derived stem cells into type 2 diabetes mice." *Biochemical and Biophysical Research Communications* 443, no. 2 (2014): 775-781.

[120] Moriscot, Christine, Florence De Fraipont, Marie-Jeanne Richard, Mélanie Marchand, Pierre Savatier, Domenico Bosco, Marie Favrot, and Pierre-Yves Benhamou. "Human bone marrow mesenchymal stem cells can express insulin and key transcription factors of the endocrine pancreas developmental pathway upon genetic and/or microenvironmental manipulation in vitro." *Stem cells* 23, no. 4 (2005): 594-603.

[121] Xie, Qiu-Ping, Hai Huang, Bin Xu, Xin Dong, Shun-Liang Gao, Bo Zhang, and Yu-Lian Wu. "Human bone marrow mesenchymal stem cells differentiate into insulin-producing cells upon microenvironmental manipulation in vitro." Differentiation 77, no. 5 (2009): 483-491.

[122] Wu, Li-Fang, Ni-Na Wang, Yuan-Sheng Liu, and Xing Wei. "Differentiation of Wharton's jelly primitive stromal cells into insulin-producing cells in comparison with bone marrow mesenchymal stem cells." *Tissue Engineering Part A* 15, no. 10 (2009): 2865-2873.

[123] Jiang, Ranhua, Zhibo Han, Guangsheng Zhuo, Xiaodan Qu, Xue Li, Xin Wang, Yuankang Shao, Shimin Yang, and Zhong Chao Han. "Transplantation of placenta-derived mesenchymal stem cells in type 2 diabetes: a pilot study." *Frontiers of medicine* 5, no. 1 (2011): 94-100.

[124] Aylin, Kucukarslan, Daskapan Arzu, Sayinalp Sabri, Tuzun Emine Handan, and Alaca Ridvan. "The effect of combined resistance and home-based walking exercise in type 2 diabetes patients." *International journal of diabetes in developing countries* 29, no. 4 (2009): 159.

[125] Sigal, Ronald J., Glen P. Kenny, David H. Wasserman, and Carmen Castaneda-Sceppa. "Physical activity/exercise and type 2 diabetes." *Diabetes care* 27, no. 10 (2004): 2518-2539.

[126] Umpierre, Daniel, Paula AB Ribeiro, Caroline K. Kramer, Cristiane B. LeitŃo, Alessandra TN Zucatti, Mirela J. Azevedo, Jorge L. Gross, Jorge P. Ribeiro, and Beatriz D. Schaan. "Physical activity advice only or structured exercise training and association with HbA1c levels in type 2 diabetes: a systematic review and meta-analysis." *Jama* 305, no. 17 (2011): 1790-1799.

[127] Jeon, Christie Y., R. Peter Lokken, Frank B. Hu, and Rob M. Van Dam. "Physical activity of moderate intensity and risk of type 2 diabetes: a systematic review." *Diabetes care* 30, no. 3 (2007): 744-752.

[128] Boulé, Normand G., Elizabeth Haddad, Glen P. Kenny, George A. Wells, and Ronald J. Sigal. "Effects of exercise on glycemic control and body mass in type 2 diabetes mellitus: a meta-analysis of controlled clinical trials." *Jama* 286, no. 10 (2001): 1218-1227.

[129] Ishii, Tomofusa, Tetsuya Yamakita, Toshihiko Sato, Shiro Tanaka, and Satoru Fujii. "Resistance training improves insulin sensitivity in NIDDM subjects without altering maximal oxygen uptake." *Diabetes care* 21, no. 8 (1998): 1353-1355.

[130] Cuff, Darcye J., Graydon S. Meneilly, Alan Martin, Andrew Ignaszewski, Hugh D. Tildesley, and Jiri J. Frohlich. "Effective exercise modality to reduce insulin resistance in women with type 2 diabetes." *Diabetes care* 26, no. 11 (2003): 2977-2982.

[131] Hegde, Shreelaxmi V., Prabha Adhikari, Shashidhar Kotian, Veena J. Pinto, Sydney D'Souza, and Vivian D'Souza. "Effect of 3-month yoga on oxidative stress in type 2 diabetes with or without complications: a controlled clinical trial." *Diabetes care* 34, no. 10 (2011): 2208-2210.

[132] Yang, Kyeongra, Lisa M. Bernardo, Susan M. Sereika, Molly B. Conroy, Judy Balk, and Lora E. Burke. "Utilization of 3-month yoga program for adults at high risk for type 2 diabetes: a pilot study." *Evidence-Based Complementary and Alternative Medicine* 2011 (2011).

[133] Malhotra, V., S. Singh, K. P. Singh, S. B. Sharma, S. V. Madhu, P. Gupta, and O. P. Tandon. "*Effects of yoga asanas and pranayama in non-insulin dependent diabetes mellitus.*" (2004).

[134] Shantakumari, Nisha, Sheifa Sequeira, and Rasha Eldeeb. "Effect of a yoga intervention on hypertensive diabetic patients." *Journal of Advances in Internal Medicine* 1, no. 2 (2012): 60-63.

[135] Singh, Savita, V. Malhotra, K. P. Singh, S. V. Madhu, and O. P. Tandon. "Role of yoga in modifying certain cardiovascular functions in type 2 diabetic patients." *JAPI* 52 (2004): 203-206.

[136] Nielsen, Jörgen V., and Eva A. Joensson. "Low-carbohydrate diet in type 2 diabetes: stable improvement of bodyweight and glycemic control during 44 months follow-up." *Nutrition & metabolism* 5, no. 1 (2008): 1-6.

[137] Garg A, Bantle JP, Henry RR, Coulston AM, Griver KA, Raatz SK, Brinkley L, Chen YI, Grundy SM, Huet BA, Reaven GM. "Effects of varying carbohydrate content of diet in patients with non—insulin-dependent diabetes mellitus." *JAMA* 271, no. 18 (1994): 1421-1428.

[138] Risérus, Ulf, Walter C. Willett, and Frank B. Hu. "Dietary fats and prevention of type 2 diabetes." *Progress in lipid research* 48, no. 1 (2009): 44-51.

[139] Barnard, Neal D., Joshua Cohen, David JA Jenkins, Gabrielle Turner-McGrievy, Lise Gloede, Amber Green, and Hope Ferdowsian. "A low-fat vegan diet and a conventional diabetes diet in the treatment of type 2 diabetes: a randomized, controlled, 74-wk clinical trial." *The American journal of clinical nutrition* 89, no. 5 (2009): 1588S-1596S.

[140] Barnard, Neal D., Joshua Cohen, David JA Jenkins, Gabrielle Turner-McGrievy, Lise Gloede, Brent Jaster, Kim Seidl, Amber A. Green, and Stanley Talpers. "A low-fat vegan diet improves glycemic control and cardiovascular risk factors in a randomized clinical trial in individuals with type 2 diabetes." *Diabetes care* 29, no. 8 (2006): 1777-1783.

[141] Meyer, Katie A., Lawrence H. Kushi, David R. Jacobs Jr, Joanne Slavin, Thomas A. Sellers, and Aaron R. Folsom. "Carbohydrates, dietary fiber, and incident type 2 diabetes in older women." *The American journal of clinical nutrition* 71, no. 4 (2000): 921-930.

[142] Chandalia, Manisha, Abhimanyu Garg, Dieter Lutjohann, Klaus Von Bergmann, Scott M. Grundy, and Linda J. Brinkley. "Beneficial effects of high dietary fiber intake in patients with type 2 diabetes mellitus." *New England Journal of Medicine* 342, no. 19 (2000): 1392-1398.

[143] Fairfield, Kathleen M., and Robert H. Fletcher. "Vitamins for chronic disease prevention in adults: scientific review." *Jama* 287, no. 23 (2002): 3116-3126.

[144] Montonen, Jukka, Paul Knekt, R. I. T. V. A. Jarvinen, and Antti Reunanen. "Dietary antioxidant intake and risk of type 2 diabetes." *Diabetes care* 27, no. 2 (2004): 362-366.

[145] Palomer, X., J. M. González-Clemente, F. Blanco-Vaca, and Didac Mauricio. "Role of vitamin D in the pathogenesis of type 2 diabetes mellitus." *Diabetes, Obesity and Metabolism* 10, no. 3 (2008): 185-197.

[146] Song, Yiqing, Lu Wang, Anastassios G. Pittas, Liana C. Del Gobbo, Cuilin Zhang, JoAnn E. Manson, and Frank B. Hu. "Blood 25-hydroxy vitamin D levels and incident type 2 diabetes: a meta-analysis of prospective studies." *Diabetes care* 36, no. 5 (2013): 1422-1428.

[147] Mitri, Joanna, Bess Dawson-Hughes, Frank B. Hu, and Anastassios G. Pittas. "Effects of vitamin D and calcium supplementation on pancreatic β cell function, insulin sensitivity, and glycemia in adults at high risk of diabetes: the Calcium and Vitamin D for Diabetes Mellitus (CaDDM) randomized controlled trial." *The American journal of clinical nutrition* 94, no. 2 (2011): 486-494.

[148] Pittas, Anastassios G., Bess Dawson-Hughes, Tricia Li, Rob M. Van Dam, Walter C. Willett, Joann E. Manson, and Frank B. Hu. "Vitamin D and calcium intake in relation to type 2 diabetes in women." *Diabetes care* 29, no. 3 (2006): 650-656.

[149] Aljabri, Khalid S., Somoa A. Bokhari, and Murtadha J. Khan. "Glycemic changes after vitamin D supplementation in patients with type 1 diabetes mellitus and vitamin D deficiency." *Annals of Saudi medicine* 30, no. 6 (2010): 454-458.

[150] Liu, Simin, I-Min Lee, Yiqing Song, Martin Van Denburgh, Nancy R. Cook, JoAnn E. Manson, and Julie E. Buring. "Vitamin E and risk of type 2 diabetes in the women's health study randomized controlled trial." *Diabetes* 55, no. 10 (2006): 2856-2862.

[151] Lonn, Eva, Salim Yusuf, Byrcon Hoogwerf, Janice Pogue, Qilong Yi, Bernard Zinman, Jackie Bosch, Dagenais, Mann, Gerstein. "Effects of vitamin E on cardiovascular and microvascular outcomes in high-risk patients with diabetes: results of the HOPE study and MICRO-HOPE substudy." *Diabetes care* 25, no. 11 (2002): 1919-1927.

[152] Harding, Anne-Helen, Nicholas J. Wareham, Sheila A. Bingham, KayTee Khaw, Robert Luben, Ailsa Welch, and Nita G. Forouhi. "Plasma vitamin C level, fruit and vegetable consumption, and the risk of new-onset type 2 diabetes mellitus: the European prospective investigation of cancer–Norfolk prospective study." *Archives of internal medicine* 168, no. 14 (2008): 1493-1499.

[153] Paolisso, Giuseppe, Anna D'Amore, Vinico Balbi, Clelia. Volpe, Domenico Galzerano, D. Giugliano, Sgambato, Michele Varricchio, and Felica D'Onofrio. "Plasma vitamin C affects glucose homeostasis in healthy subjects and in non-insulin-dependent diabetics." *American Journal of Physiology-Endocrinology and Metabolism* 266, no. 2 (1994): E261-E268.

[154] Pandey, Manisha, Rohit K. Verma, and Shubhini A. Saraf. "Nutraceuticals: new era of medicine and health." *Asian J Pharm Clin* Res 3, no. 1 (2010): 11-15.

[155] Khan, Alam, Mahpara Safdar, Mohammad Muzaffar Ali Khan, Khan Nawaz Khattak, and Richard A. Anderson. "Cinnamon improves glucose and lipids of people with type 2 diabetes." *Diabetes care* 26, no. 12 (2003): 3215-3218.

[156] Allen, Robert W., Emmanuelle Schwartzman, William L. Baker, Craig I. Coleman, and Olivia J. Phung. "Cinnamon use in type 2 diabetes: an updated systematic review and meta-analysis." *The Annals of Family Medicine* 11, no. 5 (2013): 452-459.

[157] Baker, William L., Gabriela Gutierrez-Williams, C. Michael White, Jeffrey Kluger, and Craig I. Coleman. "Effect of cinnamon on glucose control and lipid parameters." *Diabetes care* 31, no. 1 (2008): 41-43.

[158] Augusti, K. T., and C. G. Sheela. "Antiperoxide effect of S-allyl cysteine sulfoxide, an insulin secretagogue, in diabetic rats." *Experientia* 52, no. 2 (1996): 115-119.

[159] Parastouei, K., S. H. Ravanshad, H. Mostaphavi, and E. Setoudehmaram. "Effects of garlic tablet on blood sugar, plasma lipids and blood pressure in type 2 diabetic patients with hyperlipidemia." *Journal of Medicinal Plants* 5, no. 17 (2006): 48-54.

[160] Ashraf, Rizwan, Kausar Aamir, Abdul Rashid Shaikh, and Talat Ahmed. "Effects of garlic on dyslipidemia in patients with type 2 diabetes mellitus." *J Ayub Med Coll Abbottabad* 17, no. 3 (2005): 60-64.

[161] Kalsi, Arshpreet, Shivangi Singh, Nancy Taneja, Samiksha Kukal, and Shalini Mani. "Current treatments for type 2 diabetes, their side effects and possible complementary treatments." *International Journal* 10, no. 3 (2017).

[162] Zhang, Yifei, Xiaoying Li, Dajin Zou, Wei Liu, Jialin Yang, Na Zhu, Li Huo. "Treatment of type 2 diabetes and dyslipidemia with the natural plant alkaloid berberine." *The Journal of Clinical Endocrinology & Metabolism* 93, no. 7 (2008): 2559-2565.

Chapter 6

Oral Antidiabetic Agents

Vijay Mishra[1,*]
Abhigyan Ranjan[1]
and Murtaza M. Tambuwala[2]
[1]School of Pharmaceutical Sciences, Lovely Professional University, Phagwara (Punjab), India
[2]Lincoln Medical School, University of Lincoln, Brayford Pool, Lincoln, England, UK

Abstract

The most successful care of diabetes mellitus (DM) necessitates an interdisciplinary strategy that includes pharmacologic therapy when appropriate to achieve specific glycemic objectives in addition to dietary and activity adjustments. Type 2 diabetes mellitus (T2DM) is the primary target of oral hypoglycemic drugs. The present chapter discusses the overview of different oral antidiabetic agents.

Keywords: diabetes mellitus, hyperglycemia, blood sugar, oral hypoglycemics

1. Introduction

The accidental findings of hypoglycemia as a side effect of numerous investigational compounds and the first oral hypoglycemic medicines were

---

* Corresponding Author's Email: vijaymishra2@gmail.com.

In: Management of Diabetes Mellitus Based on Natural Products
Editors: Yachana Mishra and Vijay Mishra
ISBN: 979-8-88697-853-7

developed. C. K. Watanabe discovered that guanidine may produce hypoglycemia under specific circumstances in 1918 while researching the biological effects of guanidine. According to Watanabe, injecting guanidine subcutaneously into rabbits initially caused hyperglycemia, followed by hypoglycemia within a few hours. These discoveries motivated E. Frank, M. Nothmann, and A. Wagner to attempt to alter the guanidine molecule. Numerous guanidine derivatives, such as monoguanidines and biguanidines, were investigated. The most hypoglycemic impact was discovered to be with the biguanidines. Decamethyl-diguanidine, the first commercially accessible guanidine derivative, was initially introduced in 1928 and marketed in Europe as Synthalin. Phenylethyl-biguanidine, often known as Phenformin, was first made accessible for therapeutic usage in the United States in 1959 after being launched in 1957 to treat diabetes. Because Synthalin proved harmful to the liver and kidneys, its use was stopped [1].

In 1939, Argentine scientists Celestino Ruiz and L. L. Silva noticed that several sulfonamide compounds have hypoglycemic effects. M. J. Janbon, a professor of pharmacology at Montpellier University, discovered that the sulfonylurea drug developed for the treatment of typhoid fever exhibited strange lethal side effects in 1942 when France was still under occupation. Confusion, cramping, and unconsciousness were among the symptoms that Janbon rightly ascribed to hypoglycemia. Patients with diabetes were subsequently given this chemical, which helped to reduce their blood sugar levels. The researchers investigated the chemical's putative mode of action and discovered that pancreatectomized test animals rendered the substance useless. Sulfonylureas became the subject of an in-depth investigation following widely reported findings by German researchers Hans Franke and Joachim Fuchs. During the testing of the novel long-acting sulfonamide antibiotic, Franke and Fuchs identified the hypoglycemic properties of sulfonylureas. A substance called D 860 was created by Hoechst chemists and sold as tolbutamide in the US in 1956. This substance was the first sulfonylurea agent to be sold commercially [1,2].

Numerous chemicals have been investigated for their hypoglycemic effects, but very few of them have reached the market. For instance, Boehringer-Mannheim and Hoechst examined 8000 distinct compounds for hypoglycemic qualities between 1962 and 1977; 6000 of these substances led to hypoglycemia in experimental animals. Only five of them advanced to clinical testing, and only one, HB 419 (glibenclamide/glyburide), was finally approved for marketing [3].

2. Biguanides

Currently, the only biguanide utilized in most nations is metformin (dimethyl biguanide). *Galega officinalis*, often known as goat's rue or French lilac, is a guanidine-rich plant with a long history of usage in Europe as a traditional remedy for diabetes [4]. Several guanidine derivatives were used to treat diabetes in the 1920s because guanidine had a glucose-lowering action [5]. With the development of insulin, these medications vanished, but in the late 1950s, three biguanides—metformin, phenformin, and buformin—were developed. Due to a high frequency of lactic acidosis, phenformin and buformin were removed from the market in numerous nations in the late 1970s [6, 7].

Since its introduction in the USA in 1995, metformin has been the most frequently prescribed antidiabetic medication globally. The medicine also protects against vascular problems independently of its antihyperglycemic impact [8,9]. Metformin works in various ways to combat insulin resistance and decrease blood sugar. Metformin affects glucose metabolism at the cellular level in both ways, depending on insulin levels. Metformin appears to affect food metabolism and energy generation independently of insulin through the activation of adenosine 5′monophosphate-activated protein kinase (AMPK). It also appears to moderately increase insulin sensitivity through post-receptor signaling pathways for insulin. Metformin does not imitate or activate the genetic effects of insulin; therefore, for it to be effective in decreasing blood sugar levels, at least some insulin must be present [10].

Furthermore, when administered as monotherapy, metformin does not appear to produce frank hypoglycemia; rather, its primary glucose-lowering impact appears to be a decrease in hepatic glucose synthesis. By improving hepatic insulin sensitivity and reducing hepatic extraction of some gluconeogenic substrates, such as lactate, metformin lowers gluconeogenesis. Additionally, hepatic glycogenolysis is diminished. By enhancing the translocation of insulin-sensitive glucose transporters (GLUT-4) into the cell membrane and raising glycogen synthase activity, which encourages glycogen formation, metformin can improve insulin-stimulated glucose uptake in skeletal muscle. For individuals with hypertriglyceridemia, metformin has the potential to lower triglyceride levels by inhibiting the oxidation of fatty acids without the need for insulin. This limits the energy source for hepatic gluconeogenesis and restores equilibrium to the glucose-fatty acid (Randle) cycle, allowing for higher usage of glucose as a cellular source of energy compared to fatty acids. Metformin can inhibit the mitochondrial respiratory chain at complex 1 if it builds up to a high cellular concentration (for example, in the gut). By accelerating glucose-lactate turnover, this may support the drug's ability to reduce blood sugar levels and prevent weight gain.

2.1. Pharmacokinetics

Because metformin is quickly but inefficiently absorbed, has minimal binding to plasma proteins, and is not digested, it does not interact with concurrently given medications. Although metformin is broadly dispersed at plasma-like quantities (about 5-10 mol/L), substantially larger amounts are maintained in the walls of the gastrointestinal system. With unmodified drug clearance in the urine often occurring within 12 hours, the plasma half-life ($t_{1/2}$) is roughly 6 hours. Metformin is not recommended for individuals with substantial glomerular filtration impairment, despite the fact that tubular secretion rather than glomerular filtration is more important for renal clearance. The only medication known to compete for clearance to the extent that it raises plasma metformin concentrations to clinically relevant amounts is cimetidine [11].

2.2. Indications and Contraindications

Although it has equal antihyperglycemic effectiveness in patients of normal weight, metformin is frequently favored for overweight and obese adults with type 2 diabetes mellitus (T2DM) since it does not promote weight gain [12]. If there is any indication of compromised renal function (e.g., serum creatinine >130 mol/L, creatinine clearance 60 mL/min, or estimated glomerular filtration rate [eGFR] 45 mL/min/1.73 m^2), patient appropriateness should be carefully addressed to prevent drug build up. Significant liver illness, alcoholism, or a history of metabolic acidosis are further contraindications, as are any other conditions that increase the risk of hypoxia or impaired tissue perfusion (such as hypotension or septicemia). It is not practical to pinpoint specific cut-off points for beginning or terminating metformin medication since it is important to consider the possibility of abrupt worsening in renal, cardiac, and hepatic function. In light of this, senior patients who do not have renal impairment or other exclusions can take metformin. In the absence of diabetes, ovulation can return in women with the ovulatory polycystic ovarian syndrome (PCOS), which is an unapproved medication use [13].

Metformin standard (so-called immediate release [IR]) tablets or liquid formulation should be taken with meals or right before meals to reduce potential gastrointestinal adverse effects. Start with 500 or 850 mg once a day or 500 mg twice daily (divided between the morning and evening meals). When the desired level of blood glucose management is reached, the dosage is gradually raised by one tablet at a time, spaced roughly one to two weeks apart. Return to the initial dose if the aim is not reached and an additional dose has no further positive effects. Consider combination therapy in the case of monotherapy by including a second medication (e.g., an insulin secretagogue or thiazolidinedione).

The maximum daily dose of metformin, given in separate doses with meals, is around 2000 mg; in some countries, it may be 2550 or 3000 mg. Most nations have slow-release metformin formulations (XR/SR/ER), which can be taken once daily in the morning or twice a day if necessary. Several fixed-dosage combination pills combine metformin with either a sulfonylurea, thiazolidinedione or dipeptidyl peptidase 4 (DPP - 4) inhibitor. Metformin can also be used in conjunction with any other type of antidiabetic medication, including insulin. Remember that metformin administered with an insulin-releasing drug or insulin can result in significant hypoglycemia, even though metformin used alone is unlikely to cause this.

When taking metformin for a long time, it is advised to check at least once a year for the development of any contraindications, notably renal (as a minimum, serum creatinine). Yearly hemoglobin measurement is advised, especially for people with known or suspected nutritional deficiencies, because metformin can decrease the gastrointestinal absorption of vitamin B12. Even though this is seldom the cause of frank anemia, this is a rare cause of anemia. Metformin should be temporarily halted when utilizing intravenous radiographic contrast agents, during general anesthetic surgery, or in any concurrent circumstances when the exclusion criteria could be invoked. In some situations, insulin substitution may be necessary.

2.3. Efficacy

Optimally titrated metformin often lowers fasting plasma glucose by 2 to 4 mmol/L, which translates to a reduction in HbA1c by around 1 to 2% (11 to 22 mmol/mol) in individuals whose diabetes is not well managed by lifestyle management. As long as some -cell activity is still intact; this is independent of body weight, age, and diabetes duration. It is anticipated that dosage titration and the inclusion of a second drug will be necessary to maintain glycemic control over the long term to account for the progressive nature of T2DM [14].

Metformin carries a low risk of serious hypoglycemia or weight gain when taken as monotherapy. It could decrease basal insulin levels, especially in hyperinsulinemic individuals, enhancing insulin sensitivity. In hyperlipidemic individuals, plasma concentrations of triglycerides, fatty acids, and low-density lipoprotein (LDL) cholesterol tend to decline. In contrast, plasma concentrations of high-density lipoprotein (HDL) cholesterol tend to rise following metformin treatment. Although a reduction in triglycerides and free fatty acids is anticipated to aid increase insulin sensitivity and boost the glucose-fatty acid cycle, these benefits appear to be independent of the antihyperglycemic impact [12].

In the UK Prospective Diabetes Study (UKPDS), obese individuals who began metformin-based oral diabetes medication had a 39% lower risk of myocardial infarction than those who received standard care ($P = 0.01$). The lack of a clear correlation between the dose of metformin and the outcomes suggests that patients who can only take a modest dose of the medication may still benefit from taking it, even if other medications are needed to maintain appropriate glycemic control. The magnitude of metformin's glucose-lowering action or its effects on traditional cardiovascular risk variables like blood pressure or plasma lipids were not associated with the decline in myocardial infarction. Metformin has reportedly been shown to have positive effects on a number of atherothrombotic risk factors and indicators, including decreased carotid intima-media thickness (CIMT), improved fibrinolysis, and decreased levels of the antithrombolytic factor plasminogen activator inhibitor-1 (PAI-1). There is evidence that combining metformin with sulfonylurea may initially raise cardiovascular mortality, which takes away slightly from the overall positive cardiovascular risk findings. The greater cardiovascular risk brought on by more severe metabolic disorders in individuals who require therapy with the combo is one possible complicating factor [15]. Large databases' evidence supporting the use of a sulfonylurea and metformin combination treatment has been encouraging. Subsequent findings from the UKPDS post-trial follow-up study (without the continuance of randomized groups) demonstrated that metformin's cardiovascular effects were sustained [16, 17].

Metformin's potential to increase insulin sensitivity typically necessitates a reduction in insulin dose when it is introduced to the regimens of patients taking insulin treatment. Similar to this, adding insulin to individuals who are already on metformin typically results in less weight gain and needs lower insulin doses. Less insulin is also linked to less frequent and less severe hypoglycemia episodes [18].

It is noteworthy that the US Diabetes Prevention Program found that metformin reduced the incidence of new cases of diabetes in overweight and obese subjects with impaired glucose tolerance by 33%, compared to a reduced risk of 58% using an intensive diet regimen and exercise. This is even though metformin is not indicated for the prevention of diabetes. The younger, more obese patients who took metformin showed the greatest benefit in terms of prevention [19].

2.4. Adverse Effects

Abdominal pain and other gastrointestinal side effects, including diarrhea, are metformin's primary tolerability problems. These are frequently momentary and can be reduced by titrating the dosage gently and taking the medication with meals. If the dose is decreased, symptoms could go away, but 10% or so of people are unable to tolerate the medication at any level. Lactic acidosis is the most severe side effect linked to metformin; it is uncommon (approximately 0.03 incidences per 1000 patients/years), but roughly half of cases are deadly. Some instances previously linked to metformin were probably brought on by other causes because the baseline prevalence of lactic acidosis among T2DM patients has not been determined. The majority of documented occurrences of lactic acidosis in metformin-using individuals were brought on by incorrect prescriptions, specifically failing to consider renal impairment. Metformin will inevitably build up as a result, boosting lactate production and worsening any hypoxic or liver-dysfunctional conditions. Metformin may be an accidental influence in some instances since hyperlactatemia is a complication of cardiogenic shock and other conditions that reduce tissue perfusion. Regardless of the reason, metformin should be discontinued right once in any situation where lactic acidosis is suspected or confirmed [19,20].

A higher blood lactate content (e.g., >5 mmol/L), a drop in arterial pH, and/or a bicarbonate concentration with an expanded anion gap ($[Na^+]$ [Cl + HCO_3] >15 mmol/L) are common signs of lactic acidosis. Presenting symptoms are often non-specific, however, they frequently include stomach pain, malaise, and hyperventilation. Without waiting to see if metformin is the reason, treatment should start right once; bicarbonate is still the standard treatment, but there isn't much proof of its effectiveness. Hemodialysis can be beneficial in removing excess metformin and may aid with fluid and electrolyte restoration following therapy with high-dose intravenous bicarbonate [21, 22].

3. Sulfonylureas

Sulfonylureas have been widely employed as insulin secretagogues for the treatment of T2DM since their inception in the 1950s. After sulfonamides were shown to induce hypoglycemia, sulfonylureas were created as structural alternatives. The term "first generation" is frequently used to describe early sulfonylureas such as carbutamide, tolbutamide, acetohexamide, tolazamide, and chlorpropamide. More effective "second generation" sulfonylureas, such as glibenclamide (glyburide), gliclazide, glipizide, and most recently, glimepiride, have essentially replaced them [23].

3.1. Mode of Action

To increase insulin production, sulfonylureas directly activate the β - cells of the islets of Langerhans. They enter the β-cell and attach to the cytosolic surface of the sulfonylurea receptor 1 (SUR1), which is a complex transmembrane member of the potassium channel Kir6.21 that is ATP-sensitive (K^+ATP channels) [24, 25]. Sulfonylurea binding blocks the K^+ATP channel, limiting potassium outflow and allowing membrane depolarization. Localized membrane depolarization activates nearby voltage-dependent L-type calcium channels, boosting calcium inflow and the level of cytosolic free calcium. The contraction of microtubules and microfibrillaments, which regulate the exocytotic release of insulin granules, are controlled by calcium-dependent signaling proteins that are activated as a result. First-phase insulin release refers to the rapid release of preformed insulin granules close to the plasma membrane. The second phase of insulin release starts roughly 10 minutes later. Preformed and freshly formed insulin granules are moved to the plasma membrane for secretion during the "second phase" of insulin release. As long as the - cells are functionally capable, sulfonylureas continue to promote insulin release when bound to the SUR1. However, prolonged, repetitive stimulation might lead to some desensitization. Sulfonylureas are capable of producing hypoglycemia, mostly because of insulin's ability to block hepatic glucose synthesis when glucose concentrations are below the typical threshold for glucose-stimulated insulin release (about 5 mmol/L) [26, 27].

There is some evidence that sulfonylureas can reduce blood sugar levels somewhat without causing an increase in insulin production. Although there has been some evidence of a slight decrease in glucagon levels, enhanced peripheral glucose transport, and increased hepatic glucose deposition, these effects are not considered clinically significant [28, 29].

3.2. Pharmacokinetics

The pharmacokinetic characteristics of sulfonylureas vary widely, impacting their therapeutic usefulness for various individuals. They typically absorb well, reaching their maximal plasma concentration in 2 to 4 hours [30]. Due to their strong affinity for plasma proteins, sulfonylureas can interact with other medications that are also protein-bound, including salicylates, sulfonamides, and warfarin. Additionally, the risk of hypoglycemia might be increased by the displacement of protein-bound sulfonylurea. To variable degrees, sulfonylureas are metabolized in the liver to produce a variety of active and inactive metabolites that are excreted with the medication itself through the bile and urine. Although longer-lasting sulfonylureas can be used once daily, there is a higher risk of hypoglycemia, particularly when active metabolites are present. Sites and rates of metabolism and elimination are also crucial factors to take into account, particularly in elderly patients, those who have concurrent liver or renal illness, or those who are taking several drugs [31].

Some sulfonylureas have changed their formulas to change how long they last before acting. For instance, glibenclamide (glyburide) is available in the USA in a micronized version that accelerates gastrointestinal absorption for a quicker beginning of the action. For once-daily dosage, two new formulations of glipizide—an "extended-release" formulation and a "modified release" (MR) formulation—have been launched. Interestingly, the 30 mg dosage of gliclazide MR has comparable effectiveness to 80 mg of unmodified gliclazide and lowers the danger of life-threatening hypoglycemia.

3.3. Indications and Contraindications

Sulfonylureas are frequently used alone or in conjunction with thiazolidinediones or metformin. Additionally, they can be used with a -glucosidase inhibitor, and some people may benefit from taking a sulfonylurea together with an incretin, a DPP-4 inhibitor, or insulin. The efficacy of decreasing blood sugar when sulfonylurea is used with another form of antidiabetic medication is often additive, at least initially, although there is an increased risk of hypoglycemia. A sulfonylurea's additive effectiveness with another kind of insulin secretagogue depends on how it affects the β-cell (Meglinide prandial insulin secretagogues act through the SUR1 complex similarly to sulfonylureas, so they typically provide no additional benefit beyond up titrating the sulfonylurea, except a few rare cases where the two types of agent are carefully timed to coincide with unusual or unpredictable meal patterns) [30].

Sulfonylureas (or other insulin secretagogues) are added to insulin therapy for T2DM patients based on the pharmacologic notion that subcutaneous insulin injections do not accurately simulate the typical endogenous transport of more insulin to the liver than to the peripheral. Therefore, stimulation to boost endogenous insulin supply to the liver should help to reduce hepatic glucose generation, especially during mealtime digestion, where there is residual endogenous-cell action. As a result, daytime sulfonylurea is occasionally administered along with nighttime insulin, which can significantly lower the necessary insulin dose if only momentarily. When metformin is ineffective or not tolerated, current guidelines suggest sulfonylureas as an alternate first-line oral treatment. Sulfonylurea treatment is linked to weight gain; hence these medications have customarily been preferred for patients who are not overweight.

Start the sulfonylurea treatment with a modest dose, preferably with the patient testing their blood sugar at least once a day throughout the first several weeks. This is especially advised in cases of grave worry over the potential negative effects of hypoglycemia (e.g., in elderly patients, those living alone, operating machinery, or driving). Patients who have somewhat (but insufficiently) reacted to lifestyle changes and have less pronounced fasting hyperglycemia are more likely to have hypoglycemia when using sulfonylureas. If necessary, increase the dose at intervals of 2 to 4 weeks. Hypoglycemia is the most significant barrier to sulfonylurea dosage increase, especially early hypoglycemic symptoms. It is advised to go back to the original dose if hypoglycemia symptoms appear before the glycemic target is reached or if a dosage increase has no additional glycemic effect. Altering the delivery schedule may help, or a different class of insulin secretagogue may be more appropriate. The standard course of action is to add a medication to lower insulin resistance or α -glucosidase inhibitor when the sulfonylurea is used as monotherapy and the glycemic target is not met. The fact that sulfonylurea's blood-glucose-lowering impact is typically seen at doses much below the maximum advised dose suggests that the insulin secretion has already been stimulated to its fullest extent [32].

3.4. Efficacy

Sulfonylureas can be predicted to lower fasting plasma glucose by roughly 2 to 4 mmol/L when used as monotherapy in individuals whose conditions are not sufficiently managed by lifestyle changes, translating to a drop in HbA1c of 1 to 2% (11 to 22 mmol/mol). Sulfonylureas immediately reduce blood sugar levels and are particularly effective in the short term. However, effectiveness depends on a significant reserve of β-cell activity, which must be balanced against the inevitable reduction in β-cell function as T2DM progresses naturally. As a result, it is anticipated that the dose will need to be increased to combat the gradual loss of β-cell activity, which may decrease the longevity of the glucose-lowering effectiveness.

In between 5 and 10% of patients every year, glycemic control rapidly deteriorates while receiving sulfonylurea medication (also known as "secondary sulfonylurea failure"). While there is a chance that this will differ amongst compounds, it mostly represents the development of cell failure. In contrast to late intervention in patients with substantially impaired - cell function, early intervention in individuals with a higher reserve of - cell activity typically causes a better and longer response to sulfonylureas, but not without risk of hypoglycemia. Blood lipids are often not significantly affected by sulfonylureas. On rare occasions, their usage will result in a small rise in HDL cholesterol or a drop in plasma triglycerides [29, 33].

3.5. Adverse Effects

After starting sulfonylurea medication, the weight increase is commonplace, ranging from 1 to 4 kg, and stabilizes after 6 months. The higher plasma insulin concentrations and decreased excretion of glucose in the urine have likely anabolic effects, which are reflected in weight gain [33, 34].

Hypoglycemia is the most frequent and perhaps most significant side effect of sulfonylurea medication. Even minor impairment of brain or motor function might jeopardize the patient and others and may lead to a poor prognosis following a myocardial infarction, while it is seldom life-threatening in T2DM patients. Sulfonylurea-treated patients should be educated on avoiding hypoglycemia, recognizing it when it occurs, and taking quick corrective action.

About 20% of patients receiving sulfonylurea treatment in the UKPDS reported experiencing hypoglycemia symptoms at least once per year. Similar rates have been reported by other investigations. In the UKPDS, severe hypoglycemia (requiring third-party intervention) occurred in roughly 1% of patients per year, and lower rates (about 0.2-2.5 incidents per 1000 patients/years) have been recorded elsewhere. According to reports, there is a 0.014 to 0.033 chance of death from sulfonylurea-induced hypoglycemia for every 1000 patients/year. Longer lasting sulfonylureas, irregular eating patterns, additional diabetes medications, particularly insulin, heavy alcohol use, already close to normal fasting glycemia, advanced age, and interfering medications might raise the risk of hypoglycemia [35].

Sulfonylurea-induced hypoglycemia necessitates urgent hospital admission. To prevent a recurrence of hypoglycemia when long-acting sulfonylureas are involved, treat with glucose by continuous intravenous infusion, presumably for longer than 1 day. Forcible alkaline diuresis may improve renal elimination if the buildup of chlorpropamide is expected. In severe sulfonylurea-induced hypoglycemia, the vasodilator diazoxide and the somatostatin analog octreotide have been used effectively (albeit with considerable care). Since glucagon is an insulin secretagogue in and of itself, it should not be used by T2DM patients.

Sulfonylureas very rarely cause sensitivity responses, which are often brief skin rashes. The erythema multiforme is uncommon. Fever, jaundice, acute porphyria, photosensitivity, and blood dyscrasias are also uncommon. Chlorpropamide, a drug no longer widely used, was once recognized for its tendency to make people flush their faces when they drank alcohol and to make their kidneys more sensitive to antidiuretic hormone, which might occasionally result in water retention and hyponatremia. It is said that glibenclamide has a slight diuretic effect. Although stimulating insulin secretion is necessary for sulfonylureas to work, this seldom causes plasma insulin concentrations to rise above those of healthy (non-diabetic) and people with impaired glucose tolerance (IGT). There is no evidence to support the claim made in the 1960s by the University Group Diabetes Program research that tolbutamide-induced hyperinsulinemia might harm the cardiovascular system.

The discovery that two isoforms of the sulfonylurea receptor, SUR2A and SUR2B, are expressed in cardiac muscle and vascular smooth muscle, respectively, stimulated more research on the cardiovascular safety of sulfonylureas. These isoforms still have a benzamido binding site but lack the sulfonylurea binding site. SUR2A/B can only bind sulfonylureas that have a benzamido group, as a result (glibenclamide, glipizide, glimepiride). Tolbutamide, chlorpropamide, and gliclazide are examples of sulfonylureas without a benzamido group that has relatively low interaction with the cardiac and vascular SUR receptors. Sulfonylureas containing a benzamido group limit the effects of the K^+ATP channel opening nicorandil, an anti-anginal medication having cardioprotective characteristics. There is no conclusive proof that therapeutic concentrations of sulfonylureas cause such an effect, despite the possibility that substances with a benzamido group could theoretically interfere with ischemic preconditioning and increase vascular contractility at a time when this might be undesirable (such as in severe myocardial ischemia). Ischemia preconditioning does not seem to occur in hyperglycemic situations, yet some experts still recommend that sulfonylurea usage be restricted in individuals with overt coronary artery disease [36].

4. Meglitinides

Following the discovery in the 1980s that meglitinide, the non-sulfonylurea moiety of glibenclamide that includes the benzamido group, might stimulate insulin secretion similarly to a sulfonylurea, meglitinide analogs were examined as possible antidiabetic drugs. These chemicals' pharmacokinetic characteristics made them suitable for treatment with meals to increase prandial insulin release since they had a quick but fleeting insulin secretory impact 60. These medicines aid in partially restoring the first phase of glucose-induced insulin response that is lost in T2DM by causing a quick rise in insulin to coincide with meal digestion. Targeting postprandial hyperglycemia specifically may also help lower the risk of interprandial hypoglycemia and the vascular risk associated with postprandial glucose excursions. Targeting postprandial hyperglycemia specifically may also help lower the risk of interprandial hypoglycemia and the vascular risk associated with postprandial glucose excursions. As "prandial insulin releasers," two substances—the meglitinide derivative repaglinide and the structurally similar phenylalanine derivative nateglinide—were launched in 1998 and 2001, respectively. Even though they mostly have an impact during the pre-prandial and early postprandial periods, notably with repaglinide, their effects are long-lasting enough to result in some decrease in fasting hyperglycemia [37].

4.1. Mode of Action

The benzamido site on the sulfonylurea receptor SUR1 in the plasma membrane of islet β-cells is where postprandial insulin releasers bind. Although this site is different from the sulfonylurea site, the K^+ATP channel is closed due to binding, much like with sulfonylureas. The two agonist kinds do not, therefore, have therapeutically additive advantages, although the expert may be able to mix a meglitinide and a sulfonylurea to suit an odd meal pattern due to differences in their binding affinities and duration of action [38].

4.2. Pharmacokinetics

Repaglinide is quickly and virtually completely absorbed, reaching its peak plasma concentrations after about an hour. In the liver, it is swiftly converted to inactive metabolites that are primarily eliminated in the bile. Repaglinide causes an immediate insulin response that lasts for around 3 hours when taken roughly 15 minutes before a meal, matching the time it takes for food to digest. Nateglinide's onset is a little quicker and its activity lasts a little less time [39].

4.3. Indications and Contraindications

Prandial insulin releasers may be administered as monotherapy in individuals whose condition has not been effectively managed by non-pharmacological treatments. They may be particularly effective for people who experience post-meal hyperglycemia excursions while maintaining close to normal fasting glycemia. As rapid-acting insulin releasers, they may be useful for those who have erratic or missed-meal lifestyles. Although the requirement for numerous daily dosages may be a deterrent, the decreased risk of hypoglycemia also presents a valuable option for some older individuals, particularly if other medicines are contraindicated.

It is best to take repaglinide 15 to 30 minutes before a meal. Before each main meal, titrate treatment at a low dose (for example, 0.5 mg) while monitoring glycemic control every two weeks up to a maximum of 4 mg. Repaglinide should not be taken in the same amount when a meal is skipped. Repaglinide can be used for individuals with mild renal impairment when certain sulfonylureas and metformin are contraindicated with the proper care and monitoring.

Repaglinide and nateglinide can be used as monotherapies, while nateglinide tends to be quicker and shorter acting and needs to be taken with caution in individuals with hepatic illness. It should be noted that nateglinide is only approved for use in combination treatment in specific nations, such as the UK.

Consider introducing combo treatment early if a prandial insulin releaser does not achieve the targeted glycemic aim (e.g., with an agent to reduce insulin resistance). Additionally helpful supplements to metformin or a thiazolidinedione monotherapy are postprandial insulin releasers [37, 38].

4.4. Efficacy

Taking repaglinide (0.5–4 mg) or nateglinide (60–180 mg) before meals results in dose-dependent increases in insulin concentrations and lower postprandial hyperglycemia, which is consistent with its usage to promote prandial insulin production. Usually, there is a little decrease in fasting hyperglycemia. Due to sulfonylureas' shorter duration of action, HbA1c reductions are comparable to or less than those seen with those medications. They can lower HbA1c by an extra 0.5 to 1.5% (6 to 17 mmol/mol) when taken in addition to metformin.

4.5. Adverse Effects

Compared to sulfonylureas, hypoglycemic episodes are less frequent and less severe with prandial insulin releasers. Sensitivity responses are rare and often brief. Repaglinide plasma levels may rise when gemfibrozil is also administered. When used as initial monotherapy, prandial insulin releasers may slightly increase body weight; however, when used in combination with metformin or patients switching from sulfonylureas, there is minimal impact on body weight [39].

5. Thiazolidinediones

Early in the 1980s, a thiazolidinedione (ciglitazone) was discovered to have antidiabetic properties. The peroxisome proliferator-activated receptor (PPAR) family was discovered to be a member of nuclear receptor superfamily 1 in the early 1990s, and it was found that thiazolidinediones were powerful PPAR-γ agonists [40]. Troglitazone was the first thiazolidinedione to be approved for routine clinical use in the USA, having been released in 1997. Thiazolidinediones have been found to increase whole-body insulin sensitivity through PPAR-γ mediated transcriptional actions. However, the medication was removed from the market in 2000 when it was linked to fatal cases of idiosyncratic hepatotoxicity. In 1997, Troglitazone was very briefly accessible in the UK. In the USA in 1999 and Europe in 2000, two other thiazolidinediones—rosiglitazone and pioglitazone—that did not exhibit hepatotoxicity were made available. There are other fixed-dose combinations of each medication and metformin available [41].

5.1. Mode of Action

Thiazolidinediones tend to have the most antidiabetic effectiveness when PPAR is stimulated, which increases insulin sensitivity. Adipose tissue has a high level of PPAR-γ expression, while liver and muscle have a lower level of expression. It binds to a nucleotide sequence known as the peroxisome proliferator response element (PPRE) found in the promoter regions of PPAR-γ responsive genes (AGGTCAXAGGTCA) when activated, forming a heterodimeric complex with the retinoid X receptor. This modifies a variety of insulin-sensitive and other genes' transcriptional activity in combination with co-activators like Peroxisome proliferator-activated receptor-gamma co-activator (PGC-1). Many of these genes are involved in the metabolism of lipids and carbohydrates. A thiazolidinedione's stimulation of PPAR-γ encourages the differentiation of pre-adipocytes into mature adipocytes: these new small adipocytes are particularly sensitive to insulin and show increased uptake of fatty acids with increased lipogenesis. This in turn lowers the level of free fatty acids in the blood, resetting the glucose-fatty acid (Randle) cycle in a way that makes it easier for the body to use glucose and limits the availability of fatty acids for hepatic gluconeogenesis. Ectopic lipid deposition in muscle and the liver is decreased by lowering circulating fatty acids, which further leads to improvements in glucose metabolism [42, 43].

Through an increase in the availability of GLUT 4 glucose transporters, thiazolidinediones also boost the absorption of glucose into adipose tissue and skeletal muscle. Reduced production of numerous adipocyte-derived pro-inflammatory cytokines, including tumor necrosis factor (TNF - α), which has been linked to muscle insulin resistance, is expected to help improvements in insulin sensitivity. Additionally, thiazolidinediones boost adiponectin synthesis, which improves insulin action and may have positive effects on vascular reactivity. Thiazolidinediones can alter responsive genes at these places since PPAR-γ is very weakly expressed in many tissues, which gave origin to the term "pleotropic effects" for these actions.

Like metformin, thiazolidinediones are antihyperglycemic drugs and need enough insulin in the body to have an impact on decreasing blood sugar levels. Thiazolidinediones often reduce plasma insulin concentrations, and there is evidence that they may even increase the long-term survival of islet β-cells [44].

5.2. Pharmacokinetics

When taken with meals, the absorption of rosiglitazone and pioglitazone is somewhat slowed but still rapid and almost complete. The liver extensively metabolizes both medications. The major cytochrome P450 isoform CYP2C8 metabolizes rosiglitazone to inactive or only very weakly active metabolites with a plasma half-life of 100 to 160 hours; these are primarily excreted in the urine. The enzymes CYP2C8 and CYP3A4 convert pioglitazone mostly into active metabolites that are excreted in the bile. Gemfibrozil may interact with rosiglitazone. Other medications processed by CYP3A4, such as oral contraceptives, do not appear to be clinically significantly affected by pioglitazone in terms of their plasma concentrations. Although both thiazolidinediones are virtually entirely linked to plasma proteins, their quantities are insufficient to prevent other protein-bound medications from working as intended [45].

5.3. Indications and Contraindications

Patients with T2DM who are non-obese or obese and whose lifestyle does not provide appropriate glycemic control can utilize thiazolidinediones as a monotherapy. Thiazolidinediones are positioned differently in different treatment algorithms, although they are typically used as monotherapy when metformin is ineffective or poorly tolerated and for individuals for whom an insulin secretagogue is not as preferred. They are frequently used with other antidiabetic medications, especially metformin, to achieve additive effectiveness. It is difficult to go from a sulfonylurea or metformin to a thiazolidinedione without a transient worsening in glycemic control due to their late start of the action. Thiazolidinediones and insulin work together to enhance glycemic control while lowering insulin doses, especially in obese individuals, but they must be used with additional care since they might cause peripheral edema is more common.

Thiazolidinediones tend to cause fluid retention, which can increase plasma volume by up to 500 mL, a drop in hematocrit, and a decrease in hemoglobin concentration of up to 1 g/dL. Thiazolidinediones are thus not recommended for those who have heart failure symptoms. The cardiac status-based exclusion criteria differ from country to country; for instance, New York Heart Association classifications I through IV are excluded in Europe whereas III and IV are excluded in the USA. In particular, for individuals thought to be at increased risk of cardiac failure and those exhibiting considerable early weight gain, appropriate clinical surveillance is crucial. The subject of the current debate is a meta-analysis that found rosiglitazone increased myocardial infarction risk in the first 6 to 12 months of treatment. Even though this study has drawn much criticism, the labeling has been strengthened to draw attention to the problem. Thiazolidinediones do not raise blood pressure despite an increase in fluid content; in fact, they typically cause a small drop [46].

Although neither rosiglitazone nor pioglitazone has been associated with hepatotoxicity, the troglitazone experience encouraged caution regarding liver function by testing blood alanine aminotransferase (ALT) before commencing medication and regularly subsequently. Thiazolidinediones should not be used if there is pre-existing liver disease, a developing clinical hepatic dysfunction, or increased ALT values >2.5 times the upper limit of normal. Interestingly, new research has revealed that this type of medication may even be helpful for treating non-alcoholic steatohepatitis due to the effects of thiazolidinediones on hepatic fat metabolism.

The elderly can take rosiglitazone and pioglitazone if there are no contraindications. They can also be taken into account for individuals with modest renal impairment who are aware that edema is a possibility. Thiazolidinedione usage can restore ovulation in women with anovulatory PCOS, although it is not advised to continue using those while pregnant [47].

5.4. Efficacy

The antihyperglycemic action of thiazolidinediones develops gradually and often takes two to three months to reach its peak. Because the therapeutic response might differ significantly across people, this usually causes the dose titration procedure to take longer. If there is no clinically significant benefit after three months, it is fair to consider the patient a non-responder and move to another medication. The two thiazolidinediones reduce HbA1c by around 0.5 to 1.5% (6 to 17 mmol/mol) and have comparable effects on blood sugar levels. The ADOPT research compared rosiglitazone's long-term monotherapy with metformin or a sulfonylurea and found that rosiglitazone had a more gradual but longer-lasting impact on decreasing blood sugar levels over the course of more than 3 years. Clinical trial data indicate that patients with a larger-cell reserve and more overweight persons may respond better to thiazolidinedione therapy, but a definite predictor of the best responders has not yet been identified. As a monotherapy, thiazolidinediones do not result in hypoglycemia [41].

Both thiazolidinediones significantly lower circulating non-esterified (free) fatty acids, however, there is disagreement about how they can affect other elements of the plasma lipid profile. The total cholesterol concentration is more likely to slightly increase after taking rosiglitazone, although this usually settles out within three months. Appropriate statin medication may help to reduce this effect. The LDL: HDL cholesterol ratio and the total: HDL cholesterol ratio appear to have altered little or slightly as a result of the impact, which appears to represent an increase in both LDL and HDL cholesterol. In clinical studies, Pioglitazone typically lowers triglyceride concentrations and generally seems to have no impact on total cholesterol levels. The fraction of the smaller, denser (more atherogenic), LDL particles is decreased by both thiazolidinediones [48].

Following the start of thiazolidinedione medication, weight gain of a magnitude comparable to that seen with sulfonylurea therapy (generally 1 to 4 kg) and stabilizing over 6 to 12 months is frequently seen. Numerous research suggests that the body's fat distribution has changed. The subcutaneous adipose depot grows as new, tiny, insulin-sensitive adipocytes are produced, whereas the visceral adipose depot undergoes no change or is diminished.

Several atherothrombotic risk indicators, measures of vascular reactivity, and elements of the "metabolic syndrome" have been shown to respond favorably to thiazolidinediones. Thiazolidinediones, for instance, downregulate the expression of PAI-1, lower urine albumin excretion than anticipated for an improvement in diabetic management, lower cIMT, and coronary restenosis, and lower circulating indicators of chronic low-grade inflammation. In those with IGT or those with a history of gestational diabetes, thiazolidinediones also lessen the likelihood of new-onset diabetes [49].

5.5. Adverse Effects

The primary issues with thiazolidinediones are the cardiovascular effects of edema, decreased hemoglobin levels, and congestive heart failure despite improvements in a number of atherothrombotic risk factors. In addition, a meta-analysis revealed a higher risk of myocardial infarction during the first few months of rosiglitazone therapy, albeit neither extensive study of treatment databases nor long-term prospective studies have been able to corroborate this. Nevertheless, pioglitazone decreased long-term vascular events in a sizable prospective trial.

After combining a thiazolidinedione with a sulfonylurea, hypoglycemia may develop many weeks later. Self-monitoring blood sugar levels can assist determine whether the dosage of the sulfonylurea has to be decreased. It has been recommended that rosiglitazone be started with sulfonylurea at half the maximum dosage. Recent research has also found that post-menopausal women using thiazolidinediones had an almost doubled risk of bone fracture, particularly at distal sites, and that males may also have a slightly higher risk. Those who are more at risk shouldn't be included in a bone density test. Theoretically, familial polyposis coli is a contraindication to thiazolidinediones since stimulation of PPAR-γ in colonic cells has been shown to both enhance and decrease the incidence of malignancies in animals and cell models [50-52].

6. Gliptins

Gliptins are dipeptidyl peptidase (DPP)-4 inhibitors that raise incretin levels. By delaying the fast breakdown of the incretin hormones glucose-dependent insulinotropic polypeptide (GIP) and glucagon-like peptide 1, they function as selective inhibitors of the enzyme DPP-4 to increase endogenous incretin activity (GLP-1). The development, composition, and use of incretin hormones, as well as the potential medical applications of incretin, mimics as exenatide and liraglutide. Incretin hormones are released from the gut in response to food digestion; one of its main effects is to stimulate the pancreatic islet β- cells production of glucose-induced insulin, which lowers postprandial glucose excursions. Additionally, GLP-1 reduces the islet α- cell's ability to secrete glucagon [53, 54].

Incretin impact was shown to be diminished in T2DM in the 1980s, and this was attributed, at least in part, to decreased GLP-1 secretion. Contrarily, the physiologic activities of GLP-1 remained largely unaltered in T2DM, indicating that therapeutic use of further GLP-1 treatment may be possible. Due to the peptide's quick degradation (t1/2 2 minutes), this wasn't an easy choice. Studies from the early 1990s demonstrated that the enzyme DPP-4 was mostly responsible for the breakdown. As a result, GLP-1 analogs and DPP-4 resistant constructions have been created [55, 56].

Inhibiting the activity of DPP-4 is a different treatment strategy. Inhibitors of DPP-4 were originally investigated in the late 1990s, but they lacked sufficient specificity for practical use. Following the creation of numerous distinct inhibitors, sitagliptin (2007) and vildagliptin (2008) were made available in a number of nations. Saxagliptin, a new DPP-4 inhibitor, was only released in 2009, and other DPP-4 inhibitors are now under development [57].

6.1. Mode of Action

DPP-4 is an enzyme that is free in circulation and bound to endothelial and other epithelial cells in most tissues, particularly in the intestinal mucosa. DPP - 4 inhibitors work to stop the enzyme's aminopeptidase activity. Peptides with either an alanine or a proline residue penultimate to the N-terminus are cleaved by DPP-4 to provide the N-terminal dipeptide [58]. DPP-4 inhibitors more than double the concentrations of the incretins GLP-1 and GIP in the blood, but they do not increase them to levels comparable to those of incretin mimetics that are injected subcutaneously. Increased insulin production and increased β-cell mass have been seen in animal experiments, and endogenous incretin concentrations have been shown to promote nutrient-induced insulin release. High GLP-1 levels also improve the inhibition of glucagon secretion 88. There is little chance of causing serious hypoglycemia because these effects are glucose-dependent. Body weight typically fluctuates little, and the increase in GLP-1 levels brought on by DPP-4 inhibitors is typically insufficient to generate a palpable satiety effect or a significant delay of stomach emptying.

The action period of these drugs is mostly preprandial because the incretin-mediated impact of DPP-4 inhibitors potentiates glucose-dependent insulin production. A significant carryover effect benefits the management of interprandial glycemia despite their special effectiveness in decreasing postprandial hyperglycemia. DPP-4 inhibitors, on the other hand, do not start insulin secretion, and as a result, they do not boost baseline insulin secretion. Additionally, there is no chance of interprandial "over-shoot" into hypoglycemia since they exclusively decrease glucagon secretion in the hyperglycemic state [59].

6.2. Pharmacokinetics

Vildagliptin and sitagliptin are reversible, competitive, and selective DPP-4 inhibitors (IC_{50} approximately 18 and 3.5 nmol, respectively). Both sitagliptin (a derivative of the piperazine) and vildagliptin (a derivative of the cyanopyrrolidine) are highly bioavailable (about 87% and 85%, respectively), quickly absorbed (t_{max} 1-4 and 2 hours, respectively), and have relatively low plasma protein binding (about 38% and 9%, respectively). Sitagliptin has a plasma half-life of 8 to 14 hours, and CYP3A4 and CYP2C6 metabolize a small amount of it in the liver. With the help of the organic anion transporter (OAT3), the majority of a sitagliptin dosage (about 79%) is removed intact in the urine by renal tubular secretion. A single 100 mg sitagliptin dosage results in an approximately 12 hours period of nearly full DPP-4 activity inhibition and about 80% inhibition up to 24 hours. Vildagliptin has a shorter plasma half-life of 1.5 to 4.5 hours; the majority (about 69%) is mostly metabolized by the kidneys to inactive metabolites with minimal participation from CYP450 isoforms, and the majority (roughly 85%) is excreted in the urine. A dosage of 50 to 100 mg of vildagliptin inhibits DPP-4 almost completely for 12 hours and around 40% for 24 hours.

6.3. Indications and Contraindications

Although this is not an approved indication in all countries where accessible, gliptins can theoretically be used as monotherapy in patients with T2DM who have reacted insufficiently to lifestyle interventions. Gliptins are now chosen as "add-on" therapies in individuals whose blood sugar levels are insufficiently managed by metformin or thiazolidinedione. As their mode of action on the beta cell differs from that of sulfonylureas and meglitinides, they could theoretically be used with any other class of oral agents or insulin. Additionally, due to their ability to lower glucagon levels, they may be useful as an adjunct therapy to insulin even in the absence of β-cell function. In reality, however, the substantial β-cell reserve is necessary for complete efficiency in T2DM. Gliptins are suitable for overweight and obese patients due to their lack of weight gain. Their low risk of hypoglycemia, when used as monotherapy (and in combination with non-insulin releasing agents), encourages the use of these medications in patients with only mildly elevated basal glycemia, those who are close to their glycemic target, and those who have unpredictable meal times [60].

Vildagliptin is often taken twice daily, whereas sitagliptin is typically given once daily (100 mg) in the morning (50 mg). The risk of any major glucose-lowering impact is reduced by the glucose-dependent mode of action unless there is hyperglycemia, which eases anxiety about skipping meals. As a result, there is no dosage titration; however, it is advised to reassess fasting and postprandial glycemia after roughly 2 weeks of therapy, particularly when introduced as a second agent.

For patients with moderate renal insufficiency (creatinine clearance 30 to 50 mL/min), a reduced dose (50 mg once daily) is advised; for patients with severe renal insufficiency (creatinine clearance 30 mL/min) or with an end-stage renal disease requiring hemodialysis or peritoneal dialysis, consider a dose of 25 mg once daily. If renal function is sufficient, sitagliptin can be used in individuals with mild to moderate liver function impairment because it does not appear to induce or inhibit P450 isoforms.

Vildagliptin is not advised for use in individuals with moderate or severe renal impairment (e.g., creatinine clearance 50 mL/min) due to the renal metabolism and removal of the drug. A liver function test should be performed both before commencing medication and on a regular basis moving forward since certain instances of reversibly increased ALT or aspartate aminotransferase (AST) have been noted in individuals receiving vildagliptin. Treatment is not recommended if there is a significant increase in liver enzymes (e.g., ALT or AST >3 upper limits of normal) or other symptoms of hepatic impairment.

Neither gliptin has been associated with any notable medication interactions. Due to the paucity of clinical data, it is advised to take these medications with caution in heart disease patients and to discontinue gliptin therapy during pregnancy.

6.4. Efficacy

6.4.1. Sitagliptin

After 24 to 52 weeks, sitagliptin 100 mg/day frequently decreased HbA1c (from a baseline of around 8% [64 mmol/mol]) by about 0.7 to 0.8% (8 to 9 mmol/mol). This effect was seen with both monotherapy and add-on treatment. People with high baseline HbA1c often had decreases in HbA1c of >1% (11 mmol/mol). Fasting plasma glucose levels decreased by 1.0 to 1.5 mmol/L, while postprandial glucose levels, which were assessed two hours after a typical mixed meal, typically decreased by 3 mmol/L. A sitagliptin + metformin combination was linked to fewer hypoglycemic episodes than a combination of glipizide + metformin despite equal levels of HbA1c. Sitagliptin medication did not result in a clinically meaningful increase in the incidence of hypoglycemia. Sitagliptin did not increase body weight compared with placebo in any trials [61].

6.4.2. Vildagliptin

When administered as a monotherapy or as an add-on to metformin or a thiazolidinedione in clinical studies, vildagliptin demonstrated similar effectiveness and tolerability to sitagliptin at a single daily dosage of 50 to 100 mg. Even though vildagliptin showed somewhat better HbA1c reductions in several studies, this was mostly due to slightly higher average beginning HbA1c levels (>8.5% [>69 mmol/mol]). Again, neither hypoglycemia nor body weight was affected [62].

6.5. Adverse Effects

Gliptins haven't shown any significant side effects in clinical studies yet. Measures of tolerance and adverse events in clinical studies (usually lasting 6 to 12 months) were frequently compared to placebo or comparison. With a 100 mg dosage of vildagliptin, there were some increases in liver enzymes, but not with the 50 mg level that is commercially available. The ability to impede stomach emptying is unlikely to have a clinically meaningful effect, according to nominal increases in the signs or symptoms of abdominal pain that have been described.

Gliptins have the potential to affect the hunger-satiety system, gastrointestinal motility, growth, and vascular function because there are numerous natural substrates for DPP-4, including bradykinin, enkephalins, neuropeptide Y, peptide YY1-36, gastrin-releasing polypeptide, substance P, insulin-like growth factor I, vasostatin 1, the chains of thyrotropin, lute, However, neither CD26 knockout mice nor the DPP - 4 - specific inhibitors employed in animals or people have yet demonstrated any appreciable adverse immune-related consequences. DPP-4 is also the CD26 T-cell activation antigen. Because inhibiting similar enzymes like DPP-8 and DPP-9 has caused blood dyscrasias and skin lesions in certain species but not in humans, it is important to selectively inhibit DPP-4. However, it is wise to look for any signs of skin lesions [58].

7. α-Glucosidase Inhibitors

Studies from the late 1970s found that intestine-glucosidase inhibitors might slow the absorption of sugars by delaying the last stages of carbohydrate digestion. It was established that this strategy might lower postprandial hyperglycemia in diabetes by the early 1980s. Early in the 1990s, the first -glucosidase inhibitor, acarbose, was made available. Two more agents, miglitol and voglibose, were subsequently introduced in various nations. Patients who eat meals high in complex carbohydrates can benefit from the successful reduction of postprandial glucose excursions by using -glucosidase inhibitors. These medications likewise have a strong safety record, although gastrointestinal side effects have restricted their use [61].

7.1. Mode of Action

In the brush border of the enterocytes lining the intestinal villi, α-glucosidase inhibitors compete with one another to block the activity of α-glucosidase enzymes. They have a strong binding affinity for the enzymes and stop them from breaking down oligosaccharides and disaccharides into monosaccharides. This postpones the process of digesting carbohydrates to completion and may postpone it farther down the digestive tract, delaying glucose absorption.

The affinities of various α-glucosidase inhibitors for various α-glucosidase enzymes vary. This results in somewhat varied activity profiles (e.g., miglitol is a more potent inhibitor of sucrase than acarbose, which has a greater affinity for glycoamylase, sucrase, maltase, and dextrinases). It is noted that patients must consume complex, digestible carbohydrates for α-glucosidase inhibitors to be effective. The absorption of glucose itself is not considerably impacted by these substances. α-Glucosidase inhibitors may change the release of glucose-dependent intestinal hormones like GIP and GLP-1, which boost nutrient-induced insulin secretion, by relocating glucose absorption more distally throughout the intestinal tract. Thus, -glucosidase inhibitors may decrease the release of GIP, which comes mainly from the jejunal mucosa while increasing the secretion of GLP-1, primarily from the ileal mucosa. The reduced risk in postprandial glucose levels is likely how glucosidase inhibitors lower postprandial insulin concentrations [62].

7.2. Pharmacokinetics

Less than 2% of the medication is absorbed intact, along with some intestinal degradation products, since amylases break down acarbose in the small intestine and intestinal bacteria. Within 24 hours, the majority of ingested substances are removed from the urine. Nearly all of the miglitol is absorbed, and it is excreted unaltered in the urine [63].

7.3. Indications and Contraindications

α-Glucosidase inhibitors can be used as a monotherapy, often for T2DM patients with postprandial hyperglycemia but only modestly elevated fasting glycemia; however, they are most frequently used as a supplement to other medications, again to target postprandial hyperglycemia. In those using sulfonylurea and/or insulin, α-glucosidase inhibitors can also be used to prolong the postprandial phase in order to decrease interprandial glycemic troughs or hypoglycemia. Although not an approved application, acarbose has also been demonstrated to stop the development of IGT to T2DM [64].

However, they are most usually used as a complement to other drugs to target postprandial hyperglycemia. Glucosidase inhibitors can be used as a monotherapy, frequently for T2DM patients with postprandial hyperglycemia but only mildly raised fasting glycemia. In order to lessen interprandial glycemic troughs or hypoglycemia in those using sulfonylurea and/or insulin, glucosesidase inhibitors can also be administered to lengthen the postprandial phase. Acarbose has also been shown to halt the progression of IGT to T2DM, despite not being an authorized use.

Since high doses of acarbose can occasionally cause an increase in liver enzyme concentrations and α-glucosidase inhibitors are contraindicated for patients with a history of chronic intestinal disease, it is advised to periodically measure transaminase concentrations in patients receiving the maximum dosage (200 mg acarbose three times daily). As the dose is decreased, elevated liver enzymes should subside; otherwise, alternative reasons for hepatic dysfunction should be taken into account.

7.4. Efficacy

The success of α-glucosidase inhibitors depends on dietary adherence since they target postprandial glucose excursions during meals containing complex carbohydrates. These medications can lower peak postprandial glucose levels by 1 to 4 mmol/L when used alone. Some people see a more than halving of the incremental area under the postprandial plasma glucose curve, and there is typically a longer duration of impact to just slightly reduced basal glycemia up to roughly 1 mmol/L. If a high dose of the medication is taken and dietary compliance is maintained, the reduction in HbA1c is typically between 0.5 and 1.0% (6 and 11 mmol/mol) [65].

Although there are very moderate overall decreases in HbA1c, α-glucosidase inhibitors have several advantages, including the fact that they do not lead to weight gain or severe hypoglycemia and may lessen interprandial hypoglycemia. α-glucosidase inhibitors frequently lower plasma triglyceride levels and, when used in conjunction with other antidiabetic medications, can lessen postprandial hyperinsulinemia. When used in combination treatment, the α-glucosidase inhibitor can cause small changes in the intestinal absorption of other α-glucosidase inhibitors, although β-glucosidase inhibitors often result in additive effectiveness increases when combined with any other kind of α-glucosidase inhibitor. Acarbose may prevent serious cardiac events like myocardial infarction; however, this has not been shown. It is also unknown if this results from the drug's ability to target postprandial hyperglycemia or if it is a separate impact [66].

7.5. Adverse Effects

The biggest issue with -glucosidase inhibitors is their gastrointestinal adverse effects. For instance, in the STOP - NIDDM study, 31% of patients receiving acarbose quit therapy early compared to 19% of patients receiving a placebo. Undigested oligosaccharides enter the large intestine if the dosage is too high (in comparison to the number of complex carbohydrates in the meal). These are fermented and can cause flatulence, gastrointestinal pain, and occasionally diarrhea; however, these side effects often go away over time and with slower titration. Although it is not advised to use cholestyramine or medicines that influence gastrointestinal motility in combination with each other, hypoglycemia is not prevalent and there are no clinically relevant medication interactions [64].

8. Combination Therapy

The use of mixtures of two or more oral medications with diverse mechanisms of action has become prevalent as the target-driven early and intensive approach to controlling hyperglycemia in T2DM gains traction. Several fixed-dosage, single-tablet combinations have been made available to help with combination treatment. These are created to offer bioequivalence and correspondingly equivalent efficacy, while slight formulation changes could also permit a little more blood glucose-lowering activity. Compared to similar combinations of individual tablets, fixed dosage combinations can be more convenient, lower the "pill burden," make administration regimens simpler, and perhaps boost patient adherence. It may also be possible to obtain effectiveness while avoiding dosage-related adverse effects by using lower doses of two different types of drugs as opposed to a large dose of one agent. Metformin is now used in fixed dosage combinations with sulfonylurea, a thiazolidinedione, gliptin, or meglitinide, as well as combinations of thiazolidinedione and sulfonylurea. The majority of the frequently used dose combinations have been accommodated, notwithstanding the possibility that single pills might limit titration flexibility. It should be emphasized that any type of combination therapy must adhere to the same warnings and restrictions that each active ingredient entails [67].

8.1. Efficacy

The first justification for combination therapy is its improved efficacy, whether it involves using oral medications alone, oral medications plus insulin, or oral medications and additional injectable medications such as incretin mimetics. Randomized controlled studies of antidiabetic drugs have shown, among other things, that adding or combining therapy is more effective than moving from one medicine to another. Patients receiving maximal doses of glyburide but still had insufficient glycemic control were randomized to continue receiving that monotherapy, receive metformin monotherapy that was titrated gradually to maximal doses (850 mg orally three times a day), or receive a combination of glyburide and metformin. Fasting plasma glucose (FPG) did not significantly improve with either treatment, but combination therapy with an insulin secretagogue and metformin showed a remarkable improvement.

Similar to this, research on other combination medicines found slight advantage in moving to a different agent class but improved glucose-lowering effectiveness when combined with an agent that works through a different mechanism. Using some drugs that treat preprandial hyperglycemia and other compounds that treat postprandial hyperglycemia may increase effectiveness as the last benefit of combination therapy. It could be crucial to balance the use of both strategies, much like with basal and bolus insulin.

Combining oral medications may appear more difficult than monotherapy, yet there are times when their convenience can be increased. A single dosage of a long-acting sulfonylurea, such as glimepiride, combined with one or two metformin pills may be more beneficial than three or four metformin tablets alone.

There are now combo tablets for metformin and secretagogues, like glyburide, glipizide, and repaglinide. Metformin-thiazolidinedione combo tablets (metformin-rosiglitazone, metformin-pioglitazone) are also offered. The combination medications rosiglitazone and glimepiride and pioglitazone and glimepiride have just been made accessible. Some more recent medications, including sitagliptin, are marketed as combination pills and have been authorized for use with metformin. Future years will probably see a rise in the use of combo medications.

Many people and medical professionals may find appeal in drug formulations that include two substances with dual effects. While many individuals may benefit from the independent titration of different medicines, combination formulations may be preferable for other people. The individual agent in a combination pill may usually be accurately identified by the adverse symptoms that are frequently specific to that agent (e.g., sulfonylureas with hypoglycemia, metformin with gastrointestinal side effects, glitazones with fluid retention). Rarer or idiosyncratic adverse effects may occasionally be harder to link to a particular medication. This strategy may be particularly appealing to individuals who need to take additional drugs to manage their blood pressure, lipid abnormalities, heart disease, and other conditions in addition to two or more agents for glycemic control [68, 69].

9. Miscellaneous Drugs

9.1. Hydroxychloroquine

Antimalarials are widely used therapeutic treatments for conditions including rheumatoid arthritis and systemic lupus erythematosus (SLE) because they are well-tolerated and safe. Patients taking these medications for immune illnesses have shown their benefits for diabetic management. One of the uncommon side effects of these medication classes is hypoglycemia. Particularly in Sulfonylurea (SU)-resistant individuals, hydroxychloroquine (HCQ) has been demonstrated to decrease HbA1c levels. The need for insulin is significantly reduced when HCQ is added to insulin treatment.

The main mechanism is a decrease in insulin metabolism, which is achieved by direct contact with the insulin receptor, a slower rate of insulin receptor dissociation, a lengthened half-life of the insulin-receptor complex, and, therefore a longer insulin action. The stimulation of islet cells to produce more insulin and a decrease in hepatic gluconeogenesis are two additional modes of action.

HCQ has a beneficial effect on lipid metabolism acting by reducing triglycerides, low-density lipoprotein (LDL)-cholesterol, apo-B, and increasing HDL-cholesterol. Moreover, a recently published study from India showed a favorable effect of HCQ at a dose of 400 mg/day on both glycemic and lipid profiles in type 2 diabetes patients who were inadequately controlled with a combination of SUs and metformin.

Intriguingly, HCQ is successful in reducing the incidence of newly developed diabetes mellitus in addition to its impact on lowering blood sugar in diabetic patients. In prospective, randomized research of 4,905 RA patients, it was discovered that those who used HCQ for more than 4 years had a 77% lower chance of acquiring diabetes mellitus.

Ocular toxicity is one of the less frequent side effects of long-term HCQ treatment. Depending on the total dose and length of treatment, every patient with HCQ should undergo routine screening for retinal toxicity [70].

9.2. Sodium-Glucose Cotransporter 2 (SGLT2) Inhibitors

An FDA-approved group of prescription drugs known as SGLT2 inhibitors is combined with diet and exercise to decrease blood sugar levels in persons with T2DM. SGLT2 inhibitors include canagliflozin, dapagliflozin, and empagliflozin as medications. They can be found as one-ingredient formulations or in mixtures with other diabetic medications like metformin. By encouraging the kidneys to eliminate sugar from the body through the urine, SGLT2 inhibitors reduce blood sugar levels. The FDA has not authorized SGLT2 inhibitors for use in individuals with T1DM because their safety and effectiveness in these patients have not been shown.

A normal adult's glomeruli filter around 180 g of glucose daily, and virtually all that glucose is reabsorbed from the glomerular filtrate and put back into the bloodstream. The active transport of sodium out of the basolateral cells by the Na/K-ATPase pump causes this cotransport of glucose and sodium. 4 Along with the concentration gradient, glucose is also moved out of the cell and into circulation via glucose transporters. Renal glucose processing and transport are enhanced in T2DM, most likely due to SGLT2 upregulation. Increasing glucose excretion is inhibited, which decreases the reabsorption of filtered glucose and lowers blood glucose levels [71].

9.3. Canagliflozin

In 2013, the FDA authorized the first SGLT2 inhibitor, canagliflozin. In individuals with T2DM, it is now recommended as a supplement to diet and exercise. Studies have demonstrated the advantages of glycemic management, weight loss, and decreased systolic blood pressure (SBP), whether used alone or in conjunction with other antihyperglycemic medications. It has also been demonstrated that canagliflozin 100 mg and 300 mg significantly lower weight, SBP, and fasting plasma glucose (FPG). It is administered once daily and is available as 100 mg and 300 mg tablets [72, 73].

9.4. Dapagliflozin

Dapagliflozin, a second SGLT2 inhibitor, received FDA approval in January 2014. Studies on dapagliflozin monotherapy and in combination with other antihyperglycemic drugs have shown improvements in glycemic management, weight loss, and SBP decrease. Dapagliflozin has been investigated in combination with metformin, glimepiride, pioglitazone, and insulin, even though it is only presently licensed for monotherapy. Dapagliflozin reduced pioglitazone-induced weight gain and edema when combined with pioglitazone monotherapy. When dapagliflozin 5 mg and 10 mg were added to oral antihyperglycemic medications or insulin treatment, the total daily insulin dosage was reduced by 6 U/day. It is administered once daily and comes in 5 mg/10 mg pills.

The main benefits of this family of medications are that they are straightforward, non-specialized types of therapy that are effective and independent of B-cell activity and enhance insulin-dependent processes. These medicines may result in weight loss and a drop in blood pressure, and they are less susceptible to hypoglycemia. Patients with end-stage renal illness, ketonuria, or ketonemia should not use these medications. Lower urinary tract infections and a slightly higher rate of genital infections are among the medications' reported adverse effects. Electrolyte abnormalities and polyuria are also uncommonly reported [74, 75].

9.5. Bromocriptine

In 2009, the US FDA granted bromocriptine approval to treat diabetes. It is a centrally acting antidiabetic drug that, if administered first thing in the morning, would normalize the excessively increased sympathetic drive in T2DM patients' hypothalamus. This would thus lead to a decrease in hepatic glucose production. Additionally, studies have demonstrated that it increases insulin sensitivity in peripheral tissues and insulin release. A reduction in

HbA1c of 0.5 to 0.7 is seen in people with poorly managed T2DM who use bromocriptine in addition to diet alone, metformin, SUs, or thiazolidinediones [76].

Apart from nausea, the medication is well tolerated and is used at significantly lower levels (up to 4.8 mg per day) for treating diabetes than for treating Parkinson's disease. It is a desirable choice for the treatment of type 2 diabetes due to its new method of action, favorable side effect profile, and ability to lower the rates of cardiovascular events [77].

9.6. Liraglutide

An agonist of the glucagon-like peptide-1 (GLP-1) receptor is liraglutide. It is an injectable formulation that is sold at a dosage of 3 mg for the treatment of obesity and a separate dose (1.8 mg) for the treatment of type 2 diabetic patients. As a part of the SCALE initiative, four phases 3 studies in various overweight/obese populations have been or are being carried out. According to published data, individuals treated with liraglutide lost much more weight than those given a placebo, and the majority of them did so at a rate of 5% of their body weight. Additionally, liraglutide therapy was linked to statistically significant reductions in HbA1c, fasting plasma glucose, and fasting insulin.

Clinical investigations revealed the most frequent adverse effects of nausea, hypoglycemia, diarrhea, constipation, vomiting, headaches, reduced appetite, dyspepsia, exhaustion, disorientation, abdominal discomfort, and elevated lipase. Liraglutide was authorized with REMS due to prior findings so that medical professionals are aware of the potentially significant hazards of medullary thyroid cancer and acute pancreatitis. A personal or family history of medullary thyroid cancer or type 2 multiple endocrine neoplasia syndrome is, therefore, a contraindication. Additionally, liraglutide should not be used by pregnant women or those with a history of hypersensitivity to the drug or any of its ingredients [78, 79].

9.7. Lorcaserin

A specific 5HT2c receptor antagonist is lorcaserin. Although the specific processes are still being investigated, it reduces the urge to eat. Currently, 10 mg administered twice daily is the recommended dosage. The main evidence used to support lorcaserin's approval in the United States came from three clinical trials. In the patients receiving lorcaserin in these studies (BLOOM, BLOSSOM, and BLOOM-DM), there was a small amount of weight reduction and an improvement in cardiovascular risk factors. Additionally, HbA1c and fasting glucose tests in diabetic individuals showed a considerable decrease.

If patients do not lose at least 5% of their body weight in the first 12 weeks after starting this drug, it is advised that they stop taking it. The adverse effects of lorcaserin, which include dry mouth, headaches, dizziness, lethargy, and constipation, are often minor and well-tolerated. Earlier worries about valvulopathy have been disregarded. Pregnancy continues to be prohibited by the drug [80].

9.8. Phentermine–Topiramate

A combination of phentermine and topiramate with an extended release is another medication authorized for long-term usage but requires a risk assessment and mitigation plan (REMS). This medication combines modest doses of phentermine with topiramate (initial dose: 3.75 mg/23 mg topiramate for 14 days, followed by 7.5 mg/ 46 mg topiramate). A sympathomimetic amine, phentermine elevates norepinephrine levels in the central nervous system while decreasing hunger. Gamma-aminobutyric acid (GABA) receptor modulator topiramate has an unclear effect in controlling weight. The effectiveness of the combination in patients who were overweight or obese was investigated in two phases 3 clinical studies (CONQUER, EQUIP trials), as well as one extension trial (SEQUEL trial). These studies demonstrated a dose-dependent considerable weight decrease when compared to the placebo. Additionally, changes in cardiometabolic markers and a slower onset of T2DM were seen. The mixture was highly received [81].

The most frequent side effects are dry mouth, paresthesia, and constipation. Due to topiramate's potential to create fetal oral clefts (the source of REMS) and uncommon acute glaucoma, the combination is not recommended for usage during pregnancy or in glaucoma patients. Additional contraindications include hyperthyroidism, the use of monoamine oxidase inhibitors within 14 days of treatment, and hypersensitivity to sympathomimetic amines [82].

Conclusion

Only non-insulin dependent diabetes is successfully treated in adults by oral hypoglycemic medications. The four main classes of oral diabetes medications are: (1) secretagogues (meglitinides, sulfonylureas), which increase the availability of insulin; (2) biguanides (metformin), which reduce excessive hepatic glucose release; (3) thiazolidinediones or glitazones (pioglitazone, rosiglitazone); and (4) α-glucosidase inhibitors (miglitol, acarbose) Since oral treatments try to modulate either insulin release or sensitivity, oral hypoglycemic drugs operate on the assumption that an appropriate quantity of endogenous insulin is generated. Oral hypoglycemics may be used either alone or in combination with other agents.

References

[1] Medvei, Victor Cornelius. *The history of clinical endocrinology: a comprehensive account of endocrinology from earliest times to the present day.* CRC Press, 1993.

[2] Sanders, Lee J. "From Thebes to Toronto and the 21st century: an incredible journey." *Diabetes Spectrum* 15, no. 1 (2002): 56.

[3] White Jr, John R. *"A brief history of the development of diabetes medications."* Diabetes spectrum: a publication of the American Diabetes Association 27, no. 2 (2014): 82.

[4] Bailey, Clifford J., and Caroline Day. "Metformin: its botanical background." *Practical diabetes international 21*, no. 3 (2004): 115-117.

[5] Bailey, Clifford J. "Biguanides and NIDDM." *Diabetes care* 15, no. 6 (1992): 755-772.

[6] Bailey, Clifford J., and Robert C. Turner. "Metformin." *New England Journal of Medicine* 334, no. 9 (1996): 574-579.

[7] Bailey, Clifford J., Ian W. Campbell, Juliana CN Chan, Jaime A. Davidson, Harry CS Howlett, and Patrick Ritz. *Metformin-the gold standard: a scientific handbook.* Wiley, 2007.

[8] Bailey, Clifford J. "Metformin: effects on micro and macrovascular complications in type 2 diabetes." *Cardiovascular drugs and therapy* 22, no. 3 (2008): 215-224.

[9] Grant, P. J. "Beneficial effects of metformin on haemostasis and vascular function in man." *Diabetes & metabolism* 29, no. 4 (2003): 6S44-6S52.

[10] Gaochao Zhou, Robert Myers, Ying Li, Yuli Chen, Xiaolan Shen, Judy Fenyk-Melody, Margaret Wu, John Ventre, Thomas Doebber, Nobuharu Fujii, Nicolas Musi, Michael F. Hirshman, Laurie J. Goodyear, and David E. Moller. "Role of AMP-activated protein kinase in mechanism of metformin action." *The Journal of clinical investigation* 108, no. 8 (2001): 1167-1174.

[11] Scheen, André J. "Clinical pharmacokinetics of metformin." *Clinical pharmacokinetics* 30, no. 5 (1996): 359-371.

[12] Cusi, Kenneth, and R. A. DeFronzo. "Metformin: a review of its metabolic effects." *Diabetes Reviews* 6, no. 2 (1998): 89-131.

[13] Palomba, Stefano, Angela Falbo, Fulvio Zullo, and Francesco Orio Jr. "Evidence-based and potential benefits of metformin in the polycystic ovary syndrome: a comprehensive review." *Endocrine Reviews* 30, no. 1 (2009): 1-50.

[14] Natali, Andrea, and Eleuterio Ferrannini. "Effects of metformin and thiazolidinediones on suppression of hepatic glucose production and stimulation of glucose uptake in type 2 diabetes: a systematic review." *Diabetologia* 49, no. 3 (2006): 434-441.

[15] UK Prospective Diabetes Study (UKPDS) Group. "Intensive blood-glucose control with sulphonylureas or insulin compared with conventional treatment and risk of complications in patients with type 2 diabetes (UKPDS 33)." *The lancet* 352, no. 9131 (1998): 837-853.

[16] Rao, Ajay D., Nitesh Kuhadiya, Kristi Reynolds, and Vivian A. Fonseca. "Is the combination of sulfonylureas and metformin associated with an increased risk of cardiovascular disease or all-cause mortality? A meta-analysis of observational studies." *Diabetes care* 31, no. 8 (2008): 1672-1678.

[17] Hermansen, Kjeld, and Lene S. Mortensen. "Bodyweight changes associated with antihyperglycaemic agents in type 2 diabetes mellitus." *Drug Safety* 30, no. 12 (2007): 1127-1142.

[18] Johnson, Jeffrey A., Sumit R. Majumdar, Scot H. Simpson, and Ellen L. Toth. "Decreased mortality associated with the use of metformin compared with sulfonylurea monotherapy in type 2 diabetes." *Diabetes care* 25, no. 12 (2002): 2244-2248.

[19] Holman, Rury R., Sanjoy K. Paul, M. Angelyn Bethel, David R. Matthews, and H. Andrew W. Neil. "10-year follow-up of intensive glucose control in type 2 diabetes." *New England journal of medicine* 359, no. 15 (2008): 1577-1589.

[20] Knowler, William C., Elizabeth Barrett-Connor, Sarah E. Fowler, Richard F. Hamman, John M. Lachin, Elizabeth A. Walker, David M. Nathan P. G. Watson, J. T. Mendoza, K. A. Smith, J. Caro, B. Goldstein, C. Lark, L. Menefee, L. Murphy, C. Pepe, J. M. Spandorfer. "*Reduction in the incidence of type 2 diabetes with lifestyle intervention or metformin*." (2002): 393.

[21] Salpeter, Shelley R., Elizabeth Greyber, Gary A. Pasternak, and Edwin E. Salpeter. "Risk of fatal and nonfatal lactic acidosis with metformin use in type 2 diabetes mellitus: systematic review and meta-analysis." *Archives of internal medicine* 163, no. 21 (2003): 2594-2602.

[22] Lalau, Jean-Daniel, and Jean-Michel Race. "Metformin and lactic acidosis in diabetic humans." *Diabetes, obesity and metabolism* 2, no. 3 (2000): 131-137.

[23] Henquin, J-C. "The fiftieth anniversary of hypoglycaemic sulphonamides. How did the mother compound work?." *Diabetologia* 35, no. 10 (1992): 907-912.

[24] Ashcroft, F. M., and F. M. Gribble. "ATP-sensitive K+ channels and insulin secretion: their role in health and disease." Diabetologia 42, no. 8 (1999): 903.

[25] Gribble, F. M., and F. Reimann. "Pharmacological modulation of KATP channels." *Biochemical Society Transactions* 30, no. 2 (2002): 333-339.

[26] Rorsman, Patrik, and Erik Renström. "Insulin granule dynamics in pancreatic beta cells." *Diabetologia* 46, no. 8 (2003): 1029-1045.

[27] Ball, Andrew J., Peter R. Flatt, and Neville H. McClenaghan. "Desensitization of sulphonylurea-and nutrient-induced insulin secretion following prolonged treatment with glibenclamide." *European Journal of Pharmacology* 408, no. 3 (2000): 327-333.

[28] Lebovitz, H. E. "Insulin secretagogues: old and new." *Diabetes Review* 7 (1999): 139-153.

[29] Groop, Leif C. "Sulfonylureas in NIDDM." *Diabetes care* 15, no. 6 (1992): 737-754.

[30] Rendell, Marc. "The role of sulphonylureas in the management of type 2 diabetes mellitus." *Drugs* 64, no. 12 (2004): 1339-1358.

[31] Schernthaner, G., A. Grimaldi, U. Di Mario, J. Drzewoski, P. Kempler, M. Kvapil, A. Novials, R. Rottiers, G. E. H. M. Rutten, and K. M. Shaw. "GUIDE study: double-blind comparison of once-daily gliclazide MR and glimepiride in type 2 diabetic patients." *European journal of clinical investigation* 34, no. 8 (2004): 535-542.

[32] Yki-Järvinen, Hannele, Leena Ryysy, Kati Nikkilä, Timo Tulokas, Raimo Vanamo, and Marjatta Heikkilä. "Comparison of bedtime insulin regimens in patients with type 2 diabetes mellitus: a randomized, controlled trial." *Annals of internal medicine* 130, no. 5 (1999): 389-396.

[33] Krentz, Andrew J., and Clifford J. Bailey. "Oral antidiabetic agents." *Drugs* 65, no. 3 (2005): 385-411.

[34] UK Prospective Diabetes Study (UKPDS) Group. "Effect of intensive blood-glucose control with metformin on complications in overweight patients with type 2 diabetes (UKPDS 34)." *The Lancet* 352, no. 9131 (1998): 854-865.

[35] Krentz, Andrew J., Robin E. Ferner, and Clifford J. Bailey. "Comparative tolerability profiles of oral antidiabetic agents." *Drug Safety* 11, no. 4 (1994): 223-241.

[36] Angiolillo, Dominick J., Steven B. Shoemaker, Bhaloo Desai, Hang Yuan, Ronald K. Charlton, Esther Bernardo, Martin M. Zenni, Luis A. Guzman, Theodore A. Bass, and Marco A. Costa. "Randomized comparison of a high clopidogrel maintenance dose in patients with diabetes mellitus and coronary artery disease: results of the Optimizing Antiplatelet Therapy in Diabetes Mellitus (OPTIMUS) study." *Circulation* 115, no. 6 (2007): 708-716.

[37] Dornhorst, Anne. "Insulinotropic meglitinide analogues." *The Lancet* 358, no. 9294 (2001): 1709-1716.

[38] Davies, M. "*Nateglinide: better postprandial glucose control.*" Prescriber-London-13 (2002): 17-28.

[39] Bicklé, J. F. "Meglitinide analogues: a review of clinical data focused on recent trials." *Diabetes & metabolism* 32, no. 2 (2006): 113-120.

[40] Day, C. "Thiazolidinediones: a new class of antidiabetic drugs." *Diabetic Medicine* 16, no. 3 (1999): 179-192.

[41] Yki, Jarvinen H. "Drug Therapy: Thiazolidinediones." *N. Engl. J. Med* 351 (2004): 1106-1118.

[42] Staels, Bart, and Jean-Charles Fruchart. "Therapeutic roles of peroxisome proliferator–activated receptor agonists." *Diabetes* 54, no. 8 (2005): 2460-2470.

[43] Semple, Robert K., V. Krishna K. Chatterjee, and Stephen O'Rahilly. "PPARγ and human metabolic disease." *The Journal of clinical investigation* 116, no. 3 (2006): 581-589.

[44] Kahn, Steven E., Steven M. Haffner, Mark A. Heise, William H. Herman, Rury R. Holman, Nigel P. Jones, Barbara G. Kravitz, John M. Lachin, M. Colleen O'Neill, Bernard Zinman, and Giancarlo Viberti. "Glycemic durability of rosiglitazone, metformin, or glyburide monotherapy." *New England Journal of Medicine* 355, no. 23 (2006): 2427-2443.

[45] Bailey, C. J. "Treating insulin resistance in type 2 diabetes with metformin and thiazolidinediones." *Diabetes, Obesity and Metabolism* 7, no. 6 (2005): 675-691.

[46] Nesto, Richard W., David Bell, Robert O. Bonow, Vivian Fonseca, Scott M. Grundy, Edward S. Horton, Martin Le Winter, Daniel Porte, Clay F. Semenkovich, Sidney Smith, Lawrence H. Young and Richard Kahn. "Thiazolidinedione use, fluid retention, and congestive heart failure: a consensus statement from the American Heart Association and American Diabetes Association." *Circulation* 108, no. 23 (2003): 2941-2948.

[47] Nissen, Steven E., and Kathy Wolski. "Effect of rosiglitazone on the risk of myocardial infarction and death from cardiovascular causes." *New England Journal of Medicine* 356, no. 24 (2007): 2457-2471.

[48] Goldberg, Ronald B., David M. Kendall, Mark A. Deeg, John B. Buse, Anthony J. Zagar, Jane A. Pinaire, Meng H. Tan, Mehmood A. Khan, Alfonso T. Perez, Scott J. Jacober. "A comparison of lipid and glycemic effects of pioglitazone and rosiglitazone in patients with type 2 diabetes and dyslipidemia." *Diabetes Care* 28, no. 7 (2005): 1547-1554.

[49] Buchanan, Thomas A., Anny H. Xiang, Ruth K. Peters, Siri L. Kjos, Aura Marroquin, Jose Goico, Cesar Ochoa, Sylvia Tan, Kathleen Berkowitz, Hodis Howard N, Azen Stanley P. "Preservation of pancreatic β-cell function and prevention of type 2 diabetes by pharmacological treatment of insulin resistance in high-risk Hispanic women." *Diabetes* 51, no. 9 (2002): 2796-2803.

[50] Erdmann, Erland, John A. Dormandy, Bernard Charbonnel, Massimo Massi-Benedetti, Ian K. Moules, Allan M. Skene, and PROactive Investigators. "The effect of pioglitazone on recurrent myocardial infarction in 2,445 patients with type 2 diabetes and previous myocardial infarction: results from the PROactive (PROactive 05) Study." *Journal of the American College of Cardiology* 49, no. 17 (2007): 1772-1780.

[51] Wilcox, Robert, Marie-Germaine Bousser, D. John Betteridge, Guntram Schernthaner, Valdis Pirags, Stuart Kupfer, and John Dormandy. "Effects of pioglitazone in patients with type 2 diabetes with or without previous stroke: results from PROactive (PROspective pioglitAzone Clinical Trial In macroVascular Events 04)." *Stroke* 38, no. 3 (2007): 865-873.

[52] Loke, Yoon K., Sonal Singh, and Curt D. Furberg. "Long-term use of thiazolidinediones and fractures in type 2 diabetes: a meta-analysis." *CMAJ* 180, no. 1 (2009): 32-39.

[53] Holst, J. J. "Glucagon-like peptide-1: from extract to agent. The Claude Bernard Lecture, 2005." *Diabetologia* 49, no. 2 (2006): 253-260.

[54] Drucker, Daniel J. "The role of gut hormones in glucose homeostasis." *The Journal of clinical investigation* 117, no. 1 (2007): 24-32.

[55] Nauck, M. K., F. Stöckmann, R. Ebert, and W. Creutzfeldt. "Reduced incretin effect in type 2 (non-insulin-dependent) diabetes." *Diabetologia* 29, no. 1 (1986): 46-52.

[56] Deacon, Carolyn F. "Therapeutic strategies based on glucagon-like peptide 1." *Diabetes* 53, no. 9 (2004): 2181-2189.

[57] Gorrell, Mark D. "Dipeptidyl peptidase IV and related enzymes in cell biology and liver disorders." *Clinical Science* 108, no. 4 (2005): 277-292.

[58] Flatt, Peter R., Clifford J. Bailey, and Brian D. Green. "Dipeptidyl peptidase IV (DPP IV) and related molecules in type 2 diabetes." *Frontiers in Bioscience-Landmark* 13, no. 10 (2008): 3648-3660.

[59] Flatt, P. R., C. J. Bailey, and B. D. Green. "Recent advances in antidiabetic drug therapies targeting the enteroinsular axis." *Current drug metabolism* 10, no. 2 (2009): 125-137.

[60] Amori, Renee E., Joseph Lau, and Anastassios G. Pittas. "Efficacy and safety of incretin therapy in type 2 diabetes: systematic review and meta-analysis." *JAMA* 298, no. 2 (2007): 194-206.

[61] Nauck, M. A. "Sitagliptin Study 024 Group. Efficacy and safety of the dipeptidyl peptidase-4 inhibitor, sitagliptin, compared with the sulfonylurea, glipizide, in patients with type 2 diabetes inadequately controlled on metformin alone: a randomized, double-blind, non-inferiority trial." *Diabetes Obes Metab* 9 (2007): 194-205.

[62] Croxtall, Jamie D., and Susan J. Keam. "Vildagliptin." *Drugs* 68, no. 16 (2008): 2387-2409.

[63] Lebovitz, H. E. "α-Glucosidase inhibitors as agents in the treatment of diabetes." *Diabetes Rev* 6 (1998): 132-145.

[64] Chiasson, Jean-Louis, Robert G. Josse, Ramon Gomis, Markolf Hanefeld, Avraham Karasik, Markku Laakso, and STOP-NIDDM Trial Research Group. "Acarbose for prevention of type 2 diabetes mellitus: the STOP-NIDDM randomised trial." *The Lancet* 359, no. 9323 (2002): 2072-2077.

[65] Holman, Rury R., Carole A. Cull, and Robert C. Turner. "A randomized double-blind trial of acarbose in type 2 diabetes shows improved glycemic control over 3 years (UK Prospective Diabetes Study 44)." *Diabetes care* 22, no. 6 (1999): 960-964.

[66] Chiasson, Jean-Louis, Robert G. Josse, Ramon Gomis, Markolf Hanefeld, Avraham Karasik, Markku Laakso, STOP-NIDDM Trial Research Group, and STOP-NIDDM Trial Research Group. "Acarbose treatment and the risk of cardiovascular disease and hypertension in patients with impaired glucose tolerance: the STOP-NIDDM trial." *JAMA* 290, no. 4 (2003): 486-494.

[67] Bailey, C. J., and C. Day. "Fixed-dose single tablet antidiabetic combinations." *Diabetes, Obesity and Metabolism* 11, no. 6 (2009): 527-533.

[68] Zhang, Qian, Jingtao Dou, and Juming Lu. "Combinational therapy with metformin and sodium-glucose cotransporter inhibitors in management of type 2 diabetes: systematic review and meta-analyses." *Diabetes research and clinical practice* 105, no. 3 (2014): 313-321.

[69] Zhang, Hui-Hui, and Xiu-Li Guo. "Combinational strategies of metformin and chemotherapy in cancers." *Cancer chemotherapy and pharmacology* 78, no. 1 (2016): 13-26.

[70] Pareek, Anil, Nitin Chandurkar, Nihal Thomas, Vijay Viswanathan, Alaka Deshpande, O. P. Gupta, Asha Shah, Arjun Kakrani, Sudhir Bhandari, N. K. Thulasidharan, Banshi Saboo, Shashidhar Devaramani, N. B. Vijaykumar, Shrikant Sharma, Navneet Agrawal,M. Mahesh & Kunal Kothari. "Efficacy and safety of hydroxychloroquine in the treatment of type 2 diabetes mellitus: a double blind, randomized comparison with pioglitazone." *Current medical research and opinion* 30, no. 7 (2014): 1257-1266.

[71] Kalra, Sanjay. "Sodium glucose co-transporter-2 (SGLT2) inhibitors: a review of their basic and clinical pharmacology." *Diabetes Therapy* 5, no. 2 (2014): 355-366.

[72] Neal, Bruce, Vlado Perkovic, Kenneth W. Mahaffey, Dick De Zeeuw, Greg Fulcher, Ngozi Erondu, Wayne Shaw, Gordon Law, Mehul Desai, and David R. Matthews. "Canagliflozin and cardiovascular and renal events in type 2 diabetes." *New England Journal of Medicine* 377, no. 7 (2017): 644-657.

[73] Perkovic, Vlado, Meg J. Jardine, Bruce Neal, Severine Bompoint, Hiddo JL Heerspink, David M. Charytan, Robert Edwards, Rajiv Agarwal, George Bakris, Scott Bull, Christopher P. Cannon, George Capuano. "Canagliflozin and renal outcomes in type 2 diabetes and nephropathy." *New England Journal of Medicine* 380, no. 24 (2019): 2295-2306.

[74] Wiviott, Stephen D., Itamar Raz, Marc P. Bonaca, Ofri Mosenzon, Eri T. Kato, Avivit Cahn, Michael G. Silverman, Thomas A. Zelniker, Julia F. Kuder, Sabina A. Murphy, Deepak L. Bhatt, Lawrence A. Leiter. "Dapagliflozin and cardiovascular outcomes in type 2 diabetes." *New England Journal of Medicine* 380, no. 4 (2019): 347-357.

[75] Plosker, Greg L. "Dapagliflozin." *Drugs* 72, no. 17 (2012): 2289-2312.

[76] Luo, Shuqin, Albert H. Meier, and Anthony H. Cincotta. "Bromocriptine reduces obesity, glucose intolerance and extracellular monoamine metabolite levels in the ventromedial hypothalamus of Syrian hamsters." *Neuroendocrinology* 68, no. 1 (1998): 1-10.

[77] Cincotta, Anthony H., Shuqin Luo, Ying Zhang, Yin Liang, Keshavan G. Bina, Thomas L. Jetton, and Piotr WD Scislowski. "Chronic infusion of norepinephrine into the VMH of normal rats induces the obese glucose-intolerant state." *American Journal of Physiology-Regulatory, Integrative and Comparative Physiology* 278, no. 2 (2000): R435-R444.

[78] Moore, Katherine G., Kayce Shealy, and Jennifer N. Clements. "Liraglutide, GLP-1 receptor agonist, for chronic weight loss." *Expert Review of Endocrinology & Metabolism* 11, no. 5 (2016): 373-378.

[79] Nordisk, Novo. “Victoza (liraglutide injection), prescribing information.” Retrived from https://www.accessdata.fda.gov/drugsatfda_docs/label/2010/022341lbl.pdf (2010).

[80] Kushner, Robert F., Caroline M. Apovian, and Ken Fujioka. “Obesity consults—comprehensive obesity management in 2013: Understanding the shifting paradigm.” *Obesity* 21 (2013): S1-S15.

[81] Gadde, Kishore M., David B. Allison, Donna H. Ryan, Craig A. Peterson, Barbara Troupin, Michael L. Schwiers, and Wesley W. Day. “Effects of low-dose, controlled-release, phentermine plus topiramate combination on weight and associated comorbidities in overweight and obese adults (CONQUER): a randomised, placebo-controlled, phase 3 trial.” *The Lancet* 377, no. 9774 (2011): 1341-1352.

[82] Jordan, Jens, Arne Astrup, Stefan Engeli, Krzysztof Narkiewicz, Wesley W. Day, and Nick Finer. “Cardiovascular effects of phentermine and topiramate: a new drug combination for the treatment of obesity.” *Journal of hypertension* 32, no. 6 (2014): 1178.

Chapter 7

Molecular Targets and the Mechanisms of Antidiabetic Agents

Sumit Roy
Archita Dutta
Paranjeet Kaur
Manish Vyas
and Sanjeev Kumar Sahu*
School of Pharmaceutical Sciences, Lovely Professional University, Phagwara (Punjab), India

Abstract

Diabetes is a significant health issue that affects people all over the world. Chronically high blood glucose levels cause it because of the pancreas' beta cells' inability to produce enough insulin or the cells' inefficient insulin use. Various mechanisms exist through which existing antidiabetic drugs treat and control diabetic conditions. Several antidiabetic agents have been reported; however, designing newer potent chemical compounds is based on different molecular targets. This chapter summarizes all the possible molecular targets with their detailed study for developing antidiabetic drugs.

Keywords: diabetes mellitus, molecular targets, antidiabetic agents

---

*Corresponding Author's Email: sanjeevsahu82@yahoo.co.in.

In: Management of Diabetes Mellitus Based on Natural Products
Editors: Yachana Mishra and Vijay Mishra
ISBN: 979-8-88697-853-7

1. Introduction

Humans obtain energy from three fuel molecules: carbohydrates, lipids, and proteins. Blood glucose (carbohydrates) is the primary source of energy. Diabetes is a long-lasting (chronic) disease that occurs when blood glucose, or blood sugar, is too high. When the amount of blood glucose increases (e.g., after a meal), it triggers the release of the insulin hormone from the Beta cells of the pancreas. Insulin stimulates body cells to remove glucose from the blood (cellular glucose uptake), causing blood sugar to decrease to normal levels [1].

In diabetes, the body does not make enough insulin or does not use insulin well. Glucose then stays in the blood and does not reach body cells. Hyperglycemia is a condition where the sugar (glucose) level in the blood is too high than the normal range. Hypoglycemia is when the blood sugar (glucose) level is lower than normal. The most common forms of diabetes are type 1 diabetes (T1DM) (5%), which is an autoimmune disorder, and type 2 diabetes (T2DM) (95%), which is associated with obesity. Gestational diabetes (GD) is a form of diabetes that occurs in pregnancy, and other forms of diabetes are sporadic and are caused by a single gene mutation [2].

Effective diabetes therapy remains a major challenge despite significant improvements in contemporary medicine and successful potential therapeutic techniques. Many other measures were explored to improve insulin's impact on its target tissues, and searches were conducted for potential lead compounds that could improve insulin production by beta-cells. Researchers from several disciplines are assessing natural and synthetic derivatives on a variety of novel protein targets, including the essential therapeutic targets to obtain convenient strategies to treat diabetes [3, 4].

2. Molecular Targets for Different Antidiabetic Agents

Various antidiabetic agents are available in the market that target multiple receptors. Fewer compounds with antidiabetic activity have been identified (Figure 1). Their development toward clinical utility is being assessed in various stages of clinical studies. Different side effects associated with their

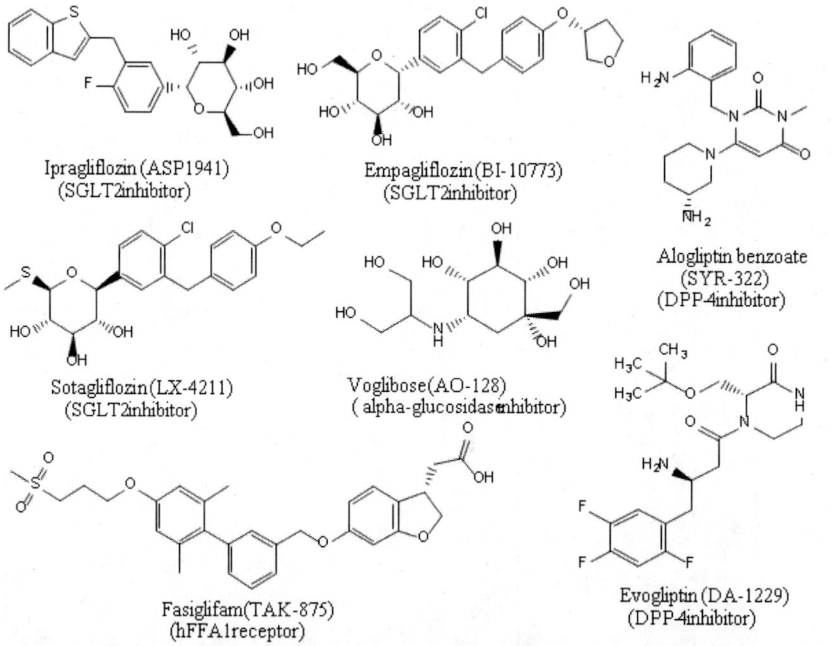

Figure 1. Small molecules as clinical candidates for Type II diabetes mellitus (T2DM) therapy.

uses (Table 1) necessitate the development of new powerful antidiabetic medicines with improved pharmacological profiles [5].

An immediate and massive effort is required to enhance diabetes prevention and treatment. In the case of diabetes and its numerous associated disorders, preventing disease progression is more important than managing symptoms. Antidiabetic medications now have unfavorable side effects and only target specific types of biomolecules. As a result, a substantial study is required to find novel disease mechanisms and molecular targets (Table 2) that could be used to treat diabetes effectively [6, 7].

Table 1. Currently available antidiabetic agents, along with their mechanism and associated sides effects

Drug/Treatment	Generic name/Chemical structure	Mechanism of action	Adverse effects
TYPE I DIABETES MELLITUS			
Insulin therapy Amylin	Insulin Pramlinitide	Improves glycemic management by modifying the rate of stomach emptying, preventing the rise in glucagon levels after meals, and heightening feelings of satiety. Stimulates the phosphorylation of insulin receptors.	Very rare but can cause allergic reactions, Nausea, appetite loss, fatigue, stomach cramps
TYPE II DIABETES MELLITUS			
Sulfonylureas	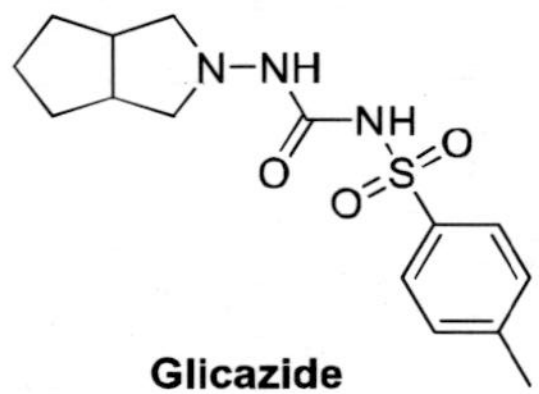 **Glicazide** 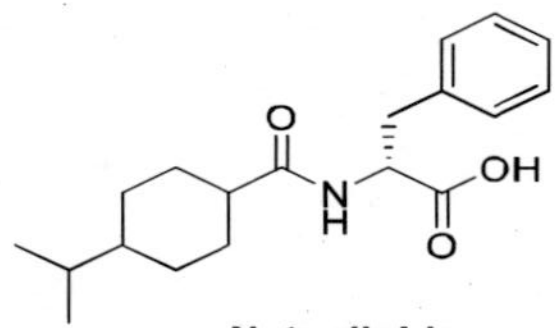 **Nateglinide**	Stimulate the pancreas to produce more insulin	Hypoglycemia (low blood sugar)

Drug/Treatment	Generic name/Chemical structure	Mechanism of action	Adverse effects
	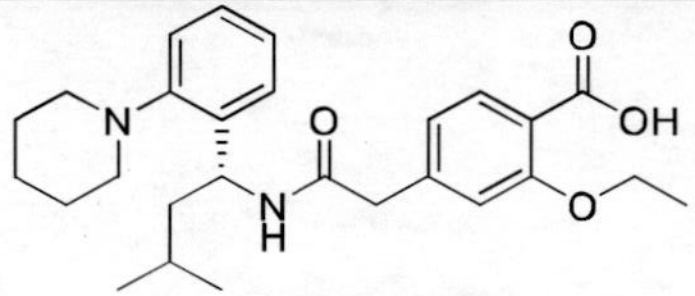 Repaglinide		
Meglitinide	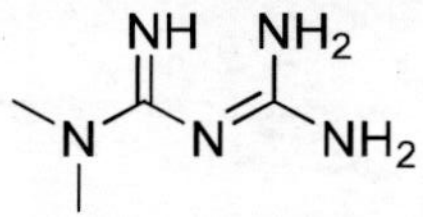 Metformin	Stimulate the pancreas to produce more insulin	Hypoglycemia
Biguanides	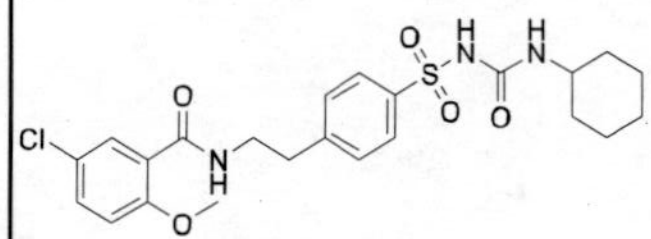 Glyburide 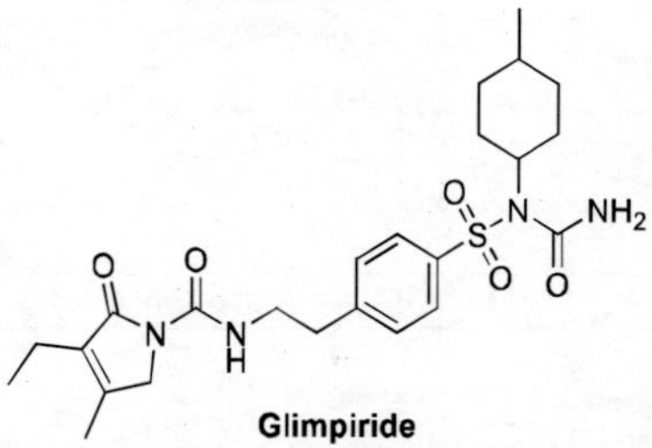 Glimpiride	Reduce the liver's ability to produce glucose, increase the body cells' sensitivity to insulin, and decrease the liver's synthesis of glucose	Diarrhea, nausea, metallic aftertaste, swelling due to water retention

Table 1. (Continued)

Drug/Treatment	**Generic name/Chemical structure**	**Mechanism of action**	**Adverse effects**
Thiazolidinediones (TZD)	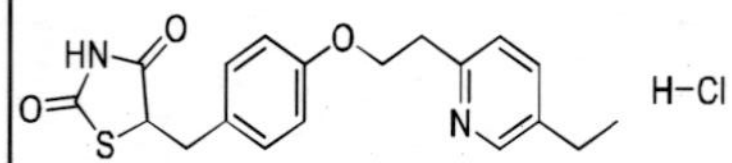 Pioglitazone 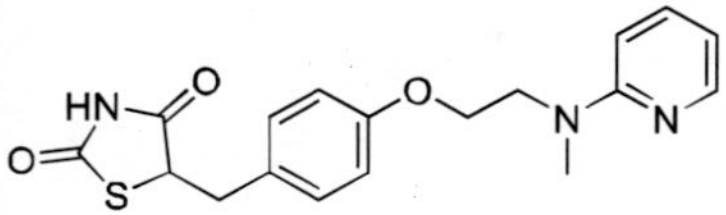 Rosiglitazone	Reduce insulin resistance and Increase glucose utilization	Weight gain, Pioglitazone- raises the chance of a nonfatal heart attack
Alpha-glucosidase inhibitors	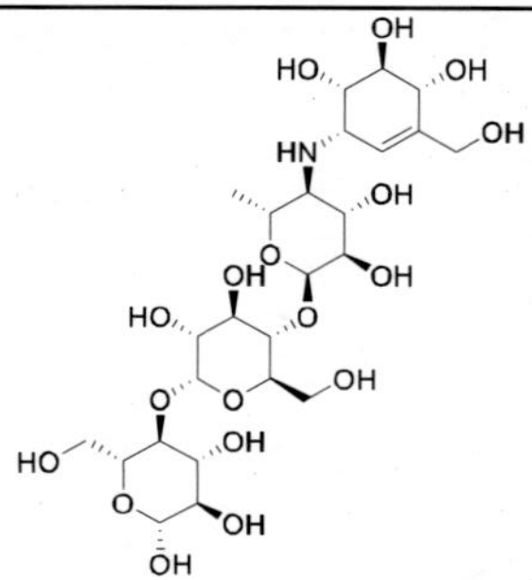 Acarbose	Reduce the rate of absorption for ingested carbohydrates (sugars)	Bloating and flatulence

Drug/Treatment	Generic name/Chemical structure	Mechanism of action	Adverse effects
Dipeptidyl-peptidase-4 (DPP-4) inhibitors	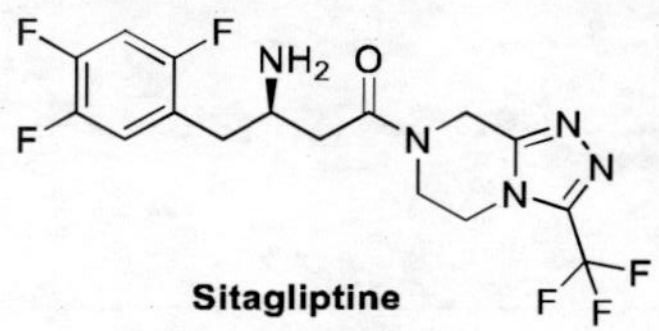 **Sitagliptine** 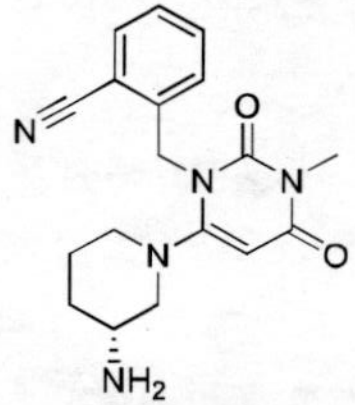 **Alogliptine** 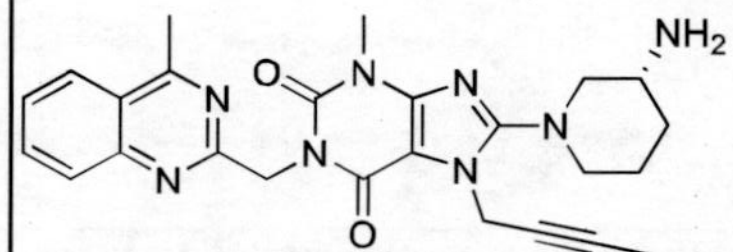 **Linagliptin**	Prolong endogenous GLP-1 action	Pharyngitis, headache

Table 1. (Continued)

Drug/Treatment	Generic name/Chemical structure	Mechanism of action	Adverse effects
Glucagon-like peptide-1(GLP-1) agonist	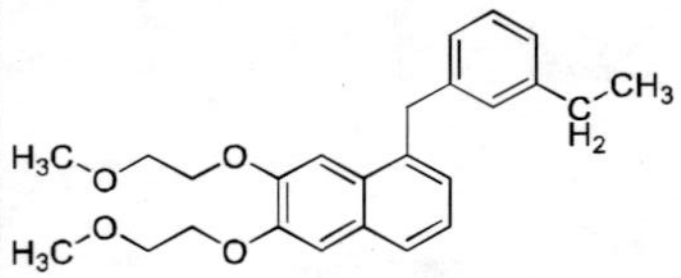 Exenatide 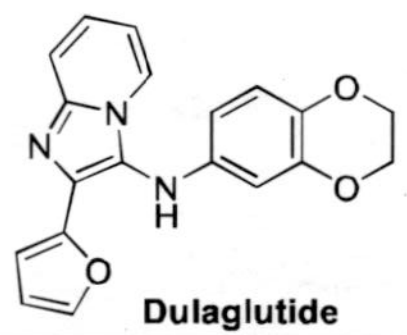 Dulaglutide	Imitate the effects of specific intestinal hormones (incretins) involved in blood sugar control	Nausea, diarrhea, vomiting
Sodium-glucose Cotransporter-2 (SGLT2) inhibitors	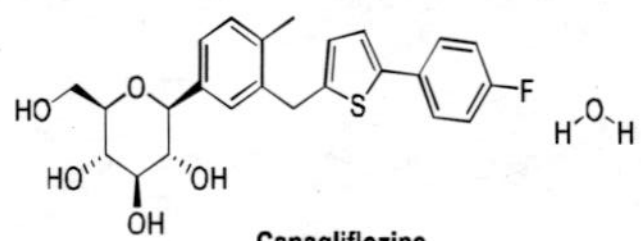 Canagliflozine	Aids in removing glucose from the urine	Genital and urinary tract infections, increased urination

Drug/Treatment	Generic name/Chemical structure	Mechanism of action	Adverse effects
	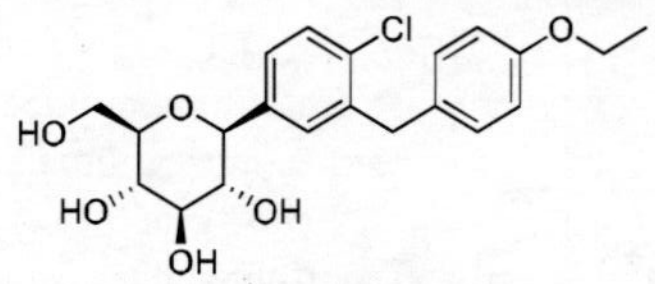 Dapagliflozine 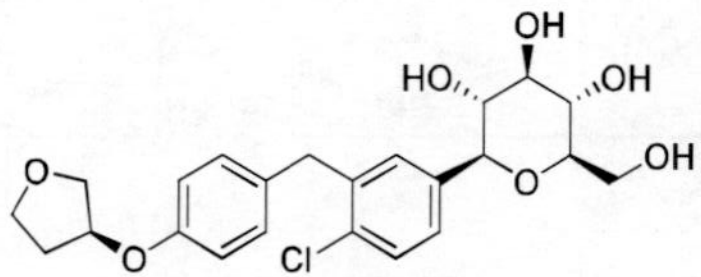 Empagliflozine		
Amylin agonists	Pramlintide	Slow gastric emptying, reduce glucagon	Nausea, vomiting, loss of appetite, or headache
Adipokines	Visfatin	Increase insulin secretion	Anxiety, burning and pain while urinating, chest pain or discomfort, decreased ability to exercise

Table 2. Different molecular targets for diabetes with their mechanism of action and example

Molecular Targets	Definition	Mechanism of action	Marketed drugs	Drugs in clinical trial
Protein Tyrosine Phosphatase 1B (PTP 1B)	Protein tyrosine phosphatase 1B (PTP 1B) is a viable therapeutic target for type II diabetes and obesity due to its crucial function as a negative modulator in insulin and leptin signaling pathways [8].	They enhance Insulin sensitivity [9].	Norathyriol 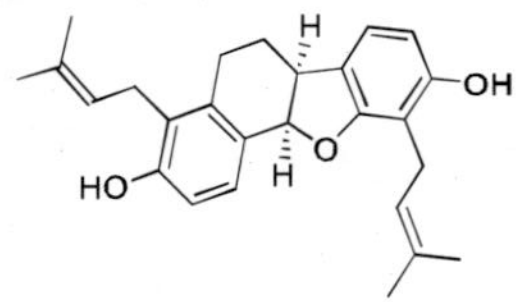 Erybraedin A	MSI-1436 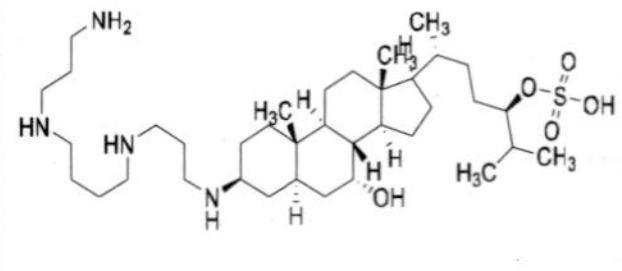
Dipeptidyl pepetidase-4-(DPP-4)	DPP IV inhibitors fall under the category of type 2 diabetes medications known as incretin-based drugs. The incretin hormones glucagon-like peptide 1 (GLP-1s) and glucose-dependent insulinotropic polypeptide are rapidly cleaved by the enzyme DPP IV (GIP) [10].	To manage hypoglycemia by stimulating the secretion of insulin [11].	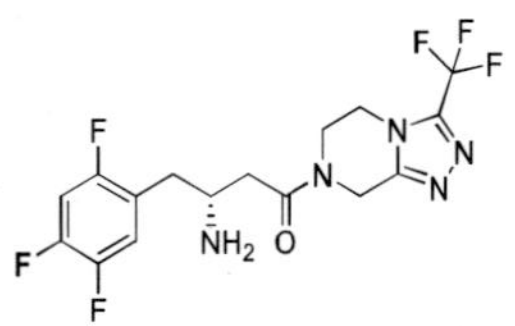 Sitagliptin	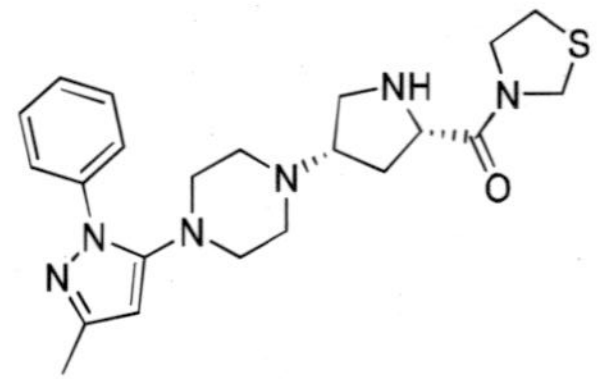 Teneligliptin (MP-513)

Molecular Targets	Definition	Mechanism of action	Marketed drugs	Drugs in clinical trial
Free fatty acid Receptors-1(FFAR1)	Free fatty acids are essential nutrients that provide energy and act as signaling molecules in several cellular processes, including the secretion of the hormone insulin [12].	FFAs activate GPR40, which increases glucose-stimulated insulin release from pancreatic cells	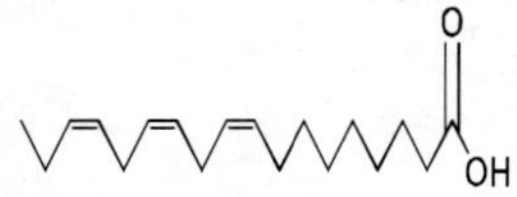 α Linolenic acid	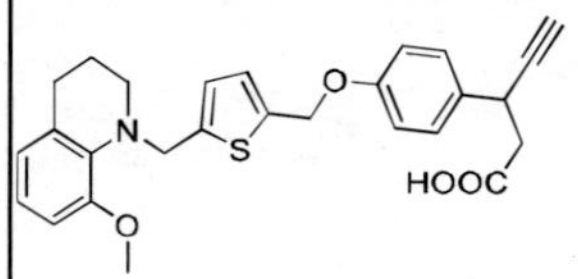 LY2922470
G protein-coupled receptors (GPCR)	GPCRs are a diverse class of plasma membrane receptors that take a role in cell signaling by binding to a range of external ligands [13].	Regulate glucose homeostasis [14].	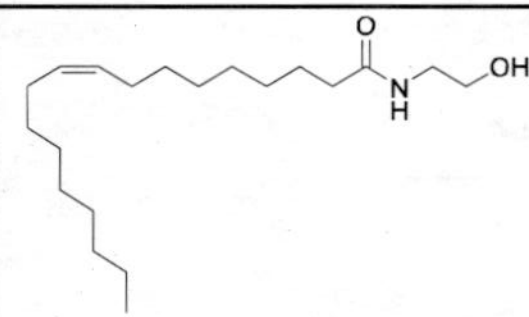 Oleoylethanolamide 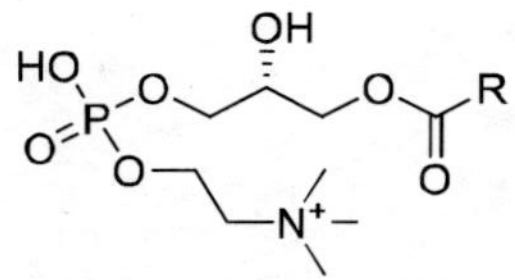 Lysophosphatidylcholine	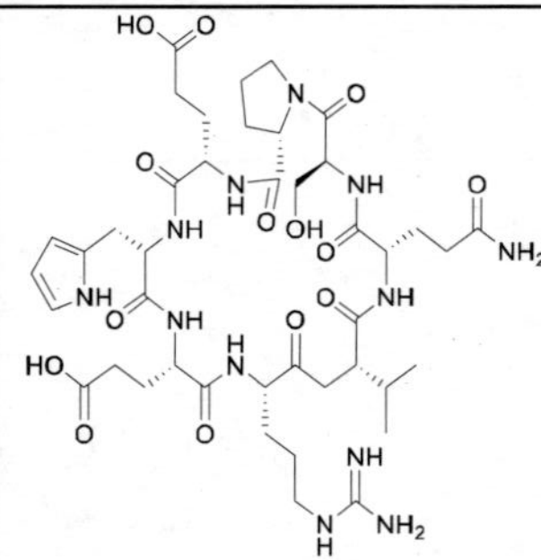 Ghrelin (azp-531)

Table 2. (Continued)

Molecular Targets	Definition	Mechanism of action	Marketed drugs	Drugs in clinical trial
Peroxisome Proliferative Activated Receptor-γ (PPAR- γ)	PPAR-nuclear receptors produce ligand-activated transcription factors, which regulate crucial metabolic processes [15].	Regulate glucose and lipid homeostasis [16].	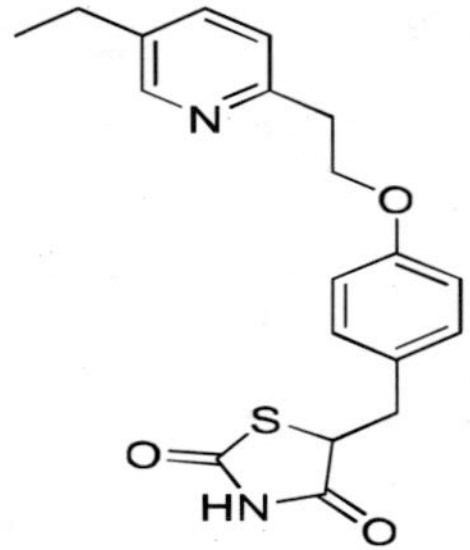 Pioglitazone	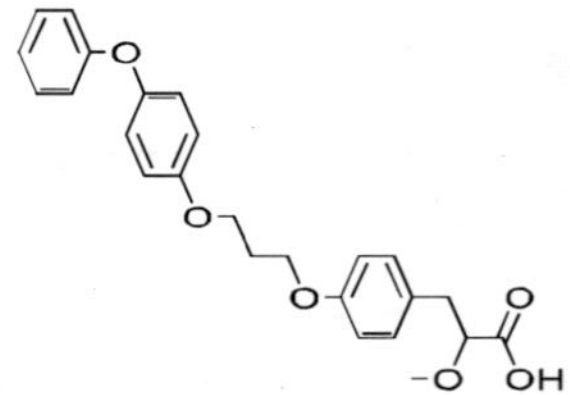 Naveglitazar
α-glucosidase inhibitors	Alpha-glucosidase inhibitors are saccharides that work as competitive inhibitors of the alpha-glucosidase enzymes in the brush border of the small intestine, which are necessary for carbohydrate digestion [17].	Glucose absorption from the intestines is inhibited [18].	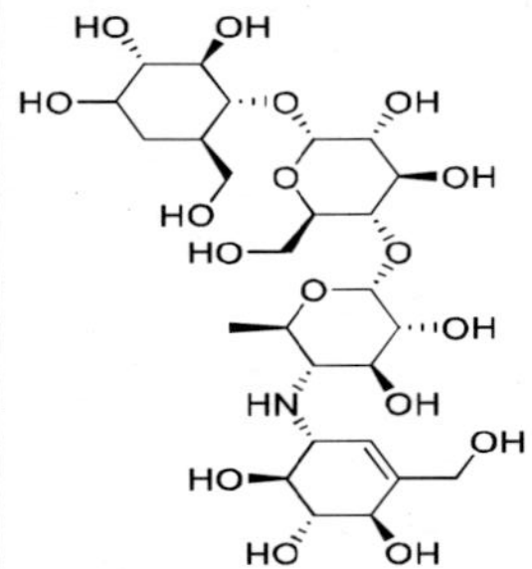 Acarbose	---

Molecular Targets	Definition	Mechanism of action	Marketed drugs	Drugs in clinical trial
			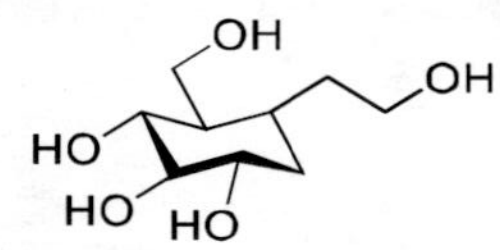 Miglitol	
Glycogen Phosphorylase Inhibitors	The muscles and the rest of the body are fueled by Glucose-1-phosphate, created by the enzyme glycogen phosphorylase (GP). The activation and inactivation of the enzyme are guaranteed by the binding of diverse ligands to catalytic or allosteric sites [19].	Lowering blood sugar levels [20].	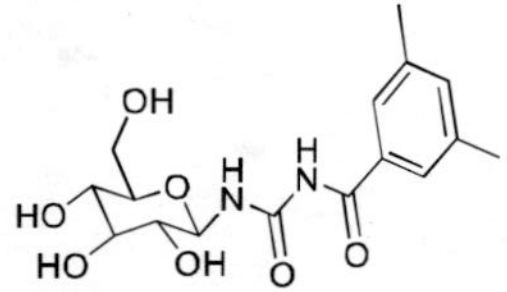 N-(3,5-Dimethyl-benzoyl)-N-(β-D-Glycopyranosyl) urea	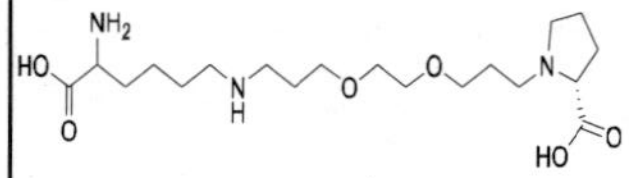 Efpeglenatide
Fructose-1,6-Biphosphatase inhibitors (FBPase)	Fructose-1,6-bisphosphatase (FBPase) inhibitors have the potential to address an unmet medical need by decreasing gluconeogenesis-mediated glucose overproduction [21].	Control the production of gluconeogenesis [22].	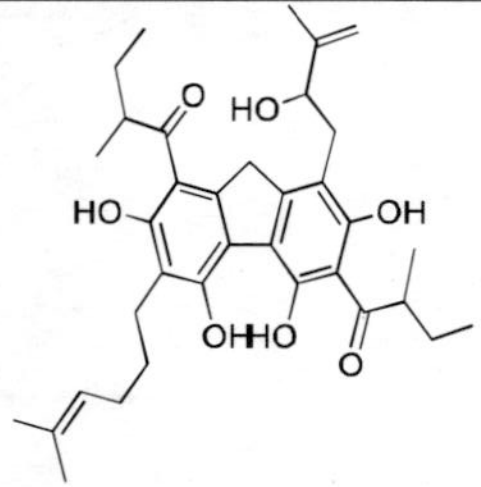 Achyrofuran	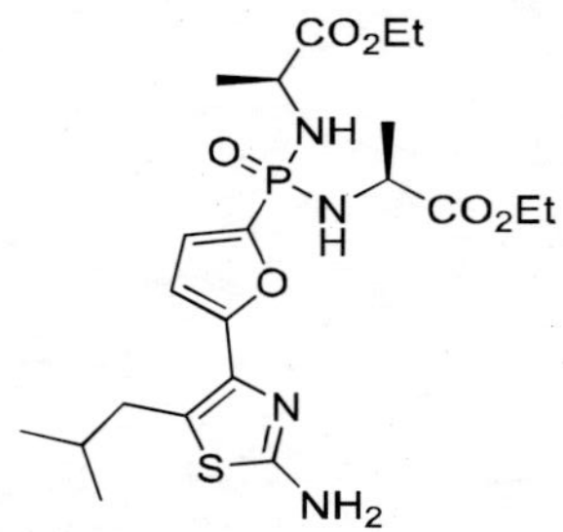 CS-917

Table 2. (Continued)

Molecular Targets	Definition	Mechanism of action	Marketed drugs	Drugs in clinical trial
Glucagon receptor inhibitor (GCGr)	Glucagon is a pancreatic hormone released into the bloodstream by the islet of Langerhans' alpha cells [23].	Increases hepatic glucose synthesis via inducing gluconeogenesis and glycogenolysis in hepatocytes [24].	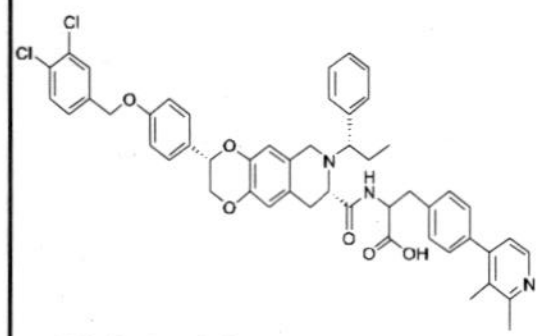 Albiglutide	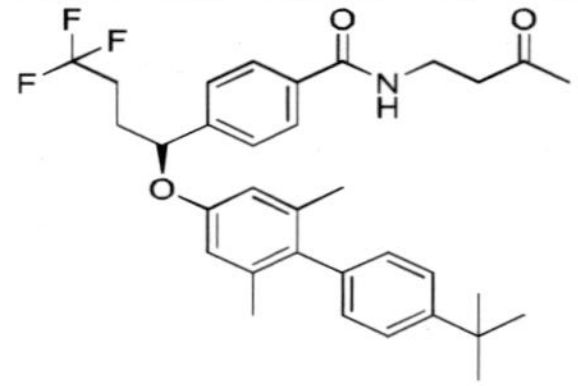 LY2409021
Phospho-enol pyruvate Carboxykinase (PEPCK)	The rate-controlling enzyme in gluconeogenesis is phospho-enol pyruvate carboxykinase (PEPCK). PEPCK inhibition in the liver [25].	Regulate gluconeogenesis in the liver	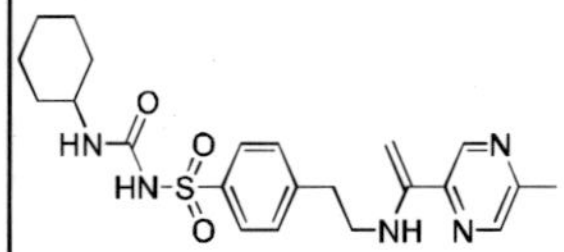 Glipizide	--
Sodium glucose-transporters	A set of membrane proteins known as SGLTs move various substances, including glucose, amino acids, vitamins, ions, and osmolytes, through the brush-border membrane of the proximal renal tubules and the intestinal epithelium [26].	Reduce hyperglycemia by lowering the renal glucose threshold and boosting glucose excretion in urine [27].	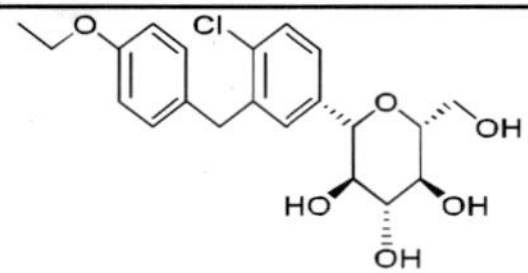 Dabagliflozin	--

Molecular Targets	Definition	Mechanism of action	Marketed drugs	Drugs in clinical trial
			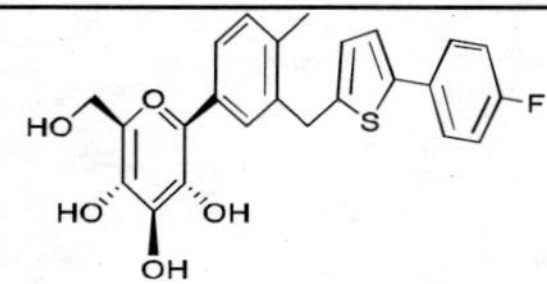 Canagliflozin 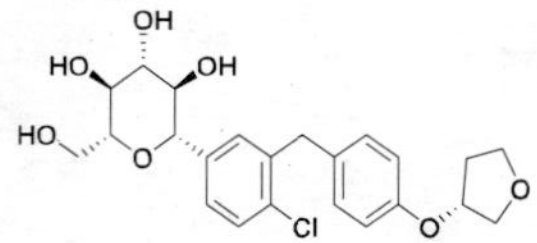 Empagliflozin	
Alpha amylase inhibitors	The 512 amino acids in a single oligosaccharide chain of the calcium-containing enzyme alpha-amylase give it a molecular weight of 57.6 kDa [28].	Lower postprandial blood glucose levels [29].	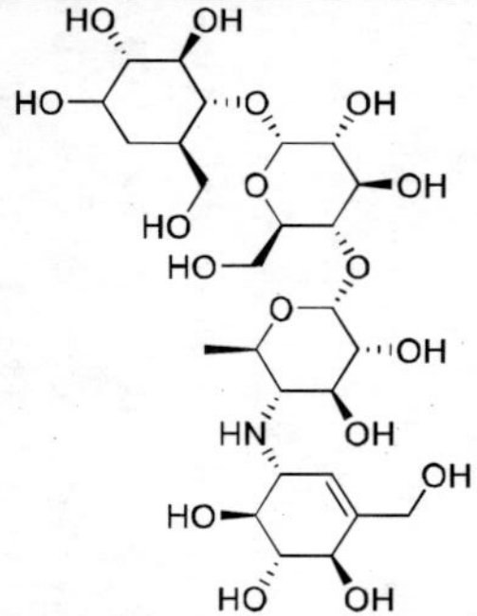 Acarbose	--

2.1. Glucagon-Like Peptide-1

Incretins are hormones that are released after meals and stimulate insulin secretion. GLP-1 is an effective incretin, and the GLP-1 signaling system is a successful drug target used for T2DM (Figure 2). GLP-1 is pre-proglucagon derivative. This hormone generally enhances insulin and interacts with the production of glucagon [30]. It also slows down gastric emptying. GLP-1 receptor agonists used as incretin mimetics include Albiglutide, Exenatide, and Lixisenatide. α cells of islets cleave proglucagon into glucagon and a large C-terminal peptide that includes GLP-1 and GLP-2 [31]. Intestinal L cells and specific hindbrain neurons process proglucagon into a large N-terminal peptide that provides glucagon or GLP-1 and GLP-2 (GLP-2 is not an insulinotropic hormone). This peptide shows incretin activity, which causes the glucose-dependent secretion of insulin. Proper blood glucose and restoration of insulin secretion can be done via giving GLP-1 at their 1st stage and can be considered essential for treating T2DM.

2.1.1. Albiglutide

Albiglutide is an agonist of the GLP-1 receptor, which is given to broaden glucose-dependent insulin release. It causes gastric elimination. It is a dipeptidyl peptidase-4 glucagon-like peptide-1 dimer. Adverse drug effects of albiglutide are hypoglycaemia, thyroid C-Cell carcinoma, acute pancreatitis, and hypersensitivity responses.

2.1.2 Exenatide

Exenatide is a known GLP-1R agonist. It is a 39-amino-destructive peptide. The initial phase of insulin release and suppression of glucagon is enhanced by administering Exenatide. Adverse drug effects associated with exenatide are hypoglycemia, increased risk of thyroid C-Cell carcinoma, and renal weakness.

2.2. Sodium-Glucose Co-Transporter 2 Inhibitors

SGLT2 inside PCT is responsible for the reabsorption of glucose. SGLT2i acts by blocking SGLT2 inside PCT, and as a result, glucose discharging occurs, improving glycemic controls. It depends on blood glucose levels. SGLT2 inhibitors cause a reduction in renal tubular glucose reabsorption, resulting in glucosuria, which will decrease glucose levels in the blood (Figure 3). They do not stimulate insulin release. GLUT is a uniporter that transports glucose, and SGLTs is a symporter that transports glucose and sodium [32]. SGLT2 inhibitor controls the glucose level in T2DM patients. SGLT2i also helps in decreasing weight because of glycosuria. SGLT2 inhibitors include Canagliflozin, Dapagliflozin, Luseogliflozin, Empagliflozin, Ipragliflozin, and Tofogliflozin.

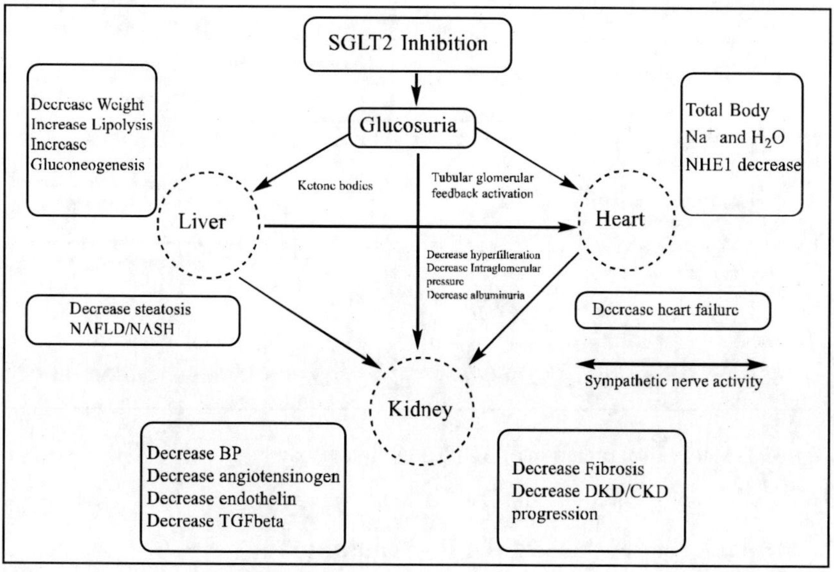

Figure 2. Mechanism of action of SGLT2 inhibitors.

2.2.1. Canagliflozin

It decreases blood glucose levels by reducing the kidney's ability to reabsorb glucose. Canagliflozin is very much tolerated in patients with the hepatic illness. Canagliflozin is contraindicated in patients with severe renal insufficiency.

2.2.2. Dapagliflozin

Dapagliflozin is used by uridine diphosphate-glucuronosyltransferase and converts into dapagliflozin 3-O-glucuronide in the kidneys and liver [33]. It is a specific inhibitor of sodium-glucose cotransporter-2. Dapagliflozin used alone or in combination with other antidiabetic drugs causes a reduction in HbA1c levels by 0.5-1.0% but does not cause hypoglycaemia. Weight loss is seen in patients with improper calorie intake. They are contraindicated in patients with renal insufficiency.

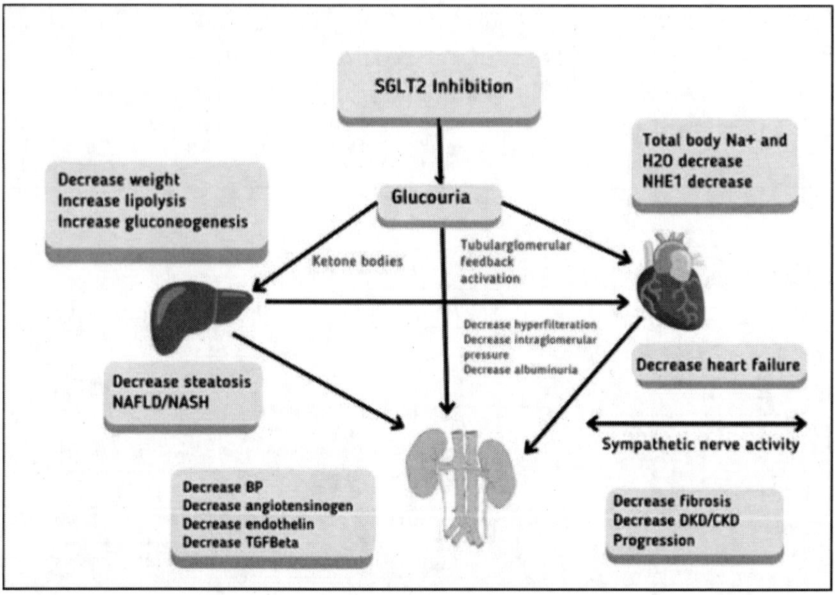

Figure 3. Mechanism of action of SGLT2 inhibitors.

2.3. Dipeptidyl Peptidase 4 [DPP-4] Inhibitors

In individuals with T2DM, Dipeptidyl peptidase-4 (DPP-4) inhibitors are used with diet and exercise to reduce blood sugar levels (Figure 4). T2DM, if left untreated, can cause significant issues like blindness, kidney and nerve damage, and heart disease [34]. The incretin hormones glucagon-like peptide-1 (GLP-1) and gastric inhibitory peptide (GIP), which increase insulin secretion and decrease glucagon secretion to maintain glucose homeostasis, are primarily affected by the ubiquitous enzyme DPP-4.

2.3.1. Sitagliptin

In 2006, Sitagliptin was first released as a competitive and selective DPP-4 inhibitor that increased postprandial insulin release, decreased glucagon levels, and lowered both mealtime and fasting blood glucose levels in T2DM [35]. There has been no noticeable impact on appetite or stomach emptying. Because GLP-1 induces little insulin release at normal plasma glucose levels, it carries a modest risk of hypoglycemia unless taken with SUs or insulin. One meta-analysis indicated that Sitagliptin reduced fasting blood glucose levels more than Vildagliptin did, even though the therapeutic efficacy of all DPP-4 inhibitors is comparable. Although nausea may occur with Sitagliptin, it is not as noticeable as with GLP-1 agonists. Sitagliptin is well tolerated. It is body-weight neutral and doesn't lead to weight loss. Some adverse effects include oedema, angioedema, exfoliative dermatitis, loose stools, headaches, rashes, and allergic responses.

2.3.2. Vildagliptin

This DPP-4 inhibitor forms a covalent bond with the enzyme. Even after the free drug has been eliminated from circulation, the complex dissociates very slowly, causing chronic DPP-4 inhibition. This explains that despite the short plasma t1/2, the action lasts the longest (12–24 hours) (2-4 hours) [36]. Only 20–25% of the substance is eliminated mainly by hepatic metabolism; the remainder is excreted in the urine. A dose decrease is recommended in moderately severe liver and renal disease. When type 2 diabetic patients take an increased dose of vildagliptin before a 75 g oral glucose tolerance test, their plasma insulin levels rise significantly. Vildagliptin restores insulin release in response to oral and intravenous glucose elevations, with no change in the effect of incretins.

2.3.3. Saxagliptin

Saxagliptin, a dipeptidyl peptidase-4 inhibitor, is used to help people with T2DM improve their glycaemia switch. Saxagliptin is administered to improve glycemic control, causing significant decreases in postprandial and blood plasma glucose levels. It exhibits clinically neutral implications for cardiovascular strain, weight gain, and phospholipid planes.

2.3.4. Teneligliptin

A brand-new DPP-4 inhibitor called teneligliptin has long-lasting DPP-4 inhibition and hypoglycaemic effects. Postprandial hyperglycemia is suppressed at all three meals of the day after a single morning dosage. Teneligliptin is given orally to adults once daily at 20 mg, increasing to 40 mg daily. Patients with renal impairment do not need to change their dosage because the metabolites of this medication are excreted through the kidneys and liver. Comparable to other DPP-4 inhibitors currently on the market, teneligliptin has a similar safety profile. Care must be taken when giving teneligliptin to people susceptible to QT prolongation.

2.3.5. Analogliptin

Another invasive inhibitor of DPP-4 is Analogliptin. It is an oral DPP-4 inhibitor and antihyperglycemic medication. Incretin hormone levels, such as glucagon-like peptide and glucose-dependent insulinotropic polypeptide, are increased by inhibiting the breakdown of the enzyme DPP-4 (GIP).

2.3.6 Linagliptin

It can be prescribed to a patient having renal or hepatic illness without any change in dose. Linagliptin acts by refining insulin discharge, lessening the creation of glucagon, easing posteriorly gastric purging, and decreasing hunger. Partiality integrates the absenteeism of life-threatening hypoglycemia and non-bias weight. Those who cannot tolerate Metformin can utilize Linagliptin as a first market for the treatment of diabetes [37].

2.3.7. Dutogliptin

Dutogliptin helps patients with T2DM maintain better glucose control. Dutogliptin is safe and beneficial for hypoglycemia. When compared to other medications in this class, it produces better results. This is a preferred water solvent with low cell absorptivity. Moderate hypoglycemia is one of the adverse effects, and it is eliminated through renal mechanisms.

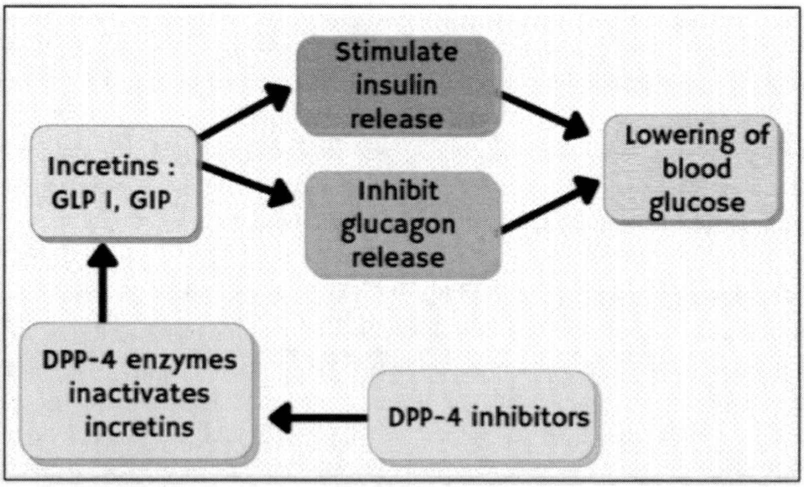

Figure 4. Mechanism of action of DPP-4 inhibitor.

2.4. Protein Tyrosine Phosphatase 1B [PTP1B]

Leptin and insulin signaling pathways are negatively regulated by the protein tyrosine phosphatase 1B (PTP1B) (Figure 5). Deletion of the PTP1B gene in mice demonstrated the crucial roles of PTP1B in diabetes and obesity. It is an illustration of a vast PTP family and has a tiny family of intracellular non-trans-membrane PTPs. PTP1B is registered for illnesses related to diabetes and hyperglycemia. PTP1B impacts various cellular processes, including glucose uptake, elongation, differentiation, apoptosis, cell-to-cell arrest, exterior lattice connections, motility, and invasion. The supplementation of PTP1B is crucial to treating diabetic foot ulcers. When it comes to controlling VEGF-induced angiogenesis, PTP1B has been essential. PTP1B regulates the insulin signaling pathway during insulin production by activating the insulin receptor and its constituents, particularly the receptor substrate proteins [38]. PTP1B dephosphorylates VEGFR2, a fundamental receptor for controlling cell duplication, movement, and cylinder arrangement. This suggests that endothelial cells with high PTP1B levels may aid in related angiogenesis and recovery from diabetic injury.

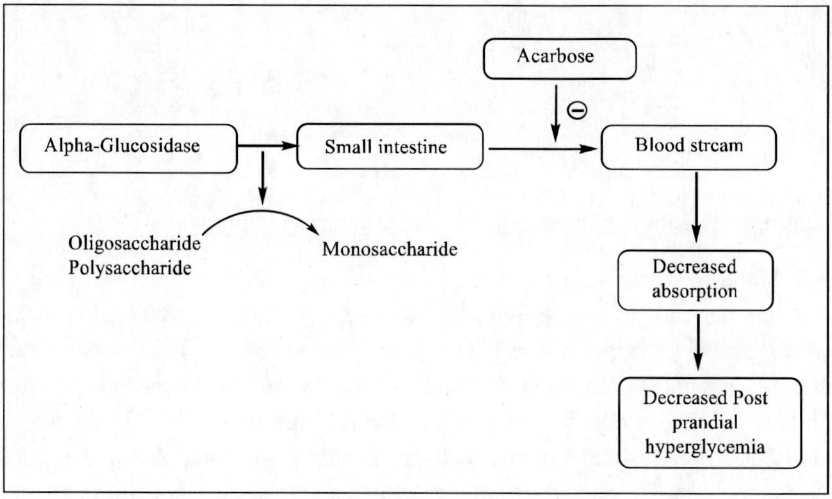

Figure 5. Mechanism of action of alpha glucosidase inhibitors.

2.5. Alpha-Glucosidase Inhibitors

Acarbose, Miglitol, and Voglibose are three common alpha-glucosidase inhibitors (AGIs) used to treat T2DM patients (Figure 6). AGIs considerably impact postprandial blood glucose and insulin levels because they slow down the generation of sugar from the digestive system. Over time, it has been clear that the most efficient way to manage postprandial hyperglycemia and its severity, particularly in T2D diabetes, is to use bioactive-glucosidase inhibitors. Glucosidase inhibitors, which hydrolyses starch, most frequently cause delayed glucose absorption in the digestive tract, which regulates glucosidase following dietary management inhibitors and efficacy [39].

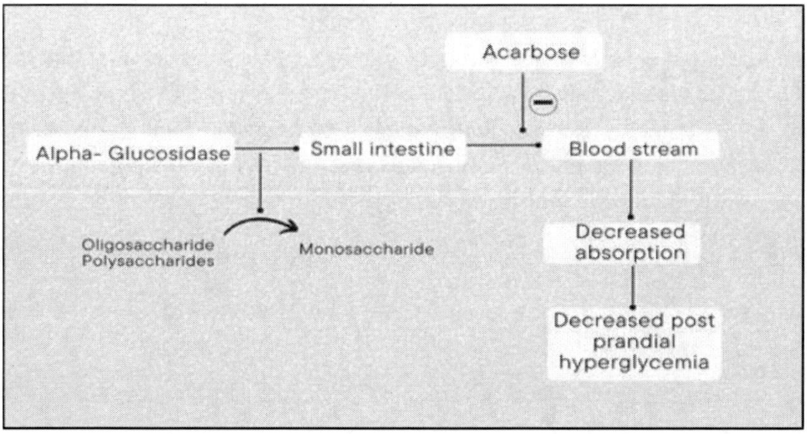

Figure 6. Mechanism of action of alpha-glucosidase inhibitors.

Alpha-glucosidase inhibitors (AGIs) are frequently utilized, particularly in Asian patients, to enable oral antidiabetic medication administration. AGIs are suggested as a second-line T2DM treatment in China if primary metformin therapy maintains reasonable glycemic control. AGIs lower postprandial glucose [PPG] levels by weakening starch digestion, with an increased likelihood of intestinal effects, and are present on the margin of the small digestive tract. A collection of proteins called alpha-glucosidase, which originates in the pancreas, helps convert 80–90% of the starch we eat into glucose. The suppression of these chemicals prevents postprandial hyperglycemia. The activity of intestinal alpha-glucosidases and catalysts in the digestive tract determines how these medicines are made. These are the oligo- and disaccharide-containing hydrolyzed starch molecules that carry glucose to the digestive tract [40]. As monosaccharides like glucose and fructose can be eaten, this hydrolysis is crucial in producing stomach starch. Acarbose, militate, or miglitol inhibit alpha-glucosidases and can reduce and reverse gastrointestinal disorders as well as postprandial hyperglycemia. There have also been reports of benzylidene-quinazolinone hybrid compounds with anti-glucosidase activity in vitro and in vivo against STZ-induced hyperglycaemic rats. Previous studies have identified a group of 2-oxindole derivatives as GSK3 inhibitors with in vivo antihyperglycemic action. However, several compounds of 3,5-disubstituted indolin-2-one were found to have strong α-glucosidase inhibitory activity.

2.6. Peroxisome Proliferator-Activated Receptors (PPARs)

Peroxisome proliferator-activated receptors (PPARs) are nuclear hormone receptor superfamily ligand-activated transcription factors that include the following three subtypes: PPARα, PPARγ, and PPARβ/δ. Triglyceride levels are reduced, and energy balance is regulated when PPAR-α is activated. While PPAR-γ activity increases glucose metabolism and makes the body more sensitive to insulin, PPAR-β/δ activation increases the metabolism of fatty acids. The use of PPARs to treat conditions like diabetes shows promise because they aid in expanding the PPAR that results from insulin inhibition. A few PPAR agonists unrelated to TZD include oxyimino-acidic corrosive helpers, which likewise function as inhibitors of diabetic movement [41]. The three types of PPARs are known as gamma, delta, and omega, respectively. These are useful in treating T2DM and metabolic disorders such as obesity and insulin resistance. Muscles' oxidation of unsaturated fat is linked to PPAR. In order to promote glucose and lipid uptake, boost glucose oxidation, lower levels of free unsaturated fat, and then reduce insulin resistance, PPAR is mainly conveyed in fat. PPAR agonists can also elicit non-hyperglycaemic impressions. Cardiovascular issues cause them, and their severity demonstrate their connection to diabetes mellitus.

Only cardiovascular issues are reduced by PPAR agonists because of diabetes. Since they aid in raising the PPARγ that results from insulin inhibition, PPARs are used to treat disorders like diabetes with great promise. A few PPAR agonists unrelated to TZD include oxyimino-acidic corrosive helpers, which likewise function as inhibitors of diabetic movement [42]. Three forms of PPARs help in treating type 2 diabetes and metabolic disorders such as obesity and insulin resistance. Unsaturated fat oxidation in muscles is connected to PPAR. In particular, PPAR is transmitted in fat to promote glucose and lipid uptake, boost glucose oxidation, lower levels of free unsaturated fat, and then reduce insulin resistance.

2.7. Adipokines

The age-related component of C3a and the selective supplementing mechanism, which work to boost beta cell insulin secretion, are controlled by adipokine (adipsin/supplement factor D) (Figure 7). In contrast to other insulin secretions, regular treatment of adipsin reduces hyperglycemia and raises insulin levels while defending beta cells by avoiding isolation and extinction in diabetic mice. Naturally, adipsin/C3a decreases the activity of the phosphatase Dusp26; Dusp26's restricted selectivity in beta cells lowers beta cell expression and accelerates cell passage. Inhibition of DUSP26 by medication causes animals with diabetes to become hyperglycaemic and shields human islet cells from cell fusion. Regarding human welfare, older persons with high adipsin adherence have a lower risk of subsequently acquiring diabetes after a change in body mass index (BMI) [43]. Targeted medicines for (Adipsin/C3a and DUSP26) may indicate a novel strategy for T2D treatment and prevention success. Although the adipokines visfatin, fetuin-A, resistin, and plasminogen activator inhibitor-1 promote insulin sensitivity, they also play a role in the development of glucose intolerance (PAI-1). Adipsin is one of the adipokines generated by fatty tissue, which is linked to maintaining the homeostasis of adipose tissue and boosting insulin production in response to glucose. As shown by additional research and clinical trials, its use as a biomarker in conjunction with the following DM analytical methods is supported by plasma adipsin concentration being low in animals and humans with DM. Additionally, the preservation of -cell bulk, enhanced -cell tolerance, and maintenance of their writing personality are all effects of adipsin on the development of hyperglycemia [44].

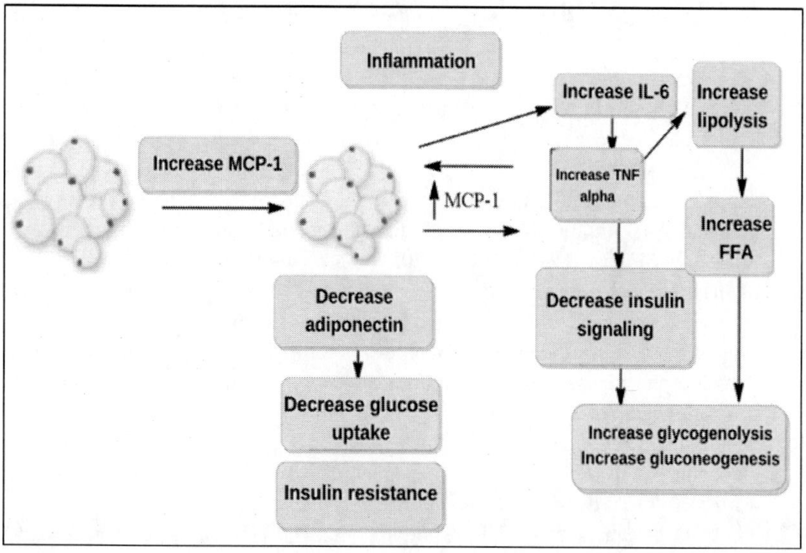

Figure 7. Mechanism of action of adipokines.

Conclusion

All the molecular targets are essential in understanding antidiabetic drugs' mechanisms. Most of the recently used approaches for drug development are based on molecular targets. A novel therapeutic target helps us to design the novel scaffold by considering the commercialized drugs as standards. Further, we can examine their interaction parameters with the proteins to better understand those compounds and their protein associations, forming the strongest framework for developing potent antidiabetic drugs.

References

[1] American Diabetes Association. Diagnosis and classification of diabetes mellitus. *Diabetes care.* 2010;33(Supplement_1): S62-9.

[2] American Diabetes Association. Diagnosis and classification of diabetes mellitus. *Diabetes care*. 2006;29(1):S43.

[3] Tiwari N, Thakur AK, Kumar V, Dey A, Kumar V. Therapeutic targets for diabetes mellitus: an update. *Clin. Pharmacol. Biopharm.* 2014;3(1):1.

[4] Kaur N, Kumar V, Nayak S K, Wadhwa P, Kaur P, Sahu S K. Alpha-amylase as molecular target for treatment of diabetes mellitus: A comprehensive review. *Chemical Biology & Drug Design.* 2021;98(4):539-60.

[5] Kerru N, Singh-Pillay A, Awolade P, Singh P. Current antidiabetic agents and their molecular targets: A review. *European Journal of Medicinal Chemistry.* 2018;152:436-88.

[6] Kaur N, Kumar V, Nayak S K, Wadhwa P, Kaur P, Sahu S K. Alpha-amylase as molecular target for treatment of diabetes mellitus: A comprehensive review. *Chemical Biology & Drug Design.* 2021;98(4):539-60.

[7] Almasi F, Mohammadipanah F. Prominent and emerging antidiabetic molecular targets. *Journal of Drug Targeting.* 2021;29(5):491-506.

[8] Maheshwari N, Karthikeyan C, Trivedi P, Moorthy NH. Recent advances in protein tyrosine phosphatase 1B targeted drug discovery for type II diabetes and obesity. *Current Drug Targets.* 2018;19(5):551-75.

[9] Hussain H, Green I R, Abbas G, Adekenov S M, Hussain W, Ali I. Protein tyrosine phosphatase 1B (PTP1B) inhibitors as potential anti-diabetes agents: patent review (2015-2018). *Expert opinion on therapeutic patents*. 2019;29(9):689-702.

[10] Gallwitz B. Small molecule dipeptidylpeptidase IV inhibitors under investigation for diabetes mellitus therapy. *Expert Opinion on Investigational Drugs*. 2011;20 (6):723-32.

[11] Crepaldi G, Carruba M, Comaschi M, Del Prato S, Frajese G, Paolisso G. Dipeptidyl peptidase 4 (DPP-4) inhibitors and their role in Type 2 diabetes management. *Journal of endocrinological investigation.* 2007;30(7):610-4.

[12] Itoh Y, Kawamata Y, Harada M, Kobayashi M, Fujii R, Fukusumi S, Ogi K, Hosoya M, Tanaka Y, Uejima H, Tanaka H. Free fatty acids regulate insulin secretion from pancreatic β cells through GPR40. *Nature.* 2003;422(6928):173-6.

[13] Sebastiani G, Ceccarelli E, Castagna MG, Dotta F. G-protein-coupled receptors (GPCRs) in the treatment of diabetes: Current view and future perspectives. *Best Practice & Research Clinical Endocrinology & Metabolism.* 2018;32(2):201-13.

[14] Hoque M, Ali S, Hoda M. Current status of G-protein coupled receptors as potential targets against type 2 diabetes mellitus. *International journal of biological macromolecules.* 2018;118:2237-44.

[15] Libby P, Plutzky J. Inflammation in diabetes mellitus: role of peroxisome proliferator-activated Receptor–α and peroxisome proliferator-activated Receptor–γ agonists. The American Journal of *Cardiology*. 2007;99(4):27-40.

[16] Rangwala SM, Lazar MA. Peroxisome proliferator-activated receptor γ in diabetes and metabolism. Trends in pharmacological sciences. 2004;25(6):331-6.

[17] Ahamad J, Naquvi KJ, Mir SR, Ali M, Shuaib M. Review on role of natural αlpha-glucosidase inhibitors for management of diabetes mellitus. *Int. J. Biomed. Res.* 2011;2(1):374-80.

[18] Van de Laar F A. Alpha-glucosidase inhibitors in the early treatment of type 2 diabetes. *Vascular health and risk management.* 2008;4(6):1189.

[19] Gaboriaud-Kolar N, Skaltsounis AL. Glycogen phosphorylase inhibitors: a patent review (2008–2012). *Expert opinion on therapeutic patents.* 2013;23(8):1017-32.

[20] Baker D J, Timmons J A, Greenhaff P L. Glycogen phosphorylase inhibition in type 2 diabetes therapy: a systematic evaluation of metabolic and functional effects in rat skeletal muscle. *Diabetes.* 2005;54(8):2453-9.

[21] van Poelje P D, Dang Q, Erion M D. Fructose-1, 6-bisphosphatase as a therapeutic target for type 2 diabetes. Drug Discovery Today: *Therapeutic Strategies.* 2007;4(2):103-9.

[22] Kaur R, Dahiya L, Kumar M. Fructose-1, 6-bisphosphatase inhibitors: a new valid approach for management of type 2 diabetes mellitus. *European journal of medicinal chemistry.* 2017;141:473-505.

[23] Kazda C M, Ding Y, Kelly R P, Garhyan P, Shi C, Lim C N, Fu H, Watson D E, Lewin A J, Landschulz W H, Deeg M A. Evaluation of efficacy and safety of the glucagon receptor antagonist LY2409021 in patients with type 2 diabetes: 12-and 24-week phase 2 studies. *Diabetes Care.* 2016;39(7):1241-9.

[24] Lotfy M, Kalasz H, Szalai G, Singh J, Adeghate E. Recent progress in the use of glucagon and glucagon receptor antago-nists in the treatment of diabetes mellitus. *The Open Medicinal Chemistry Journal*. 2014;8:28.

[25] Gómez-Valadés A G, Vidal-Alabró A, Molas M, Boada J, Bermúdez J, Bartrons R, Perales J C. Overcoming diabetes-induced hyperglycemia through inhibition of hepatic phosphoenolpyruvate carboxykinase (GTP) with RNAi. *Molecular Therapy.* 2006;13(2): 401-10.

[26] Neumiller J J, White J R, Campbell R K. Sodium-glucose co-transport inhibitors. *Drugs.* 2010;70(4):377-85.

[27] Scheen A J. Drug–drug interactions with sodium-glucose co-transporters type 2 (SGLT2) inhibitors, new oral glucose-lowering agents for the management of type 2 diabetes mellitus. *Clinical pharmacokinetics.* 2014;53(4):295-304.

[28] Sales P M, Souza P M, Simeoni L A, Magalhães P O, Silveira D. α-Amylase inhibitors: a review of raw material and isolated compounds from plant source. *Journal of Pharmacy & Pharmaceutical Sciences.* 2012;15(1):141-83.

[29] Agarwal P, Gupta R. Alpha-amylase inhibition can treat diabetes mellitus. Research & Reviews: *Journal of Medical and Health Sciences* 2016;5(4):1-8.

[30] Drucker D J, Nauck M A. The incretin system: glucagon-like peptide-1 receptor agonists and dipeptidyl peptidase-4 inhibitors in type 2 diabetes. *The Lancet.* 2006;368(9548):1696-705.

[31] Doyle M E, Egan J M. Mechanisms of action of glucagon-like peptide 1 in the pancreas. *Pharmacology & therapeutics*. 2007;113(3):546-93.

[32] Washburn W N. Sodium glucose co-transporter 2 (SGLT2) inhibitors: novel antidiabetic agents. *Expert Opinion on Therapeutic Patents.* 2012;22(5):483-94.

[33] Saeed M A, Narendran P. Dapagliflozin for the treatment of type 2 diabetes: a review of the literature. *Drug design, Development and Therapy*. 2014;8:2493.

[34] Ahrén B. Use of DPP-4 inhibitors in type 2 diabetes: focus on Sitagliptin. *Diabetes, metabolic syndrome and obesity: targets and therapy.* 2010:31-41.

[35] Plosker GL. Sitagliptin: a review of its use in patients with type 2 diabetes mellitus. *Drugs.* 2014;74(2):223-42.

[36] Ahrén B, Schweizer A, Dejager S, Villhauer E B, Dunning B E, Foley J E. Mechanisms of action of the dipeptidyl peptidase-4 inhibitor vildagliptin in humans. *Diabetes, Obesity and Metabolism*. 2011;13(9):775-83.

[37] Scheen AJ. Linagliptin for the treatment of type 2 diabetes (pharmacokinetic evaluation). *Expert Opinion on Drug Metabolism & Toxicology*. 2011;7(12):1561-76.

[38] Bandyopadhyay D, Kusari A, Kenner K A, Liu F, Chernoff J, Gustafson T A, Kusari J. Protein-tyrosine phosphatase 1B complexes with the insulin receptor in vivo and is tyrosine-phosphorylated in the presence of insulin. *Journal of Biological Chemistry*. 1997;272(3):1639-45.

[39] Lebovitz H E. Alpha-glucosidase inhibitors. *Endocrinology and metabolism clinics of North America*. 1997;26(3):539-51.

[40] Smith D L, Orlandella R M, Allison D B, Norian L A. Diabetes medications as potential calorie restriction mimetics—a focus on the alpha-glucosidase inhibitor acarbose. *GeroScience*. 2021;43(3):1123-33.

[41] Jay M A, Ren J. Peroxisome proliferator-activated receptor (PPAR) in metabolic syndrome and type 2 diabetes mellitus. *Current Diabetes Reviews*. 2007;3(1):33-9.

[42] Grygiel-Górniak B. Peroxisome proliferator-activated receptors and their ligands: nutritional and clinical implications-a review. *Nutrition journal*. 2014;13(1):1-0.

[43] Kim JE, Kim JS, Jo MJ, Cho E, Ahn SY, Kwon YJ, Ko GJ. The roles and associated mechanisms of adipokines in development of metabolic syndrome. *Molecules*. 2022;27(2):334.

[44] Saleh J, Al-Maqbali M, Abdel-Hadi D. Role of complement and complement-related adipokines in regulation of energy metabolism and fat storage. *Comprehensive Physiology*. 2011;9(4):1411-29.

Chapter 8

Sodium-Glucose Co-Transporter 2 Inhibitors in Diabetes

Yachana Mishra[1,*]
and Vijay Mishra[2]
[1]School of Bioengineering and Biosciences, Lovely Professional University, Phagwara, India
[2]School of Pharmaceutical Sciences, Lovely Professional University, Phagwara, India

Abstract

The sodium-glucose co-transporter 2 (SGLT 2) inhibitors, also known as Gliflozins, lower plasma blood glucose levels and boost renal excretion of glucose by preventing glucose absorption in the proximal renal tubules. Canagliflozin, dapagliflozin, and empagliflozin are the members of this pharmacological family. They can be used in diabetics at any stage because they don't require insulin to function. These drugs can improve beta-cell activity, increase insulin sensitivity, and minimize the consequences of glucosuria-induced glucotoxicity. The present chapter discusses the details of the SGLT 2 inhibitors.

Keywords: diabetes mellitus, pathophysiology, blood sugar level, sodium-glucose co-transporter

---

* Corresponding Author's Email: yachanamishra@gmail.com.

In: Management of Diabetes Mellitus Based on Natural Products
Editors: Yachana Mishra and Vijay Mishra
ISBN: 979-8-88697-853-7

1. Introduction

The discovery of phlorizin, an earlier medication initially made from apple tree bark, inspired its action method. Urinary glucose excretion was significantly increased as a result. In animal models, it was helpful for mechanistic investigations but too toxic for human patients. Additionally, less than 1% of people have a naturally present mutation in this co-transporter. These patients have long been well-known. In the absence of diabetes, which is uncommon in this group, they have hyperglycemia with healthy plasma glucose. They appear to lead completely normal lives, with the probable exception of more severe vaginal moniliasis brought on by glycosuria. In the 1990s, research to find less harmful phlorizin analogs started. This resulted in the medications that are now available and promoted. These medications have quickly emerged as one of the most effective tools for managing diabetes. Although there are a few smaller pilot studies, including people with type 1 diabetes (T1DM), types 2 diabetes (T2DM) trials make up the majority of the data. There is a decrease in both fasting and subsequent hyperglycemia. In the majority of patients, there is also a concomitant weight reduction, most likely due to calorie loss from exhaled glucose. There is almost little danger of hypoglycemia from them if combined with an insulin secretion or insulin itself since the action mechanism is independent of insulin itself. Other intriguing metabolic effects have been discovered, such as slightly increased plasma glucagon levels and the synthesis of ketone bodies. These three agents - canagliflozin, dapagliflozin, and empagliflozin - are now available in America and Europe. As of this writing, two are sold in Asia, and at least 2 more are in development. The effectiveness and safety data seem to be comparable for the medications now under study [1]. There aren't many direct comparative studies available, though. In most trials, the effectiveness and side effects seem to be equal. Hemoglobin A1c (HbA1c) reductions of 0.7-1.0% as therapy or combined with other antidiabetic medications, such as insulin, have often been shown in phase 3 studies.

2. Mechanism of Action

The kidney filters around 180 mg of glucose per day in nondiabetics. The sodium-glucose co-transporter 2 (SGLT 2) transports 90% of this from the renal tubules to the arterioles and back into circulation. No glucose is discharged into the urine due to the resorption of the remaining 10% in the distant collecting tubule. Diabetes makes it more difficult to remove too much blood glucose because of an apparent maladaptive rise in the tubule threshold from the typical 180 mg to 220-240 mg. The threshold for sugar elimination is lowered to around 40 mg when SGLT 2 inhibitors are present, allowing for substantially more glucose loss. Both fasting and postoperative glucose levels are often decreased [1, 2]. Weight loss is frequently observed because increased glucose excretion results in calorie loss. Most studies place this in the region of 2-3 kg. Fat loss accounts for around two-thirds of the failure, and fluid loss for the remaining third. Every glucose molecule also excretes a sodium molecule, causing a net loss of sodium in the body. As a result, there is a small drop in blood pressure, often 5 mmHg systolic. Given that the majority of patients have some salt excess, this might be advantageous. However, this might cause severe blood pressure drop and dehydration in somewhat sodium- or volume-depleted individuals. The US Food and Drug Administration (FDA) has documented about 100 occurrences of acute renal damage in individuals using these medications. Many instances are observed in elderly individuals who are on loop diuretics and have some renal impairment. Therefore, one must use caution while treating these individuals and begin with a smaller dose to gauge how they react at first.

2.1. Canagliflozin

The USFDA approved canagliflozin in March 2013 for use in people with T2DM. It is the first SGLT-2 inhibitor to be made available for purchase. If the patient tolerates the medication, the initial dose of 100 mg per day may be increased to 300 mg if the patient's GFR is less than 60 mL/min/1.73 m^2. Fixed doses of canagliflozin and metformin are available in the following ratios: 50/500, 50/1000, 150/500, and 150/1000 mg [3].

According to estimates, the glucosuric effects result in a daily excretion of around 100 g of urine glucose. Of the three SGLT-2 inhibitors that have been authorized, it has the greatest glucosuric effects. In addition to its primary SGLT-2 inhibition, canagliflozin also weakly inhibits SGLT-1, which is found in both the gastrointestinal tract and renal tubules. Although this conclusion is based on a limited number of studies, it is believed that SGLT-1 inhibition reduces hyperglycemia by postponing intestinal glucose absorption [4].

Canagliflozin's efficacy as a metformin supplement has been investigated compared to other antihyperglycemic medications such as DPP4 inhibitors and sulfonylureas [5]. In patients on metformin monotherapy (1500 mg/day), a randomized, double-blinded trial comparing the effectiveness of empagliflozin with sitagliptin was released in 2013. Both sitagliptin (100 mg) and canagliflozin (100 mg) successfully reduced hemoglobin A1C by a baseline of 0.73% after 52 weeks. Hemoglobin A1C was lowered by 0.88% with canagliflozin 300 mg. In terms of weight loss, both empagliflozin dosages (3.8% and 4.2%) performed better than sitagliptin, which had a fall of 1.3%.

In phase 3 randomized, double-blinded, 104-week research in 2015, canagliflozin and glimepiride were compared as an add-on therapy for diabetics already on therapeutic levels (1500 mg daily) of metformin. Compare canagliflozin to glimepiride, which caused an average reduction of 0.55% in hemoglobin A1C; canagliflozin reduced hemoglobin A1C by an average of 0.65% for the 100 mg dosage and 0.74% for the 300 mg dose. With a frequency of 40% in the glimepiride class and only 6% and 8% in the canagliflozin 100 and 300 mg groups, respectively, canagliflozin was also linked to decreased hypoglycemia. Patients using glimepiride had a weight increase, but canagliflozin caused weight loss, with an annual loss of 4.1% (3.6 kg) of pretreatment body weight for the 100 mg group and 4.2% (3.6 kg) for the 300 mg group [6].

Data on canagliflozin usage in individuals receiving insulin therapy are available. For 18 weeks with a 52-week follow-up, the CANVAS study compared canagliflozin, a placebo, to patients using basal or basal-bolus insulin. In this experiment, canagliflozin coupled with insulin treatment improved glycemic control. Hemoglobin A1c levels were 8.3% in both groups at the outset. Hemoglobin A1c levels decreased by 0.62% and 0.73% for canagliflozin 100 and 300 mg at 18 weeks compared to placebo. Hemoglobin A1C differences were maintained after 52 weeks, with a decrease from placebo of 0.73% for the 300 mg group and 0.58% for the 100 mg group. There were variations in both weight loss and blood pressure lowering. For each dosage of canagliflozin, a weight reduction of between 1.9% and 2.4% was seen. In each canagliflozin group, the average systolic and diastolic blood pressure dropped by 3.1 and 6.2 mmHg and 1.2 and 2.4 mmHg, respectively [7]. Patients with preexisting chronic renal disease and GFRs between 30 and 50 mL/min/1.73 m^2 have had canagliflozin safety and effectiveness tests. Differences in A1c readings from baseline were seen for the 100 and 300 mg groups, respectively (0.27% and 0.41%). Both dosages resulted in reduced body weight and blood pressure compared to the placebo [8].

2.2. Dapagliflozin

In addition to diet and exercise, dapagliflozin was authorized for use in the United States in 2014 as a therapy for people with T2DM. It is an SGLT-2 inhibitor that is very selective. The starting dose is 5 mg, and the maximum daily dose by mouth is 10 mg. It can also be used in conjunction with metformin [3]. As an adjunctive treatment to metformin, dapagliflozin is superior to DPP-4 inhibitors and non-inferior to sulfonylureas. Patients who are unaccustomed to medication have been assessed for therapy compared to metformin and dapagliflozin. The study's findings showed no distinctions between glucophage and dapagliflozin. In compared to metformin, dapagliflozin as treatment reduced haemoglobin A1C by an average of 0.55 to 0.9% [9]. When used with metformin, dapagliflozin also reduces hemoglobin A1c. Significant improvement was seen in a 52-week double-blinded experiment with patients with baseline haemoglobin A1c readings between 8 and 12%. Compared to the combination of saxagliptin and metformin (0.9%), dapagliflozin combined to metformin reduced haemoglobin A1C on average by 1.2%. Additionally, this study evaluated triple therapy using all three medications and discovered that it was superior than dual therapy by lowering hemoglobin A1c by as much as 1.5%. In comparison to the saxagliptin and metformin group (no significant change was seen), weight loss was much better in the dual-therapy dapagliflozin and metformin group with an average loss of 2.8% (2.1 kg), and in the triple therapy group with an average loss of 2.4% (2.1 kg) [10].

Dapagliflozin's efficacy has been contrasted with that of sulfonylureas. Dapagliflozin and the sulfonylurea glipizide were compared, and non-inferiority was found after 52 weeks. A consistent decrease in haemoglobin A1C was shown with dapagliflozin compared to glipizide over the 2-year extension of this study (0.32% vs 0.14%). [11].

2.3. Empagliflozin

The USFDA approved empagliflozin for use in Americans with T2DM as an antihyperglycemic medication in 2014. Starting doses range from 10 mg to 25 mg per day for people with a GFR of less than 45 mL/min/1.73 m^2. It is believed that 78 g of glucose per day is required for its glucosuric effects. It has similar effects to dapagliflozin and canagliflozin in weight reduction and decreasing blood pressure. Comparing empagliflozin to sulfonylureas and triple treatment with DPP-4 inhibitors and metformin, empagliflozin has been evaluated as an add-on medication to metformin. Patients in a double-blinded phase 3, 104-week research with poor diabetes control while using metformin as their only medication were assigned to receive either glimepiride or empagliflozin treatment. Empagliflozin 25 mg substantially reduced hemoglobin A1c levels around 7% and 10% at baseline, by a mean of 0.11% more than glimepiride. The number of adverse events was comparable between the two groups, although the empagliflozin and glimepiride groups had significantly lower rates of hypoglycemia (2% vs. 24%) [12].

In a 24-week, double-blinded experiment with poorly managed type 2 diabetes patients on linagliptin and metformin combination treatment, the inclusion of empagliflozin 10 mg and 25 mg was examined to placebo. The hemoglobin A1c levels in the empagliflozin 10 and 25 mg groups were shown to be lower than placebo by 0.79% and 0.7%, respectively. Empagliflozin was added to linagliptin and metformin, but it had no additional side effects. Both empagliflozin groups had improvements in terms of weight reduction and blood pressure control. In this experiment, the rate of hypoglycemia was higher in the empagliflozin 25 mg group than in the placebo group (2.7% vs. 0.9%) [13]. The combination of empagliflozin with other medications, including as sitagliptin, pioglitazone, and insulin treatment (both basic and basal/bolus regimens), has been associated with favourable results and improvements in glycemic control [14-17]. Clinical studies evaluating empagliflozin using GLP-1 agonists are currently being conducted [18].

3. Cardiovascular Benefits

A criterion for usually large-scale cardiovascular outcome studies has been incorporated in the approval process for the majority of new antidiabetic medications in the United States, principally to ensure that they do not raise cardiovascular risk [19]. The initial one for this new class was given in September 2015 at the European Society for the Research of Diabetes (EASD). The EMPA-REG trial for empagliflozin, in contrast to earlier studies, demonstrated a remarkable benefit, particularly in terms of cardiovascular mortality (38% relative risk reduction), congestive heart failure hospitalizations (35% relative reducing risk), and death from any cause (32% relative reducing risk). There was a 32% decrease in deaths from all causes [20]. This was far less noticeable for myocardial infarction, and none existed for stroke benefits. This experiment lasted 3.1 years on average. Surprisingly, the survival trajectories started to diverge roughly 3 months after the study started. Even if a decrease in plasma glucose was anticipated, it appears improbable that this action could rapidly produce a benefit of this size. A reduction of arterial stiffness has been suggested as a possible explanation for such quick effects. Loss of sodium and glucose lowers blood pressure and extracellular fluid volume. This enhances both systolic and diastolic functioning by lowering cardiac pre- and afterload and myocardial metabolism. All of these factors might contribute to the sudden drop in heart failure and cardiac death hospitalizations that have been noticed. Statins, proper blood pressure management, and platelet inhibitors were used to treat most individuals. As a result, the advantages seem to outweigh these conventional treatments [20-22].

These medications have been shown to reduce arterial stiffness, which was confirmed by arterial ultrasonography compression [23]. The onset of heart failure triggers a series of reactions that could result in a vicious cycle of vasoconstriction, activating the adrenergic nervous system, the renin-angiotensin-aldosterone system, and the tubular glomerular feedback in the kidney, which could change this unfortunate chain of events. The adjustments taken together most likely result in decreased cardiac preload and afterload and increased myocardial oxygenation [24].

4. Renal Effects

Increased Ketogenesis, and other metabolic effects were shown in patients with renal impairment and glomerular filtration rate (GFR) of 30-60 mL/min in a later preplanned substudy (EMPA REG Renal) [25]. When starting these medications, there is a slight decline in GFR that may be caused by diuresis and volume contraction. Nevertheless, the overall outcome was favourable for the maintaining of renal function in contrast to the placebo-treated arm, where there was a little ongoing decline of eGFR. Reductions in 29% and 38%, respectively, of the renal endpoints of newly developing or worsening nephritis and progress to macroalbuminuria, were made. Although the latter target only happened in a small number of individuals, the hard renal endpoint of double serum creatinine and requirement for renal replacement were decreased by 44% and 55%, respectively.

Angiotensin-converting enzyme inhibitors or antagonists of angiotensin receptors were given to 79-85% of these patients as part of the standard of therapy. As a result, the advantages are cumulative and outweigh those of recognized successful treatments. The potential to dramatically slow the progression of GFR reduction in chronic diabetic renal disease is promising [26]. It is uncertain if the renal advantages of SGLT-2 inhibitors are class- or empagliflozin-specific. An increase in poor renal outcomes with dapagliflozin may be possible compared to some protection with empagliflozin, according to a recent meta-analysis of adverse renal outcomes in published phase 3 clinical studies. Therefore, more research is required to determine if these advantages are shared by all medications in the class.

5. Ketogenesis

The synthesis of insulin, beta-hydroxybutyrate, and ketone bodies is known to be increased by SGLT-2 inhibitors. They appear to switch the metabolism from glucose to fatty acid oxidation. The myocardial cells easily absorb ketone substances to use as fuel. At 8 mL O_2/100 g of tissue, the myocardium has the highest myocardial oxygen consumption, followed by the kidney at 5 mL and the brain at 3 mL. It is hypothesized that metabolically stressed organs could gain from increased ketone body availability and usage [27, 28].

Experimental evidence suggests that this may lead to more effective oxygen-sparing and cardiac effort for any given demand. This could offer a different method for quicker cardiac benefit. Increased ketone body generation has caused some worry, especially in individuals who are very insulin-deficient, such type 1 diabetics. Numerous case series have brought up this issue of ketoacidosis. T2DM seems to occur at a low rate. The mechanism of action may be connected to reduced insulin levels, which cause unchecked glucagon production, lipolysis, and ketogenesis. Sepsis, dehydration, surgeries, a reduction in insulin dosage administration (for those on insulin), and a low-carbohydrate diet are risk factors and precipitants for diabetic ketoacidosis due to SGLT-2 inhibitors [29]. The risk of ketoacidosis might be reduced by informing all patients at the beginning of therapy that symptoms, including nausea, diarrhea, and hydration should be checked for ketones and should make them want to visit a doctor [30].

Conclusion

The most recent pharmacological tool for T2DM therapy is the SGLT-2 inhibitor; several trials have demonstrated both effectiveness and favorable cardiovascular effects. Their use has also improved our understanding of how fuels are metabolized and how to employ ketones as an energy source. Clinicians should be aware of the potential negative consequences of dehydrated and even nondiabetic diabetic ketoacidosis, despite the treatment being typically well tolerated. Given their notable improvements in hemoglobin A1c as well as their advantageous effect on obesity, hypertension, and cardiac outcomes, it is anticipated that usage of these medications will increase.

References

[1] Mudaliar S., Polidori D., Zambrowicz B., Henry R. Sodium-glucose co-transporter inhibitors: effects on renal and intestinal glucose transport. *Diabetes Care.* 2015;38(12):2344–53.

[2] Argento N. B., Nakamura K. Glycemic effects of SGLT-2 inhibitor canagliflozin in type 1 diabetic patients using the DexCom G4 platinum CGM. *Endocr Pract.* 2016;22(3):315–22.

[3] Plodkowski R. A., McGarvey M. E., Huribal H. M., Reisinger-Kindle K., Kramer B., Solomon M., Nguyen Q. T. SGLT-2 inhibitors for the treatment of type 2 diabetes mellitus. *Fed Pract.* 2015;32(Suppl 11):10S–7S.

[4] Polidori D., Sha S., Mudaliar S., Ciaraldi T. P., Ghosh A., Vaccaro N., Farrell K., Rothenberg P., Henry R. R. Canagliflozin lowers postprandial glucose and insulin by delaying intestinal glucose absorption in addition to increasing urinary glucose excretion: results of a randomized, placebo-controlled study. *Diabetes Care.* 2013;36(8):2154–61.

[5] Lavalle-González F. J., Januszewicz A., Davidson J., Tong C., Qiu R., Canovatchel W., Meininger G. Efficacy and safety of canagliflozin compared with placebo and sitagliptin in patients with type 2 diabetes on background metformin monotherapy: a randomised trial. *Diabetologia.* 2013;56(12):2582–92.

[6] Leiter L. A., Yoon K. H., Arias P., Langslet G., Xie J., Balis D. A., Millington D., Vercruysse F., Canovatchel W., Meininger G. Canagliflozin provides durable glycemic improvements and body weight reduction over 104 weeks versus glimepiride in patients with type 2 diabetes on metformin: a randomized, double-blind, phase 3 study. *Diabetes care.* 2015;38(3):355-64.

[7] Neal B., Perkovic V., de Zeeuw D., Mahaffey K. W., Fulcher G., Ways K., Desai M., Shaw W., Capuano G., Alba M., Jiang J. Efficacy and safety of canagliflozin,

an inhibitor of sodium-glucose co-transporter 2, when used in conjunction with insulin therapy in patients with type 2 diabetes. *Diabetes Care.* 2015;38(3):403–11.

[8] Yale J. F., Bakris G., Cariou B., Nieto J., David-Neto E., Yue D., Wajs E., Figueroa K., Jiang J., Law G., Usiskin K. Efficacy and safety of canagliflozin over 52 weeks in patients with type 2 diabetes mellitus and chronic kidney disease. *Diabetes, Obesity and Metabolism.* 2014;16(10):1016-27.

[9] List J. F., Woo V., Morales E., Tang W., Fierdorek F. Sodium-glucose cotransport inhibition with dapagliflozin in type 2 diabetes. *Diabetes Care.* 2009;32(4):650–7.

[10] Rosenstock J., Hansen L., Zee P., Li Y., Cook W., Hirshberg B., Iqbal N. Dual add-on therapy in type 2 diabetes poorly controlled with metformin monotherapy: a randomized double-blind trial of saxagliptin plus dapagliflozin addition versus single addition of saxagliptin or dapagliflozin to metformin. *Diabetes Care.* 2015;38(3):376–83.

[11] Nauck M. A., Del Prato S., Meier J. J., Durán-García S., Rohwedder K., Elze M., Parikh S. J. Dapagliflozin versus glipizide as add-on therapy in patients with type 2 diabetes who have inadequate glycemic control with metformin. *Diabetes Care.* 2011;34(9):2015–22.

[12] Ridderstråle M., Andersen K. R., Zeller C., Kim G., Woerle H. J., Broedl U. C. Comparison of empagliflozin and glimepiride as add-on to metformin in patients with type 2 diabetes: a 104-week randomised, active-controlled, double-blind, phase 3 trial. *Lancet Diabetes Endocrinol.* 2014;2(9):691–700.

[13] Søfteland E., Meier J. J., Vangen B., Toorawa R., Maldonado Lutomirsky M., Broedl U. C. Empagliflozin as add-on therapy in patients with type 2 diabetes inadequately controlled with linagliptin and metformin: a 24-week randomized, double-blind, parallel-group trial. *Diabetes Care.* 2017;40(2):201–9.

[14] Ferrannini E., Berk A., Hantel S., Pinnetti S., Hach T., Woerle H. J. Broedl U. C. Long-term safety and efficacy of empagliflozin, sitagliptin, and metformin: an active-controlled, parallel-group, randomized, 78-week open-label extension study in patients with type 2 diabetes. *Diabetes Care.* 2013;36(12):4015–21.

[15] Kovacs C. S., Seshiah V., Merker L., Christiansen A. V., Roux F., Salsali A., Kim G., Stella P., Woerle H. J., Broedl U. C. Empagliflozin as add-on therapy to pioglitazone with or without metformin in patients with type 2 diabetes mellitus. *Clin Ther.* 2015;37(8):1773–88.e1.

[16] Rosenstock J., Jelaska A., Zeller C., Kim G., Broedl U. C., Woerle H. J. Impact of empagliflozin added on to basal insulin in type 2 diabetes inadequately controlled on basal insulin: a 78-week randomized, double-blind, placebo-controlled trial. *Diabetes Obes Metab.* 2015;17(10):936–48.

[17] Rosenstock J., Jelaska A., Frappin G., Salsali A., Kim G., Woerle H. J., Broedl U. C. Improved glucose control with weight loss, lower insulin doses, and no increased hypoglycemia with empagliflozin added to titrated multiple daily injections of insulin in obese inadequately controlled type 2 diabetes. *Diabetes Care.* 2014;37(7):1815–23.

[18] De Fronzo R. *Effect of combined incretin-based therapy plus canagliflozin on glycemic control and the compensatory rise in hepatic glucose production in type 2 diabetic patients*, 2019; NCT02324842.

[19] Zaccardi F., Webb D. R., Htike Z. Z., Youssef D., Khunti K., Davies M. J. Efficacy and safety of sodium-glucose co-2 inhibitors in type 2 diabetes mellitus: systematic review and network meta-analysis. *Diabetes Obes Metab.* 2016;18:783–94.

[20] Zinman B., Wanner C., Lachin J., Fitchett D., Bluhmki E., Hantel S., Mattheus M., Devins T., Johansen O. E., Woerle H. J., Broedl U. C. Empagliflozin, cardiovascular outcomes and mortality in type 2 diabetes. *N Engl J Med.* 2015;373:2117–27.

[21] Henry R., Thakkar P., Tong C., Polidori D., Alba M. Efficacy and safety of canagliflozin, a sodium–glucose co-transporter 2 inhibitor, as add-on to insulin in patients with type 1 diabetes. *Diabetes Care.* 2015;38(12):2258–65.

[22] Abdul-Ghani M., Del Prato S., Chilton R., DeFronzo R. A. SGLT2 inhibitors and cardiovascular risk: lessons learned from the Empareg Outcome Study. *Diabetes Care.* 2016;39:717–25.

[23] Chilton R., Tikkanen I., Cannon C. P., Crowe S., Woerle H. J., Broedl U. C., Johansen O. E. Effects of empagliflozin on blood pressure and markers of arterial stiffness and vascular resistance in patients with type 2 diabetes. *Diabetes Obes Metab.* 2015;17(12):1180–93.

[24] Sattar N., McLaren J., Fristen S. L., Preiss D., McMurray J. J. SGLT2 inhibition and cardiovascular events: why did EMPA-Reg outcomes surprise and what are the likely mechanisms? *Diabetologia.* 2016;59:1333–9.

[25] Wanner C., Inzucchi S., Lachin J., Fitchett D., von Eynatten M., Mattheus M., Johansen O. E., Woerle H. J., Broedl U. C., Zinman B. Empagliflozin and progression of kidney disease in type 2 diabetes. *N Engl J Med.* 2016;375(18):1801–2.

[26] Tang H., Li D., Zhang J., Li Y., Wang T., Zhai S. Sodium-glucose transporter-2 inhibitors and risk of adverse renal outcomes in patients with type 2 diabetes: A network meta-analysis of randomized control trials. *Diabetes Obes Metab.* 2017.

[27] Ferrannini E., Mark M., Mayoux E. CV protection in the EMPAREG OUTCOME trial: a "thrifty substrate" hypothesis. *Diabetes Care.* 2016;39(7):1108–14.

[28] Mudaliar S., Alloju S., Henry R. R. Can a shift in fuel energetics explain the beneficial cardiorenal outcomes in the Empareg Outcome study? A unifying hypothesis. *Diabetes Care.* 2016;39(7):1115–22.

[29] Rosenstock J., Ferrannini E. Euglycemic diabetic ketoacidosis: a predictable, detectable, and preventable safety concern with SGLT2 inhibitors. *Diabetes Care.* 2015;38(9):1638–42.

[30] Peters A., Baschur E. O., Buse J., Cahan P., Diner J. C., Hirsch I. B. Euglycemic diabetic ketoacidosis: a potential complication of treatment with sodium-glucose co-transporter inhibition. *Diabetes Care.* 2015;38:1687–93.

Chapter 9

Chemical Scaffolds as Antidiabetic Agents

Charanjit Kaur
and Sanjeev Kumar Sahu*
School of Pharmaceutical Sciences, Lovely Professional University, Phagwara, (Punjab), India

Abstract

Diabetes mellitus is a metabolic disorder causing elevated blood sugar level due to either inadequate insulin production from beta pancreatic cells or its resistance at receptors. Several antidiabetic agents are available in the market, which are used in the treatment of diabetes mellitus. These drugs give their biological action by acting on different molecular targets. All these antidiabetic drugs are usually heterocyclic compounds like sulfonylureas, biguanides, thiazolidinediones, thiazolidine, thiazole, indoles, quinolines, quinazoline etc. This chapter is mainly focused on various chemical scaffolds with their antidiabetic activity. Further, all the potent developed derivatives under such categories of chemical scaffolds have been summarized.

Keywords: diabetes mellitus, antidiabetic drugs, chemical scaffolds

1. Introduction

Diabetes mellitus (DM) is one of the significant reasons for prolonged sickness and premature demise, 1 in every 10 seconds, and even more than

* Corresponding Author's Email: sanjeevsahu82@yahoo.co.in.

In: Management of Diabetes Mellitus Based on Natural Products
Editors: Yachana Mishra and Vijay Mishra
ISBN: 979-8-88697-853-7

HIV/AIDS [1]. The type of DM is based on the pathophysiological mechanisms behind it. Type I/insulin-dependent/juvenile-onset diabetes is an autoimmune illness involving the destruction of pancreatic cells due to the infiltration of macrophages, activated CD8+ and CD4+ T cells into the pancreatic islets [2]. In Type II DM, insulin resistance develops along with inadequate insulin production and secretion [3]. Hypoglycaemic drugs are chemical entities capable of lowering blood glucose levels by targeting various receptors involving pathophysiological pathways and are beneficial for DM. In spite of the availability of a large number of commercial drugs available in the market, the management of this ailment has been possible, but not the cure. So, there is a constant need to identify the pharmacophores in already developed and active molecules in the search for new potent antidiabetic agents with better pharmacological profiles [4]. These molecules are commonly classified as thiazole, thiazolidinediones, thiazolidine, sulfonylureas, biguanides, indoles, quinolines, quinazoline etc. These antidiabetic molecules can also be classified based on their heterocyclic structures and the targets of their interaction.

2. Chemical Scaffolds as Antidiabetic Agents

2.1. Thiazole Derivatives

Ali et al. synthesized and evaluated thiazole-pyridine hybrids against α-glucosidase. Amongst all the potent molecules, analogue **1** (Figure 1) was found most potent ($IC_{50} = 1.40 \pm 0.01$ μM). The electron-withdrawing groups showed resilient interactions with the enzyme's active site. In silico analysis showed the presence of two CH-π interactions between the dichlorobenzene ring of analogue **1** with residue His279 of the enzyme and H-bond interaction of the sulphur atom and 4-Cl with the Asp349 and Asn241 residue of the enzyme. π-hydrogen bond interaction were reported with the Phe300 residue [5].

Shah et al. designed and studied 5-chloro-2-arylbenzo[d]thiazoles against α-glucosidase. Analogues **2** (Figure 1) displayed the highest activity (IC_{50} = 22.1 ± 0.9 to 25.6 ± 1.5 μM due to the presence of -OH at C-2′ and -Br at C-5′ on aryl group (**2a**, IC_{50} = 22.1 ± 0.9 μM). *In silico* studies demonstrated the presence of Hydrogen bonding interactions between -OH and -Br at C-2′ and C-5′ position of **2a** with enzyme residues Arg312. The hydrophobic interactions were also reported between the benzothiazole ring of the **2a** forms with Glu304 and His279 residues of the enzyme [6].

Kim et al., developed and examined 4-(phenoxymethyl) thiazole derivatives as GPR119 agonists. They reported analogue **3a** (Figure 1) as the most potent hGPR119 agonist (EC_{50} = 18 nM) and was found to lower the glucose levels in the mice intolerance test. The analogues bearing a tolyl group were reported more potent as compared to F group on a benzene ring. Analogue **3a** displayed glucose level inhibition in OGTT *in vivo* (dose = 30 mg/kg) in comparison to GPR119 agonist MBX-2982 in the clinical trials [7].

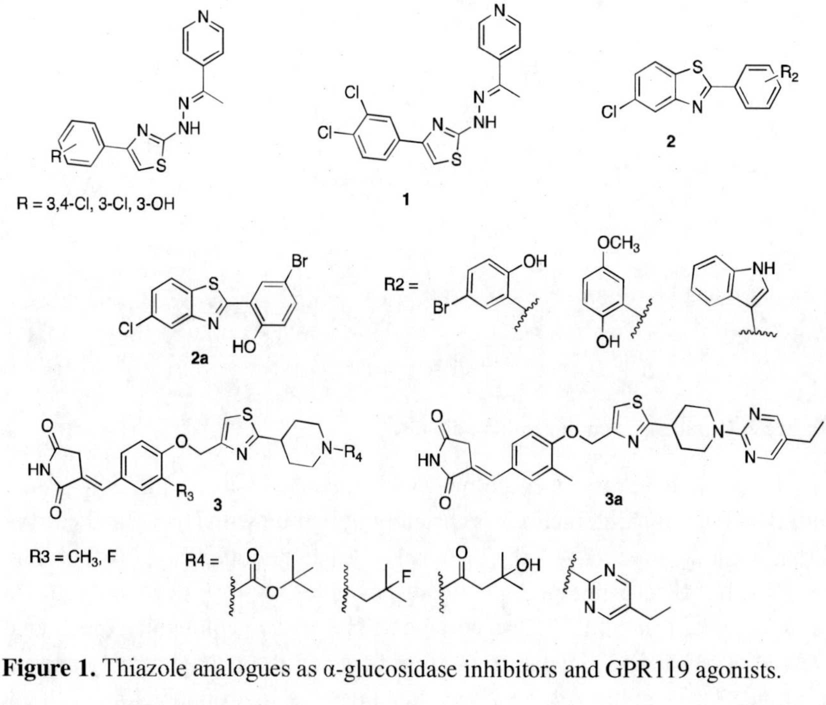

Figure 1. Thiazole analogues as α-glucosidase inhibitors and GPR119 agonists.

2.2. Thiazolidinediones

Thiazolidinediones (TZDs) are insulin sensitisers utilised for the management of type 2 diabetes mellitus (T2DM) through binding to peroxisome proliferator-activated receptors (PPAR) in fat cells, making them progressively sensitive to insulin due to their agonistic effect. Numerous thiazolidinedione derivatives were synthesised by researchers to enhance their potential or efficacy as antidiabetic drug and to lessen the adverse effects associated with them. Some of these derivatives have been discussed below with respect to their structures, the linkers used to make their hybrids and the target protein of interaction.

2.2.1. Thiazolidinedione Nucleus Bearing Heterocyclic Ring through Linkers

Clinically used drugs in market like troglitazone, rosiglitazone, pioglitazone, etc. (Figure 2) bears TZD nucleus and belong to this class with nitrogen containing heterocyclic ring connected through benzyloxy linker and alkyl chain of varying length.

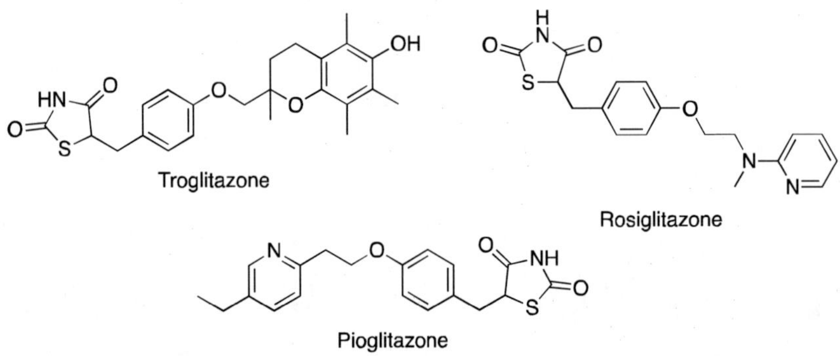

Figure 2. Clinically used thiazolidinediones.

TZDs such as rosiglitazone bind with the active site of PPAR-γ protein through H bonding interactions of the carbonyl group with His323and His449, along with residue H449 of TZD and lysine residue, K367 of protein, respectively. These interactions are responsible for 40% occupancy of the catalytic site31 in the ternary complex. The pyridine inhabits the pocket between β-sheet and H3 due to O atom between the phenyl moiety and the pyridine. The sulphur atom of the ring interacts hydrophobically with the protein and all of these interactions activate PPAR-γ.

The activated PPARs connect to the regulatory regions of the genes, initiating their transcription for glucose homeostasis pocket, consisting of F282, F363, L469 and Q286[8]. Parks et al., evaluated the rosiglitazone enantiomer's binding affinity to PPAR-γ and found the S-isomer (Figure 3) active, due to its high affinity for PPAR-γ than the R-isomer, suggesting the role of chiral ligands in better antidiabetic activity [9].

Madhavan et al., synthesized phathalazinone-thiazolidinedione analogues, and checked their agonistic action on PPAR-γ using HEK 293T cells both *in vitro* as well as *in vivo*. The synthesized compounds showed better activity in terms of lowering glucose levels as compared to the reference drugs (i.e., rosiglitazone, troglitazone and pioglitazone). Amongst the entire series, the methyl derivative of phthalazinone (**4a**) showed improvement in the triglycerides and glucose-reducing potential compared to ethyl or phenyl derivatives. Analogue **4** (Figure 3) was found to be the most active and potent PPAR-γ activator and (dose of 10 mg/kg in mice) showed 72% and 58% reduction in glucose and triglyceride levels, respectively. However, rosiglitazone (dose of 30 mg/kg in mice) showed 67% glucose reduction and 40% triglyceride reduction as per *in vivo* studies [10].

Nazreen et al., designed and evaluated oxadiazole-thiazolidinediones using *in silico*, *in vitro* as well as *in vivo* studies for their PPAR-γ transactivation activity. Based on the binding affinity of ligand and docking score on PPAR-γ (> −7.20) in comparison to standard drugs (rosiglitazone and pioglitazone), analogues **5a** and **5b** (Figure 3) also exhibited noteworthy transactivation activity of PPAR-γ *in vitro*, even 2.10- and 2.0 times more as compared to the reference drugs pioglitazone and rosiglitazone. In STZ-induced diabetic rats, compounds **5a** and **5b** lowered the levels of blood glucose to 139.6 ± 6.40 and 134.0 ± 5.09 as compared to Rosiglitazone; 144.2 ± 6.12. Moreover, elevation in weight, cardiotoxic and hepatotoxic side effects were also not reported with these compounds [11].

Yanagisava et al., reported that TZD derivatives with oxime-containing linkers with 5-benzyl-2,4-thiazolidinedione derivatives as PPAR-γ agonists. Amongst the synthesized molecules, **6a** (Figure 3) was reported to be more potent than rosiglitazone (EC_{50} = 0.19 μM). It also showed an effective lowering of blood glucose. In these derivatives, the agonistic activity was found to be enhanced due to the presence of -C_2H_5 bridge between the O atoms of the oxime and the -OPh group, and -Ar at the p-/m- position of the acetylpyridine or acetophenone oxime [12].

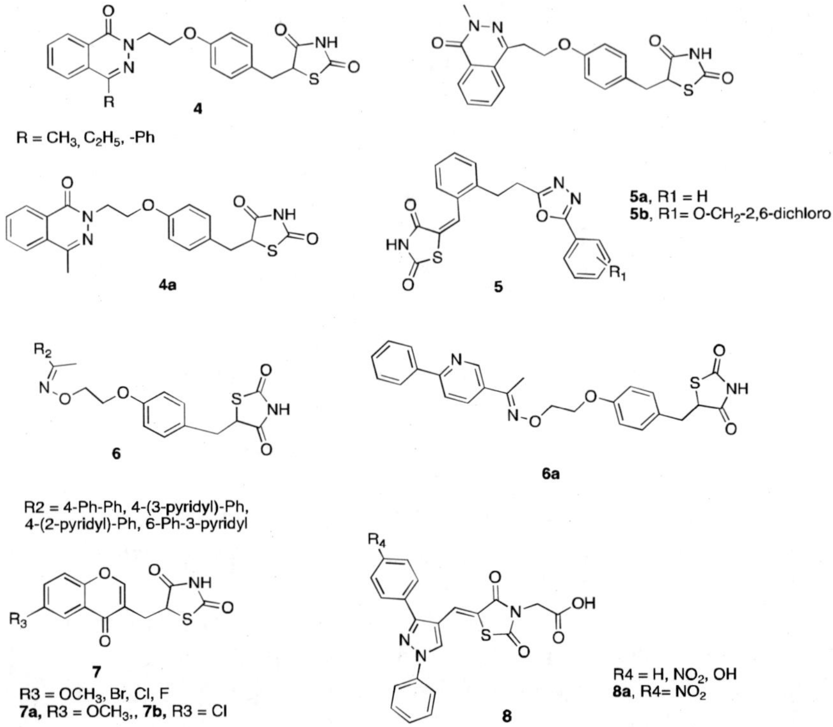

Figure 3. Thiazolidinedione analogues as PPAR-γ activators.

2.2.2. Thiazolidinedione Nucleus Bearing Heterocyclic Ring without Linkers

Nazreen et al., designed and evaluated a series of 2,4-thiazolidinediones for antidiabetic activity as PPAR-γ agonists in comparison to rosiglitazone and pioglitazone both *in vivo* and *in vitro*. Amongst them, analogues **7a** and **7b** (Figure 3) lowered the levels of blood glucose and the reduced double bond of the chromone nucleus causing the loss of activity. In a molecular docking study, these molecules exhibited superior glide scores (**7a**=−7.57, **7b**= −7.76) than pioglitazone (−5.77 against the PPAR-γ). Both the molecules were not found to cause any hepatotoxic side effects and **7b** showed 48.72% transactivation of PPAR-γ as compared to pioglitazone (62.48%) in addition to enhanced PPAR-γ expression (2.56-fold) than to the standard drug [13].

Bansal et al. designed, synthesized and checked the PPAR-γ agonistic activity of a series of thiazolidine-2,4-dione-pyrazole conjugates attached through methylene group. *In silico* studies revealed the best docking score (-17.44) of analogue **8a** (Figure 3) on PPAR-γ than pioglitazone (-12.605), which was found in accordance with *in vivo* results, with blood glucose-lowering effects 134.46 ± 0.49 in C57BL/6J mice (14th-day duration) than the standard drug (136.56 ± 0.64). Amongst the entire series, the activity was found to be dependent on the substitution on the phenyl linked to pyrazole and electron-donating groups were found with improved activity [14].

2.2.3. Thiazolidinedione Derivatives Bearing Non-Heterocyclic Ring through Linkers

Bhattarai et al., synthesized and checked the TP1B inhibitory activity of benzylidene-2,4-thiazolidinedione analogues *in vivo* using a mouse model system. The analogue **9a** (Figure 4) showed the highest potency (IC_{50} = 5.0 μM) as well as PPAR-γ agonism. The ortho substitution revealed better PTP1b inhibition than para substitution. As per *in silico* studies, Val49, Tyr46, Ala217, Ile218 and Phe182 amino acid residues at the active site of PTP1B were found involved in hydrophobic interactions, whereas Gln266 and Ser216 amino acid residues were involved in H bonding interactions with aromatic rings and the aminocarbonyl oxygen atom of compound **9a,** respectively [15].

In another series of TZD analogues synthesized by this group, **10a** (Figure 4) was reported be the most efficient PTP1B inhibitor (IC_{50} = 1.3 μM) in comparison to ertiprotafib (standard drug, IC_{50} = 1.4 μM) and was found to reduce the weight gain along with improvement of blood parameters like total cholesterol, NEFA and TG. In addition, it was also found as a potent PPAR-γ agonist [15].

Ha et al., also designed benzylidene-thiazolidine-2,4-diones for PTP1B inhibition and found the highest tyrosine inhibitory activity of compounds **11a** and **11b** (Figure 4) (IC_{50} = 13.36 and 9.87 μM, respectively) in comparison to kojic acid (reference compound, IC_{50} = 24.72 μM). **11a** and **11b** molecules were found to be 1.85 and 2.50 times more potent than kojic acid. The number and position of OH as well as OCH_3 groups was found necessary for PTP1B inhibition. The **11b** showed the highest inhibition (82.27%) due to the presence of OH at R1 and OCH_3 at R2 position [16].

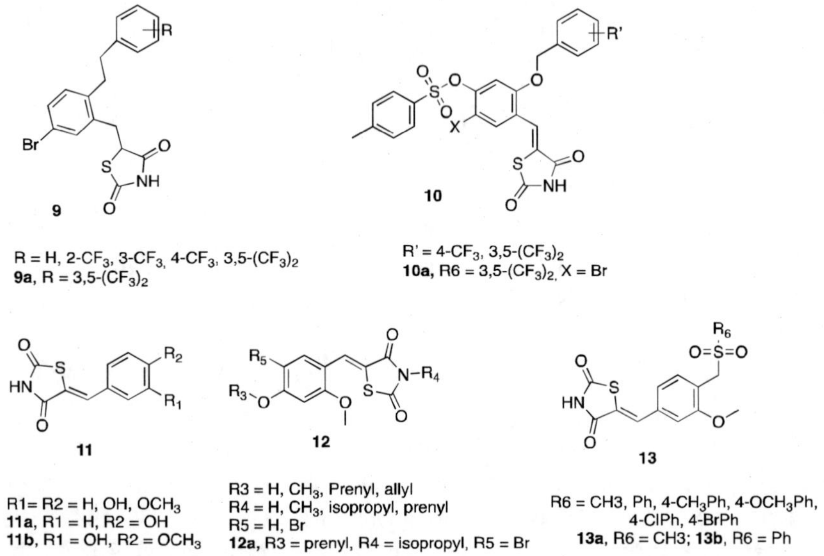

Figure 4. Thiazolidinediones as PTP1B inhibitors.

Similarly, Wang et al. described the synthesis and inhibition potency of another series of the above-discussed category. Amongst the synthesized molecules, **12a** (Figure 4) was stated to be the most potent PTP1B inhibitor (IC_{50} = 4.6 μM). The binding energy of **12a** with PTP1B was reported −7.35 kcal/mol. *In silico* analysis showed that the H bonding interactions between Gly220 residue of the enzyme and the C=O group of TZD derivatives along with hydrophobic interactions of the thiazolidinedione of **12a** are accountable for stabilization and fitting of the molecule at active site of enzyme. The molecules with prenyl group at R3, isopropyl at R4 and Br at R5 showed maximum inhibitory activity; however, allylic group at R5 reduced the enzyme inhibition [17].

Mahapatra et al. investigated another series of 5-benzylidene-thiazolidine-2,4-dione analogues, for their PTP1B inhibition and, found **13a** and **13b** (Figure 4) as the most active PTP1B inhibitor (IC_{50} = 7.31 and 8.73 μM). It was found that the analogues with bulky groups like phenylmethane, 2,4,6-trimethylphenyl presented lower PTP1B inhibition than phenyl/methanesulfonate. *In silico* evaluations revealed the H bonding interactions of the active compounds with Ser216, Ala217 and Arg221 at the active site of the enzyme. In comparison to standard pioglitazone drug, both the molecules significantly decrease the glucose level in blood 32.13% and 30.22%, respectively as per 7 days of *in vivo* studies [18].

2.2.4. Thiazolidinedione Nucleus Bearing Non-Heterocyclic Ring without Linkers

Numerous analogues of TZD has been reported as potent aldose reductase inhibitors as revealed by quantitative SAR study, according to which there is a vital role of -Ph and CH_3COOH substitution on the synthesized TZD, in the aldose reductase (ALR2) inhibition. Maccari et al., synthesized a series of 5-arylidene-2,4-thiazolidinedione analogues with variable substitution on the 5-arylidene ring as well as the N-3 position and evaluated their ALR2 inhibitory activity. The activity was found to be improved with the substitution of the 5-arylidene ring either with -Ar ring or an H-bond donor group and on the N-3 position with acetic acid. The substitution of the ring with OH group at the 4th position produced the derivative with the highest potency but the analogue with OH at 3rd position resulted in reduced potency molecule. Analogue **14**a (Figure 5) was found most active (IC_{50} = 0.15 μM) and hydrophobic as well as H bonding interactions between the cyclic imide carbonyl oxygens of compound **14a** with the residues Trp20, Pro218, Trp219 and residue Trp20 respectively are responsible for ALR2 inhibitory activity as per *in silico* studies [19].

Maccari et al., synthesized and evaluated another series of 5-arylidene-2,4-thiazolidinedione derivatives for ALR2 activity. Analogue **15a** (Figure 5) showed IC_{50} = 0.20 μM and with the highest potency due to the presence of OH or CO_2CH_3 groups, vital for binding with the enzyme. These two substituents were found responsible for inhabiting the active pocket of the enzyme as a result of weak non-covalent interactions interaction with Leu300, residue. The most potent derivatives were with substitution of OH, OCH_3, or CO_2CH_3 on 5-arylidene and replacement of the -OH with -CO_2CH_3 group enhanced the potency [20].

In addition to the above, another series of these analogues without a -COOH moiety was designed and synthesized by Maccari et al., for the ALR2 inhibitory activity. Amongst them, compound **16a** (Figure 5) presented IC_{50} = 6.52 μM as the most potent inhibitor in comparison to the standard drug sorbinil (IC_{50} = 1.41 μM). According to SAR, the presence of 4-OH at 5-arylidene contributes considerably towards inhibitory activity due to H bonding interactions with His110 and Tyr48 of ALR2 enzyme. Still, its shifting or replacement caused the loss of activity [20].

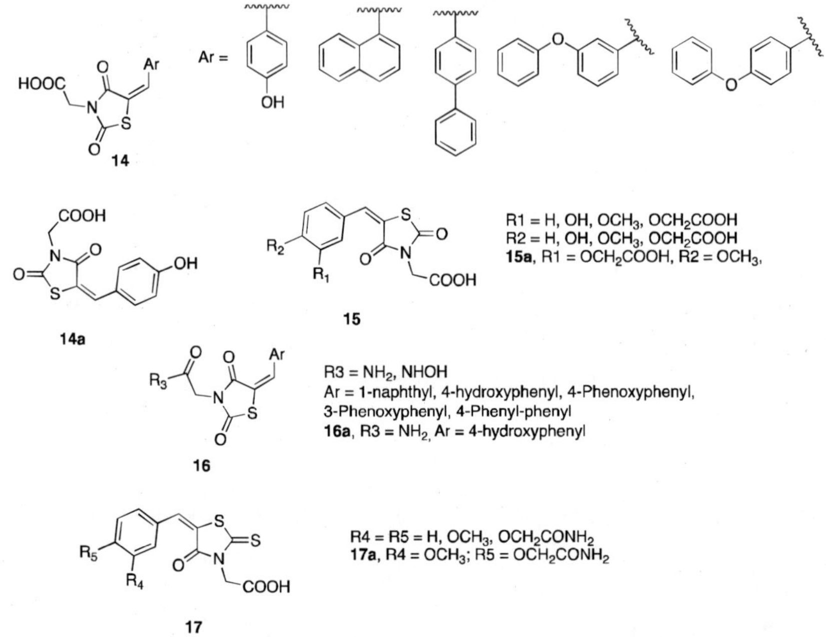

Figure 5. Thiazolidinedione analogues as ALR2 inhibitors.

Again, Maccari et al. also synthesized and evaluated benzylidene-2-oxo/thioxo-4-thiazolidinone analogues for their aldose reductase inhibitory activity. Their analogues containing -CH_3COOH exhibited improved activity than standard drugs used in the study with IC_{50} = 0.11 μM- 0.13 μM. The derivative **17a** (Figure 5) was observed with maximum inhibition potential (IC_{50} = 0.13 μM) amongst the designed molecules, along with the potential to suppress iNOS expression and NF-kB activation [21].

2.3. Thiazolidine Nucleus Bearing Heterocyclic Ring

Yoshida et al. synthesized and checked DPP-4 inhibition potency of L-prolyl piperazinyl-thiazolidines derivatives. Analogue **18a** (Figure 6) was found with the highest potency of inhibition (IC_{50} = 0.92 nmol/L in human) amongst the synthesised molecules and showed 60% plasma DPP-4 inhibition (dose=10 μmol/kg) within 9 h in Wistar rats. The 5-nitro-2-pyridine moiety in this molecule was found responsible for binding with the enzyme but the molecules with -CN substituent at 4th position of pyridine ring also showed significant enzyme inhibition [22].

Yoshida et al., also designed, synthesized, and checked the DPP-4 inhibitory activity of another series of a previously synthesized scaffold with fused bicyclic heteroaryl piperazine substituent. In this series, analogue **19a** (Figure 6) was reported to possess long-lasting inhibition along with highest potency (IC_{50} = 0.37 nM) and decreased > 40% of the plasma DPP-4 (dose-3 μmol/ kg) within 24 h in Wistar rats. This compound possesses H bonding, hydrophobic along with CH-π interactions with amino acid residues at the active site of enzyme which are responsible for its selectivity and inhibition potency as per the X-ray crystal structure. However, the derivatives with quinoline substituent at 4th position showed better inhibition potential than at 2nd position and a loss of inhibitory potential was observed on substitution of the CF_3 with a CH_3 group [23].

Yoshida et al., extended their work on the same scaffold and synthesized teneligliptin (Figure 6) for DPP-4 inhibition, prescribed in Japan. Teneligliptin showed excellent inhibition potency (IC_{50} = 0.37 nM) and lowered the glucose levels > 35% in Zucker fatty rats (dose = 0.03 mg/kg). It occupies the hydrophobic region of active site of enzyme through the thiazolidine moiety. It interacts with Glu205 residue via salt-bridge interactions of $-NH_2$ group of the proline moiety involved through H bonds between the Asn710 residue with -C=O group, CH-π interactions of pyrazolyl ring with Ser209 and hydrophobic interactions of Arg358 with the phenyl ring on the pyrazolyl moiety showing its potency in type-2 diabetes [23].

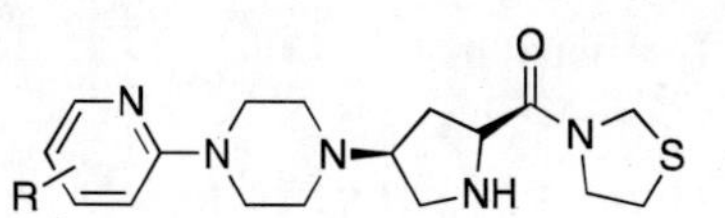

18

R = 5-NO_2, 4-CN, 3-CN
18a, R = 5-NO_2

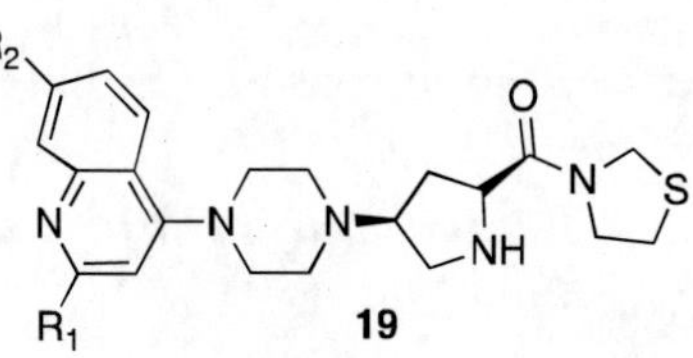

19

R1 = H, CH_3, CF_3; R2 = H, Cl
19a, R1 = CF_3; R2 = H

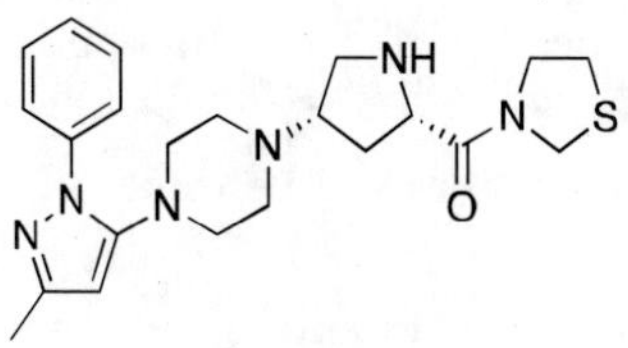

Teneligliptin

Figure 6. Thiazolidines as DPP-4 inhibitors.

2.4. Thiadiazole Derivatives

Javid et al., synthesized and evaluated 2-amino-thia-diazole and its Schiff base analogues against α-glucosidase. Amongst the two series, analogues **20a** and **21a** (Figure 7) showed maximum inhibition with same $IC_{50} = 2.30 \pm 0.1$ μM even better activity than the standard acarbose ($IC_{50} = 39.60 \pm 0.70$ μM). The SAR showed that the highest inhibitory potential of p-substituted derivatives. *In silico* evaluations showed the involvement of H bonding interactions between NH_2, -OH groups, S atom and -PhCl of compound **20a** with Glu276, Asp408, Asn347 residues and Pro309 residues, respectively. 3 arene-H-bonds were also reported with Tyr71, Phe157 and Arg312, suggesting the potential of these analogues as effective α-glucosidase inhibitors [24].

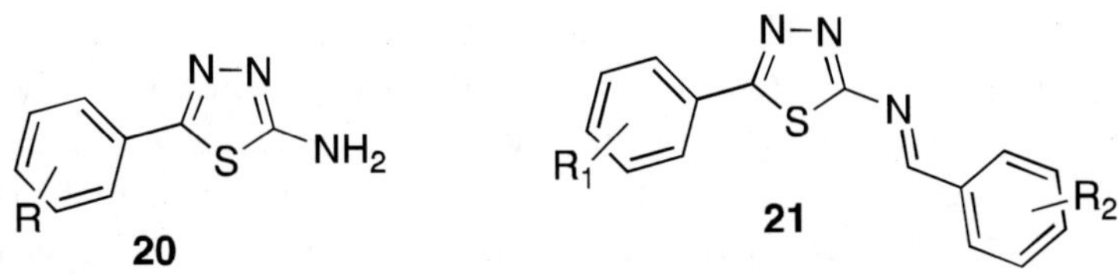

R = 4-OH, 3,4-diCl, 2-NO_2
20a, R = -OH

R1 = 4-Cl, 2,4-diCl, 2-NO_2, 4-OH
R2 = 4-OH, 4-NO_2, 2,4-diCl
21a, R1 = 4-Cl; R2 = 4-OH

Figure 7. Thiadiazole derivatives as α-glucosidase inhibitors.

2.5. Sulfonylureas and Sulphonamides Derivatives

2.5.1. Benzene Sulfonylureas Bearing Heterocyclic Ring through Pyrazoline Linkers

Sulphonyl ureas/SUR agonist stimulate the PPAR-γ transcriptional activity and act as agonists, specifically the second-generation drugs of this class (glipizide or glibenclamide). Structurally, PPAR-γ agonists were found with an acidic and hydrophobic head joined to a lipophilic tail by an aromatic scaffold through -$CONH_2$ linkers [25].

Kharbanda et al. suggested a series of benzene sulphonylurea derivatives and performed *in silico* evaluations on PPAR-γ gene in 3T3-L1 fibroblasts to check their potential. Analogue **22a** (Figure 8) was reported to with maximum potency (0.95 times enhancement in gene compatibility) than the standard drugs glibenclamide and rosiglitazone during *in vitro* study. Amongst the entire series, the molecules without substitution on phenyl ring were found more effective but replacement of urea with thiourea caused loss of antidiabetic activity [26].

They also reported another series of sulphonyl urea analogues and found compound **23a** (Figure 8) as more potent PPAR-γ agonist 42 than the standard drugs when evaluated on STZ diabetic rats. It was reported to be responsible for the PPAR-γ activation, and enhanced sensitivity to insulin without considerable increase in weight. The substitution of $-N(CH_3)_2$ on aryl group at para position enhanced the potency by 1.13 than the standard drug glibenclamide [27].

2.5.2. Benzene Sulfonylureas Bearing Non-Heterocyclic Ring through Pyrazoline Linkers

Ovais et al. developed pyrazoline-substituted benzene sulphonyl urea/thiourea derivatives and evaluated their aldose reductase inhibitory action. At a dose of 0.05 mM/kg, these derivatives showed anti-hyperglycaemic action ranging from 10 to 29.3% in normal rats. But some molecules, like **24** (Figure 8), showed both anti-hyperglycaemic and aldose reductase inhibition. It exhibited better activity than the ARI sorbinil, and benzene sulfonyl thiourea derivatives, **24a**, showed the highest aldose reductase inhibition ($IC_{50} = 0.0175$ μM). The replacement of $PhCH_2$- with cyclohexyl ring or butyl chain on thiourea was found to increase the activity. *In silico* docking studies showed the H bonding interactions between Trp111 and $-SO_2NH_2$ group of **24a**, π-interactions of phenyl ring of pyrazoline with Trp219 residue and the hydrophobic pocket of the enzyme was found to be retained by the pyrazoline [28].

2.5.3. Sulphonamide Derivatives Directly Attached to Heterocyclic Ring without Linkers

Deka et al. synthesized and examined benzene sulphonamide analogues, for the agonism on PPAR-γ (Conc=10 μM) in HEK 293 cells. Amongst the synthesized molecules, **25a** (Figure 8) had the highest transcriptional activity (E_{max} = 16%). In silico studies showed the Vander waal's and hydrophobic interaction between 9a Ile120 and Ile341, Gly63, Cys64, Arg67 residues, respectively [29].

2.5.4. Sulphonamide Derivatives Attached to Heterocyclic Ring through Linkers

Taygerly et al., designed and evaluated diaryl sulfonamide derivatives as PPAR-γ agonist. They found the **26a** molecule as the most active (IC_{50} = 18 nM and EC_{50} = 0.01 μM, Figure 8) amongst all *in vitro*. The effective blood glucose reduction was observed with analogue **26a** (dose = 1 mg/kg/day) on a KKAy diabetic mice. In addition, the substitution on compound **26a** with electron-withdrawing groups at 2,4-position of A-ring exhibited higher activity than at 4-position of A-ring [30].

2.5.5. Sulphonamide Derivatives Attached to Non-Heterocyclic Ring without Linkers

Du et al. designed and examined diethoxyphenyl methane sulphonamide derivative hybrids for PTP1B inhibitory action. Amongst the series, **27a** (Figure 8) exhibited maximum inhibition on PTP1B (IC_{50} = 0.203 μM), with 4-OCH_3 phenyl ring and 120 times selectivity over TC-PTP. However, derivatives with the 3-OCH_3 group on -Ph showed 10-fold lesser PTP1B inhibition. Analogue **27a** was found to inhibit PTP1B competitively as per kinetic studies, and increase the phosphorylation of insulin-mediated insulin receptor β (IRβ) (concentrations = 25 μM and 50 μM) [31].

Liu et al. synthesized and evaluated methane sulfonyl phenyl amino derivatives for TC-PTP and PTP1B enzyme inhibition. Out of the synthesized molecules, **28a** (IC_{50} = 0.222 μM, Figure 8) was reported to possess the highest PTP1B inhibition with 8-times selectivity over TC-PTP and enhanced glucose uptake stimulated by insulin in human skeletal muscle cells depending upon dose. However, methoxy rather than ethoxy substituent at 4th position on -Ph at R2 position caused a loss of activity [32].

Liu et al. also designed methane-sulphonamides against same enzyme as previous study. and found compound **29a** as most potent (IC_{50} = 0.05 μM) with 15-times better selectivity over TC-PTP. It was also found to enhance the glucose uptake induced by insulin at two different concentrations (15 μM and 30 μM) in transfected CHO cells. *In silico* docking studies revealed the H bonding, hydrophobic and π-π stacking interactions between 4-methyl-benzyloxy group of compound **29a** with Gly220, Ala217, Phe182, Lys120, Arg24, etc. residues of the catalytic site of PTP1B. However, the substitution of methyl group at 3rd position on benzyloxy group instead of 4th position, caused a loss of activity owing to the steric hindrance involved with the enzyme residues [33].

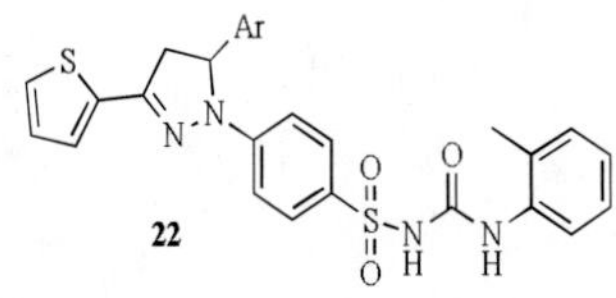

22

Ar = thiophenyl, phenyl, anthracen-9-yl
22a, Ar = Phenyl

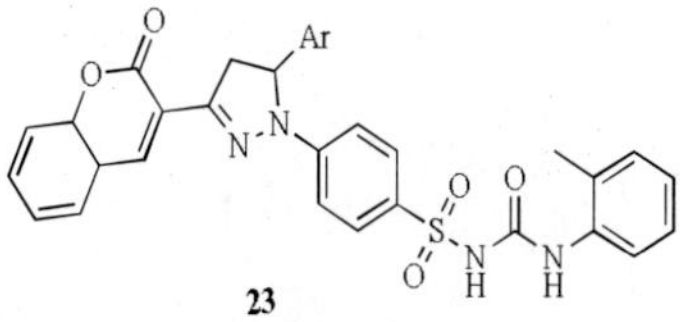

23

Ar = 4-dimethylphenyl, 4-methoxyphenyl, thiophen-2-yl
23a, Ar = 4-dimethylphenyl

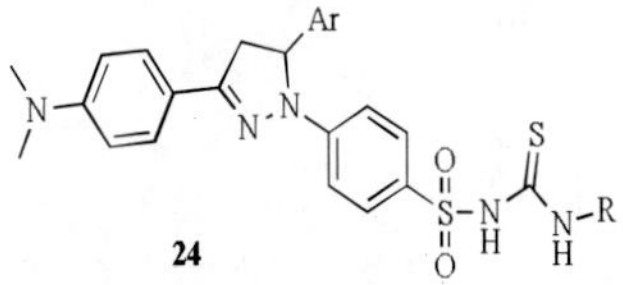

24

Ar = Ph, 4-CH_3Ph, 2-ClPh, 4-ClPh
R = -CH_2Ph, C_4H_9
24a, Ar = 4-ClPh; R = C_4H_9

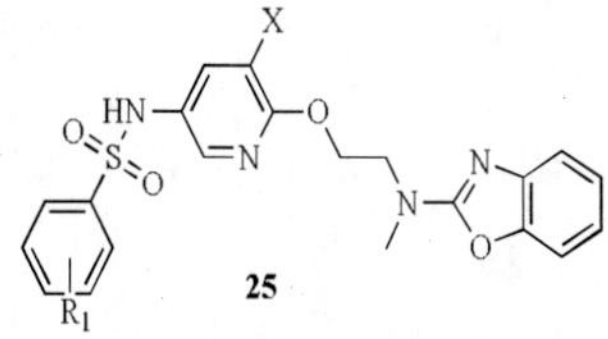

25

X = H, Cl
R1 = 2,4-diCl; 3-Cl,4-F; 2-Me
25a, X = Cl, R1 = 2,4-diCl

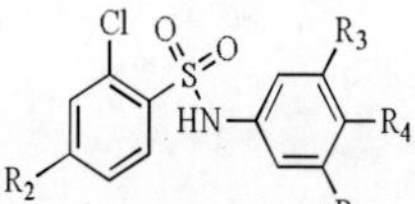

26

R2 = Cl, CF_3
R3 = H, Cl;
R4 = Cl, F, $COCH_3$

R5 =

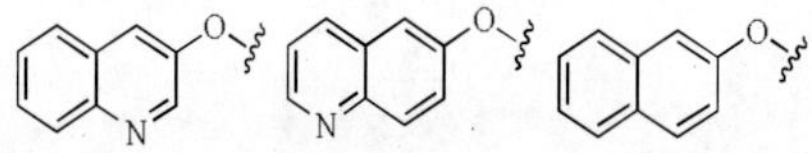

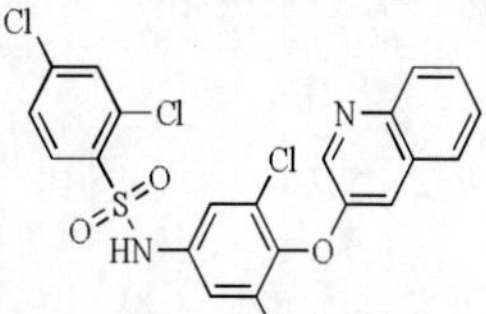

26a

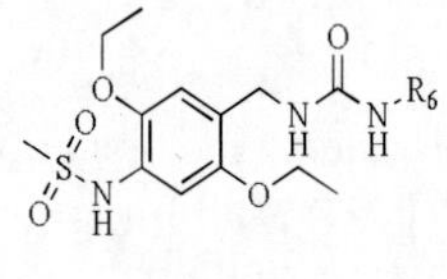

27

R6 = Ph, 4-MePh, 4-BrPh, 3-MeoPh, 4-MeoPh, 3,4-diMeoPh, benzyl
27a, R6 = 4-MeoPh

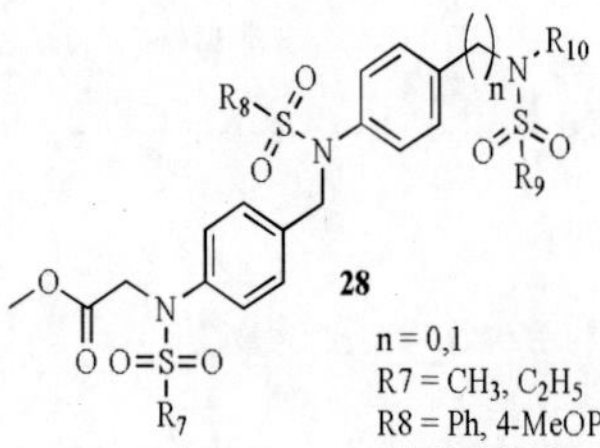

28

n = 0,1
R7 = CH_3, C_2H_5
R8 = Ph, 4-MeOPh, 4-EtOPh, 4-nPrOPh, 4-N-BuOPh, Benzyl
R9 = CH_3, EtOPh, Benzyl
R10 = Benzyl, 4-Me-Benzyl, 3-Cl-benzyl

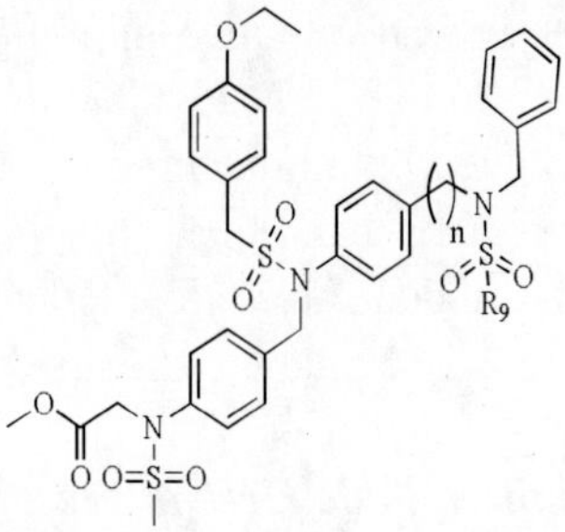

28a

Figure 8. (Continued)

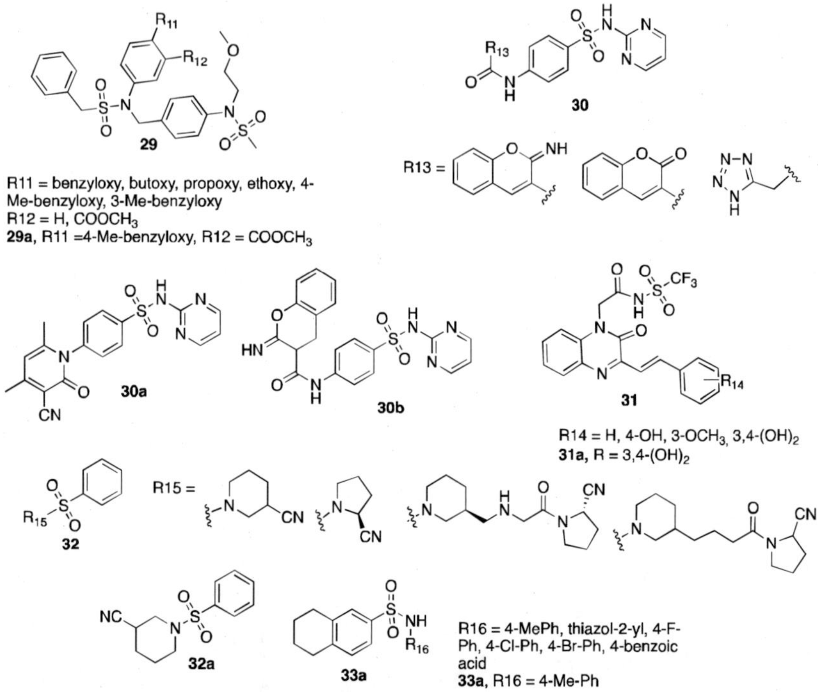

Figure 8. Sulphonyl urea and sulphonamide derivatives as PPAR-γ agonists, PTP1B, ALR2 and DPP-4 inhibitors.

Ghareb et al., also designed and examined a series of benzene-sulphonamide analogues for PTP1B inhibition.57 Two molecules **30a** and **30b** (Figure 8) showed effective inhibition (IC_{50} = 0.88 and 3.33 μM) as well reduction in body weight to 33% (dose =2 mg/kg) in rats on a high-fat diet. The derivatives with iminochromene and cyanopyridinone groups were found to be more active than others. In silico docking studies revealed H bonding, hydrophobic and electrostatic interactions between both compounds (**30a** and **30b**) and occupied catalytic site residues of the enzyme [34].

2.5.6. Sulphonamide Derivatives Attached to Heterocyclic Ring through Linkers

Ji et al., designed, synthesized and evaluated acyl sulphonamide based quinoxalinones derivatives and found **31a** (IC_{50} = 0.100 μM, Figure 8) as the most significant aldose reductase inhibitor amongst the series. *In silico* docking studies revealed the occupancy of compound 34a into catalytic pocket of the protein due to H bonding and π-π stacking interactions with Trp 111,

Thr 113, Tyr309, Trp111, Tyr48, Cys298 and His110 residues of enzyme, respectively. The presence of 2-OH at the C3 side chain and the acyl tri-fluoro methane sulphonamide at N1 are essential for activity and their replacement with other groups reduced the potency [35].

2.5.7. Sulphonamide Hybrids of Pyrrolidine and Piperidine

Sharma et al. designed and evaluated sulphonamides where amide nitrogen is shared with piperidine/pyrrolidine rings as DPP-4 inhibitors. Out of synthesized molecules, **32a** (Figure 8) exhibited the maximum potency (IC_{50} = 41.17 nM), in comparison to standard vildagliptin, which was further confirmed by *in silico* studies due to improved binding affinity (-7.4kcal/mol) with DPP-4 than the standard drug (-6.7 kcal/mol). It exhibited 59.17% DDP-4 inhibition (conc = 2 μM) in comparison to a standard drug (93.62%) due to the -CN group at the P1 site suggesting the potency of these scaffolds to develop significant antidiabetic drugs [36].

El-karim et al. designed and screened tetralin-sulphonamide analogues for their DPP-4 inhibition and reported **33a** (Figure 8) as the most efficacious DPP-4 inhibitor (IC_{50} value = 2.80 ± 0.0305 nM) with 20–40 times selective for DPP-9 and DPP-8. It was also concluded that the compounds with tetralin-sulphonamide scaffold (**33a**) and at para-substitution of phenyl with a smaller group exhibit the highest inhibition potency confirmed by significant binding affinities obtained after *in silico* analysis. The hypoglycaemic activity of **33a** was also observed after *in vivo* studies (IC_{50} = 0.09 ± 0.0173 μg/kg) in STZ-induced rats [37].

2.6. Indole Derivatives

2.6.1. Indole Scaffold Attached with Aromatic Rings

Eeda et al., designed and checked the indole analogues as PPAR-γ agonists. They found analogue **34a** (Figure 9) as the most efficacious PPAR-γ agonist (IC_{50} = 0.007 μM, Ki = 0.013 μM), using standard rosiglitazone (IC_{50} = 0.57 μM). Vanillylamine sustituted indole (**34a**) was observed with the highest agonistic activity. *In silico* evaluations showed the presence of H bonding interactions between **34a** and Ser342, Arg280, and Gln283 of the enzyme with a good docking score (−11.3 kcal/mol) [38].

2.6.2. Indole Scaffold Attached with Naphthyl Rings and Propanone Linker

Islam et al., designed and synthesized indole analogues for α-glucosidase inhibitory activity. Amongst the series, **35a** (Figure 9) was found with the maximum potency (IC_{50} = 11.8 ± 0.06 μM) due to 1-naphthyl-3-thiophene-propanone attached to the indole ring but the replacement of naphthyl group with a phenyl decrease the potency. *In silico* analysis revealed the H bonding interactions between the -NO_2 substituent of **35a** with Lys155, π-stacking of the naphthalene with His279 residue and π-cation interaction of thiophene group with His239 in the catalytic site of the α-glucosidase suggesting the stability with a good binding affinity of **35a** as a potential molecule for diabetes [39].

2.6.3. Indole Scaffold Attached to N1 Benzyl Ring

Wang et al., synthesized indole-based indolinone derivatives and evaluated their α-glucosidase inhibitory potential. Out of the synthesized molecules, **36a** (Figure 9) showed the maximum enzyme inhibition (IC_{50} = 5.98 ± 0.11 μM) due to the substituted benzyl group attached to the N1 of the indole.

In silico studies revealed its highest binding affinity to enzyme because of the attachment of two 2-fluorobenzyl groups on indole rings, as one of this group is responsible for hydrophobic interactions with the hydrophobic pocket of the α-glucosidase enzyme and the second one interacts through van der Waal interactions in the bottom pocket of the enzyme along with H bonding, arene-cation as well as π-π stacking interactions with the active sites, justifying the maximum potency of **36a** as α-glucosidase inhibitor [40].

Gollapalli et al., synthesized and examined bis-indolylmethane-sulphonohydrazide hybrids against α-glucosidase. They found **37a** (Figure 9) with highest potency (IC_{50} = 0.10 ± 0.05 μM) due to three Cl groups at 2,4,5-positions of the phenyl ring, which were found essential for the activity. *In silico* molecular docking studies showed the presence of H bonding interactions between O atoms of the SO_2, -C=O, and –NH group of **37a** with Asn241, Asp408 and Phe157, respectively. In addition, π-π stacking and hydrophobic interactions were also found with the amino acid residues at the active site of the enzyme, making it the perfect fit [41]. Nazir et al. described the synthesis of indole-oxadiazole hybrids and evaluated their antidiabetic activity as well as α-glucosidase inhibitory activity [42].

Taha et al. developed and examined tris-indole-oxadiazole hybrid analogues for α-glucosidase inhibition. The entire series of synthesized molecules exhibited significant inhibitory potential and **38a** (Figure 9) was found to be the most active ($IC_{50} = 2.00 \pm 0.01$ μM). The activity was found to improve with Cl group at R4 position but decrease on replacement with -Br group. *In silico* studies revealed the presence of H bonding, pi-pi stacking and hydrophobic interactions between **38a** and the catalytic site residue of the enzyme making it a more active molecule [43].

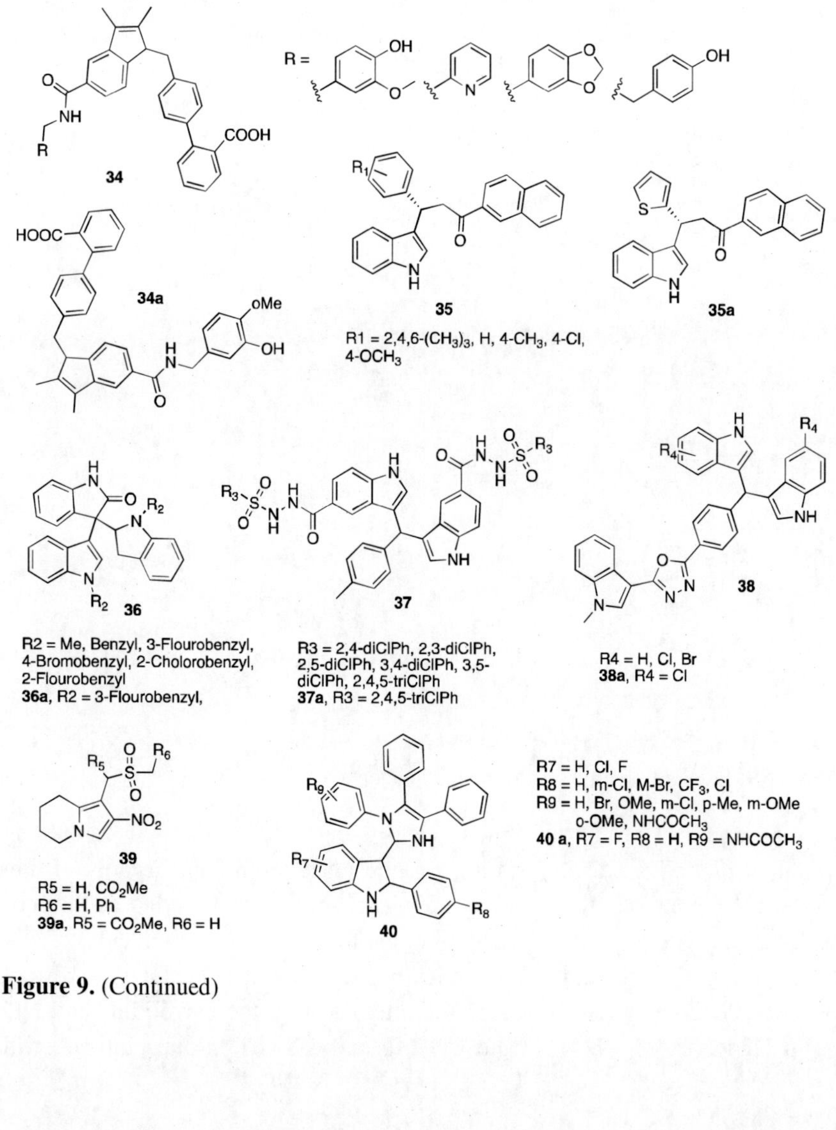

Figure 9. (Continued)

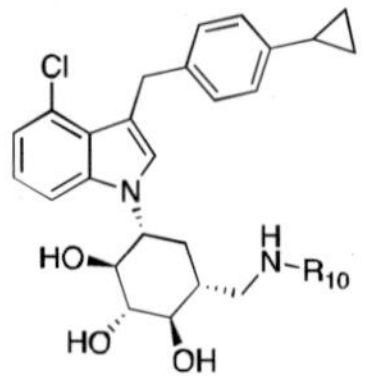

41

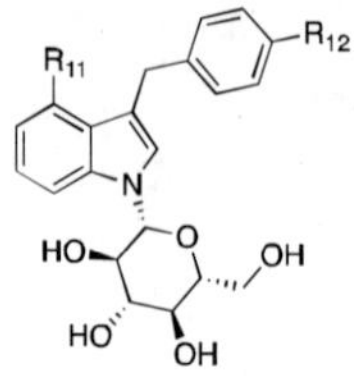

42

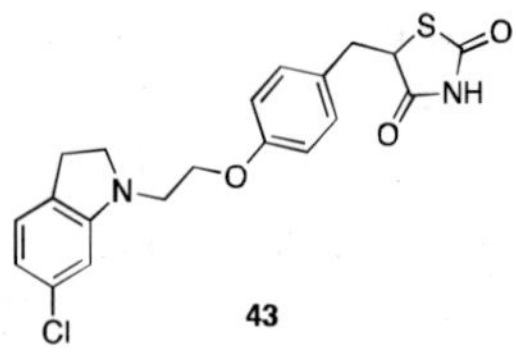

43

R10 = OH, OMe, OEt, CH_3CONH, CH_3OCONH
41a, R10 = CH_3CONH

R11 = H, F, CH_3
R12 = Et, OEt, Cl
42a, R11= CH_3, R12 = cyclopropyl

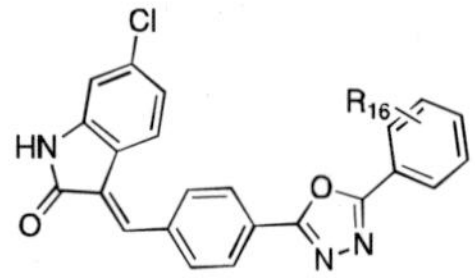

46

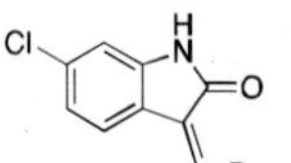

44

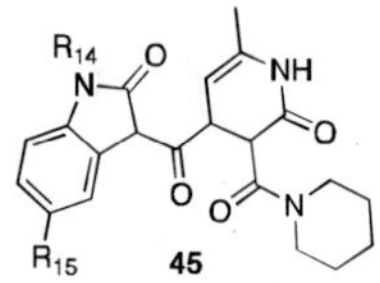

45

R13 = 3,4-diOHPh, 2-NO2Ph, 2-OH-3-OC2H5Ph, 3-OHPh, 4-OHPh, anthracenyl, 4-isopropylPh
44a, R13 = 3,4-diOHPh

R14 = H, Benzyl, Me
R15 = H, F, Br, NO_2
45a R14 = H, R15 = F

R16 = 2,4-diOH, 2,5-diOH, 3,5-diOH, 3,4-diOH
46a, R16 = 3,5-diOH,

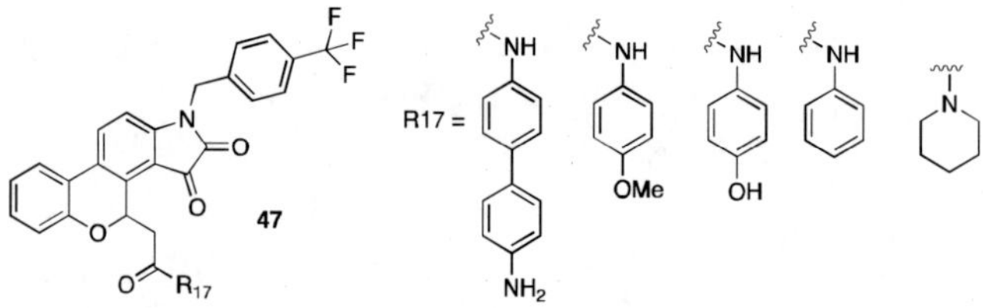

47

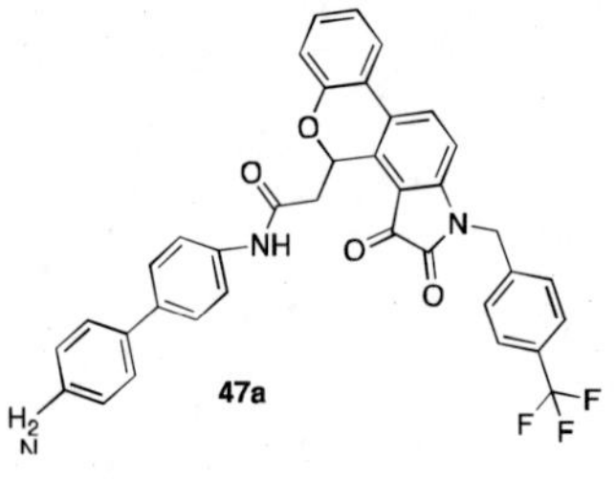

47a

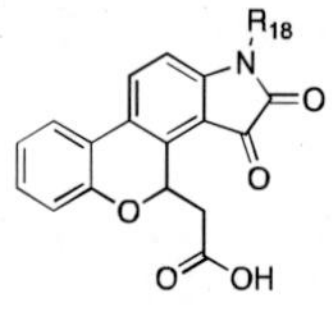

48

R18 = Me, Bn, 4-CF_3-Bn
48a, R18 = 4-CF_3-Bn

Figure 9. Indole derivatives as antidiabetic agents.

Tavani et al. designed and evaluated methyl sulphonyl tetrahydroindolizine analogues for α-glucosidase inhibition. Because of non-covalent interactions with enzyme, **39a** (Figure 9) was reported as the most efficacious (IC_{50} = 8.0 ± 0.1 μM) amongst the synthesized molecules. It was observed that unsubstituted R5 and R6 positions reduced the enzyme binding affinity. *In silico* studies revealed the interaction of the pyrrolidine and NO_2 with H245, H279, N241, while CO_2Me and SO_2CH_3 groups interact with

H239 and R312 residues of enzyme. Analogue **39a** was suggested as a mixed inhibitor and showed 25 times better inhibitory potential than the standard [44].

Naureen et al. designed and evaluated imidazole-indole hybrids for their α-glucosidase inhibition. Analogue **40a** (Figure 9) was found as the highest potency inhibitor (IC_{50} = 8.37 ± 0.11 μM) in comparison to the standard acarbose drug (IC_{50} = 37.25 ± 0.15 μM) due to the presence of $NHCOCH_3$ and F groups at R9 and R7 position rather than other substituents along free NH of the indole nucleus. All these substituents were found important for the inhibition activity amongst the synthesised molecules suggesting the potential of this class as potent antidiabetic drugs [45].

2.6.4. N-Glucosyl Indoles

Chu et al., reported and examined N-glucosyl indole derivatives as SGLT2 inhibitors. They found compound **41a** (Figure 9) as the most significant hSGLT2 inhibitor (EC_{50} = 33 nM). The presence of larger alkoxy groups in **41a** was found to decrease the inhibitory potency against hSGLT2. This molecule was found to possess lack of selectivity for hSGLT1 (EC_{50} = 37 nM) and enhanced the urinary glucose excretion (825 mg/200 g bodyweight, dose = 50 mg/kg), in comparison to the standard drug dapagliflozin (2762 mg/200 g body weight, dose =1 mg/ kg) as per *in vivo* studies [46].

Nomura et al., also reported indole-N-glucosides and found cyclopropyl derivative **42a** (Figure 9) as the strongest SGLT2 inhibitor (IC_{50} value = 1.6 nM). The replacement of chlorine with -C_2H_5 and -O C_2H_5 group as R2 enhanced the inhibition potential. In high-fat diet-fed KK (HF-KK) mice, it reduced the blood sugar AUC to 50% (dose = 3 mg/ kg) and revealed exceptional PK profiles in SD rats (F = 78%, $t_{1/2}$ = 3.9 h), suggesting its potential to the treat T2DM [47].

2.6.5. Heterocyclic Indole Derivatives

Darwish et al., designed a series of benzhydryl and indole-based TZDs as PPAR-γ/FFAR1 dual agonists and found **43** (Figure 9) as most active with the highest hPPAR-γ (EC_{50} = 4.51 μM) and FFAR1 (EC_{50} = 5.06 μM) agonistic activity in comparison to standard drug rosiglitazone. *In silico* studies showed the fitting of **43** into the active sites of PPAR-γ and FFAR1, implying this molecule for future modifications as dual PPAR-γ/FFAR1 agonists [48].

2.6.6. Indol-2one Derivatives

Khan et al., designed 6-chloro-3-oxindole analogues and evaluated only E-configurations for α-glucosidase inhibition. They reported **44a** (Figure 9) as the most potent (IC_{50} = 2.71 ± 0.007 μM) amongst series, compared to acarbose due to the presence of H bonding interactions between two OH groups with Asp349, Glu276, Asp214 of the α-glucosidase. These groups polarise the compound and make stronger interactions with the enzyme [49].

Luthra et al., also synthesized and investigated indol-2-one derivatives against this enzyme. The compound **45a** (Figure 9) was found to be the most active (IC_{50} = 0.646 ± 0.05 μM) competitive inhibitor due to the presence of the indole ring, which interacts with the enzyme. Amongst substituents, F at the C5 of indole ring and -H at R1 position enhances the interaction and activity of enzyme [50].

Taha et al., developed oxindole-based oxadiazole hybrids and evaluated their inhibitory potential against α-glucosidase. Amongst the synthesized molecules, analogue **46a** (Figure 9) was reported as the most potent (IC_{50} = 1.25 ± 0.05 μM). The presence of 2 OH groups, meta to each other as in resorcinol moiety was found better for activity. *In silico* studies showed 2 H-bonds between resorcinol of compound 53a with Lys155, Asp349, and 1 H bond between the -C=O group of the 6-chloroindolin-2-one moiety with Lys233. The arene-cation interaction was also found amongst Arg312 residue and 1,3,4-oxadiazole moiety, implying future research for identifying pharmacophores to develop better antidiabetes drugs [51].

2.6.7. Indol-2,4-Dione Nucleus

Sun et al., designed and examined tetracyclic oxindole derivatives inhibitory activity against this enzyme. The analogue **47a** (Figure 9) was observed with maximum potency as inhibitor (IC_{50} = 0.7 μM), 170 fold than standard acarbose. 4-(trifluoromethyl) benzyl in the N-1 position and aromatic amine as R showed improved inhibition. *In silico* evaluations showed the presence of H bonding and pi interactions in the 4-(trifluoromethyl) benzyl group of **47a** with Ser505 and Lys506, respectively. The benzidine ring also formed H bonds along with van der Waal interactions with the active sites, causing the perfect fit of **51a** inside the active pocket of the α-glucosidase. A σ-π interaction was also observed between **47a** and Trp329, implying its potential against α-glucosidase [52].

Han et al. synthesized and examined tetracyclic indole-2,4-dione analogues as α-glucosidase inhibitors *in vitro*. They reported compound **52a** with maximum α-glucosidase inhibition (IC_{50} = 4.8 μM) in comparison to the reference acarbose drug (IC_{50} = 115.8 μM). The 4-(trifluoromethyl) benzyl group in the N-1 position enhanced the enzyme inhibition. In silico docking studies revealed the good binding affinity of these molecules due to H bonding (K506 and W432 residues) as well as hydrophobic interactions (4-trifluoromethyl benzyl group) with the enzyme [53].

2.7. Spiro Imidazolidinones Derivatives

Iqbal et al., developed 3-arylsulphonylspiroimidazolidine-2,4-dione as aldose reductase inhibitors and found compound **48a** (Figure 10) with the highest potency (IC_{50} = 0.89 μM) as well as a better hyperglycaemic agent *in vivo*. This molecule was also found to decrease the blood glucose level in mice by 72.24% compared to the standard drug (glibenclamide; 60.92% reduction). *In silico* analysis showed the replacement of 4-Cl of the aryl group in **48a** with -CH_3, -OCH_3, or -NO_2 group reduced the inhibition activity and replacement of 4-chlorophenyl moiety with naphthyl or 2-anthraquinyl group resulted in loss of activity [54].

Iqbal et al., designed another series of arylsulfonylspiroimidazolidine-2′,4′-diones and assessed their potential against MIN6 and HEK293 (human embryonic kidney cell lines). Most of the synthesized molecules showed significant human recombinant aldose reductase enzyme inhibition and insulin release in MIN6 cells. However, compound **49a** (Figure 10) showed the highest potency (IC_{50} = 0.56 ± 0.05 μM) in comparison to the standard drug epalrestat (IC_{50} = 0.62 ± 0.35 μM). The isopropyl group on phenyl ring was found to enhance the ALR2 inhibition more than other groups. In addition, **49a** inhibited the accumulation of sorbitol in isolated erythrocytes (IC_{50} = 0.85 ± 0.04 μM) as well as in rat lens (IC_{50} = 0.65 ± 0.05 μM) depending upon dose and showed negligible cytotoxicity (14.25% inhibition, Conc = 50 μM) in HEK293 cell lines. *In silico* studies showed the presence of 3 H bonds between 31a and the His110 and Trp111 of ALR2 enzyme residues. Hydrophobic interactions and π-π stacking were also observed with the enzyme suggesting the potential of **49a** for the future development of aldose reductase inhibitor as a clinical drug [55].

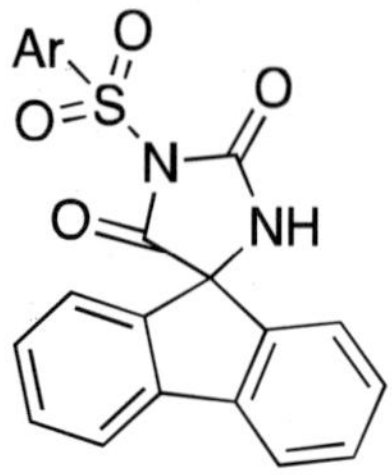

48

Ar = p-MePh, p-ClPh, p-BrPh, p-NO_2Ph, p-OMePh, Naphthyl, anthraquinon-2-yl
48a, Ar = p-ClPh

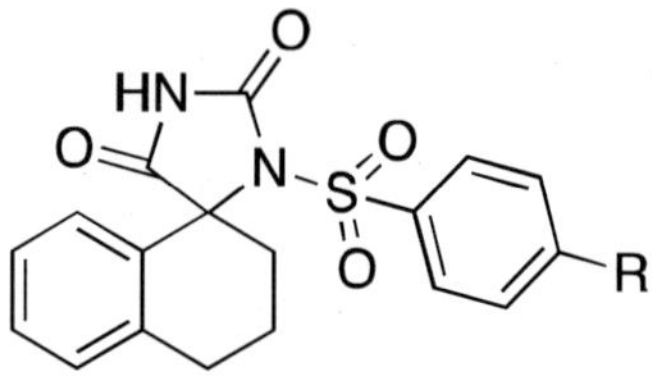

49

R = F, Cl, Br, Me, Nitro, isopropyl, acetyl, OMe
49a, R = isopropyl

Figure 10. Spiro-imidazolidines as antidiabetic agents.

2.8. Amide Hybrids

2.8.1. Non-Heterocyclic Amide Hybrids

Chen et al. synthesized GPR40 agonists with an amide linker and found compound **50a** (Figure 11) with the highest hGPR40 potency (EC_{50} = 20 nM) along with the maximum *in vitro* as well as *in vivo* potential with excellent PK profiles ($T_{1/2}$ = 5.3 h in ICR mice). Still, they exhibited a noticeable blood glucose level (dose = 2.5 g/kg) reduction in ICR mice. They found molecules with benzene or furan linker with better GPR40 agonistic activity and recommended **50a** as a favorable molecule for future development in diabetes [56].

Xie et al., found **52a** as the most active PTP1B inhibitor (Figure 11) from a series of 2-ethoxy-4-(methoxymethyl) benzamide derivatives (IC_{50} = 0.07 µM). It also increased the glucose uptake stimulated by insulin to 75% at 20 µM in HepG2 cells compared to standard pioglitazone (64.1%). It was observed that 2-ethoxy-4-(methoxymethyl)benzamide is essential for PTP1B inhibition and longer hydrophobic chains on benzamide moiety reduce the activity. These chains formed hydrophobic interactions with K121, E116, and R222 residues and occupy the hydrophobic region of the enzyme [57].

Mohammadi-khanaposhtani et al. synthesized acridine-thioacetamide derivatives against α-glucosidase. They found **53a** exhibited the maximum potency (IC_{50} = 80.0 ± 2.0 µM). In silico evaluations showed the presence of H bonding, hydrophobic and π-π interactions of **53a** with α-glucosidase enzyme. The presence of 4-CH_3 substituent on N-phenyl ring was reported to be responsible for the highest potency, while the molecules -Cl group at 3rd position were found to be more active than 3,4-dichloro followed by 4-Cl and 2-Cl. However, in case of $-OCH_3$ substitution on N-phenyl ring, the molecules with $-OCH_3$ at 3 positions were reported as more active in comparison to the molecules possessing $4-OCH_3$ and $2-OCH_3$. They observed H bonding, hydrophobic, π-cation as well as π-π interactions between $2-OCH_3$, 6-Cl and acridine ring of compound **100a** with the residues of the α-glucosidase, respectively [58].

2.8.2. Heterocyclic Amide Hybrids

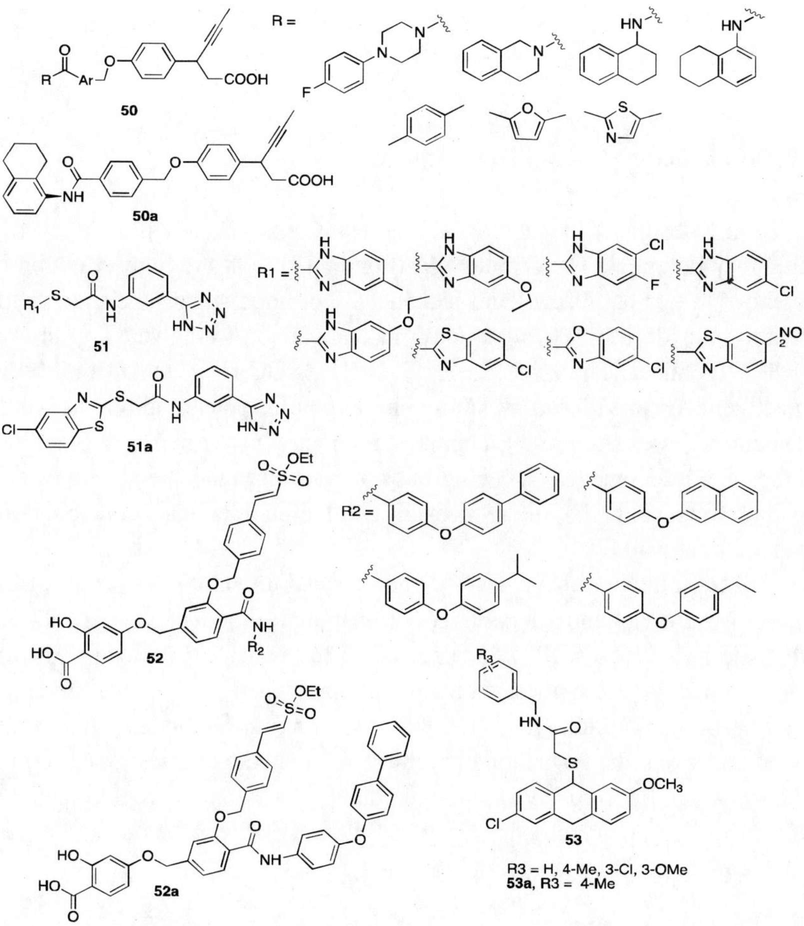

Figure 11. Amide hybrids as antidiabetic agents.

Maheshwari et al., designed tetrazole acetamide derivatives as PTP1B inhibitors and reported **51a** (Figure 11) with the highest potency (IC_{50} = 1.88 μM) in comparison to standard drug suramin ($IC_{50} \geq 10$ μM). The derivatives with benzothiazole ring exhibited higher inhibition than with benzoxazole or benzimidazole. The substituents played a vital role in case of derivatives with benzimidazole as the loss of potency was reported with electron-withdrawing and electron-rich groups on the benzo ring, while halogens enhanced the activity. For benzothiazole derivatives, $-NO_2$ and -Cl groups on the benzo ring showed increased activity. In silico studies showed the H bonding of compound 22a with Arg221 and Gln262 residues. In comparison to the standard drug glimepiride (23.61%), **51a** reduced the blood sugar level to a larger extent (30.25%, dose = 30mg/kg) in Sprague Dawley rats *in vivo* implying it as a PTP1B inhibitor [59].

2.9. Halogenated Phenol Derivatives

Li et al., designed bromophenol analogues and examined their PTP1B inhibitory potential. They found **54a** (Figure 12) with the highest inhibition potency (IC_{50} = 0.190 μM) and it reduced the blood sugar levels as well as weight gain (dose = 100 mg/kg/day) in comparison to the standard drug in BKS DB mice. The presence of $-OCH_3$, $-OC_2H_5$, and methoxyethyl substituents on phenyl ring was found important for potent inhibition, and the molecules possessing these groups also interact with the hydrophobic region of the enzyme. However, $-OC_2H_5$ groups interact through H bond with Arg254 residue suggesting the future possibility of **54a** as a lead compound for diabetic treatment [60].

Chatzopoulu et al., synthesized and checked the inhibition potency of 2-fluoro-4-pyrrolylphenol derivatives against aldose reductase (ALR2) and aldehyde reductase (ALR1) enzyme. From the series, **55a** (Figure 12) was found to possess the highest ALR2 inhibition ($IC_{50} = 0.443 \pm 0.03$ μM) and potent ALR1 inhibition ($IC_{50} = 12.10 \pm 0.46$ μM) in rat kidneys. It was also found to prevent the formation of sorbitol in isolated rat lenses. The presence of phenol or 2-fluoro phenol exhibited potent activity but the replacement of -OH with -F group decreased activity and the $-OCH_3$ group on benzoyl moiety enhanced the inhibitory potential [61].

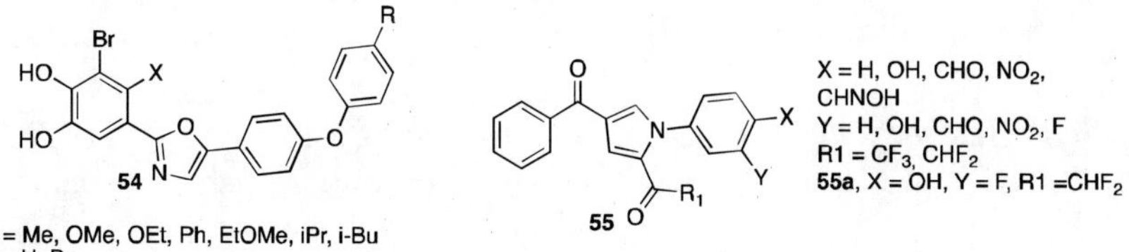

Figure 12. Phenol derivatives as antidiabetic agents.

2.10. Quinoline and Isoquinoline Derivatives

Crespo et al., designed 1-oxopyrimido[4,5-c]quinoline-2-acetic acid derivatives as aldose reductase inhibitors and found 2-acetic acid derivatives as potent human aldose reductase inhibitor than 2-amino derivatives. Amongst the series, analogue **56a** (Figure 13) exhibited the highest inhibition (IC_{50} = 0.12 ± 0.004 μM) and selectivity for AKR1B1 along with potent, selective inhibition of AKR1B10 (IC_{50} = 4.71 μM). The potency was found to enhance with the presence of alkyl chain in the R3 position due to interaction with Leu 300 enzyme residue but was lost on replacing -H with -F at R1 position [62].

Banno et al., developed and examined aminomethyl-isoquinolones as DPP-4 inhibitors. They reported **66a** (Figure 13) as the most active inhibitor from the series (IC_{50} = 0.24 μM) with an improvement in glucose tolerance in Wistar fatty rats (minimum dose = 0.3 mg/kg). The presence of hydrophilic substituents at 6-position (R15) position of 4-phenyl-1-iso-quinolone moiety enhanced the activity and the highest inhibition potency was observed with carbamoylmethoxy group at R15 position. X-ray crystal structure showed the presence of H bonding, hydrophobic and van der Waals interactions between **66a** with residue Lys554, residue Phe357, and with Tyr547 residue of the protein, respectively [63].

Pan et al. designed and checked tetrahydroisoquinoline-C-aryl glucosides analogues. From the series, analogue **67a** (Figure 13) with naphthalene group displayed the highest SGLT2 inhibitory potency (81.7%) in comparison to the standard drug dapagliflozin (85.4%). The loss of activity was observed with the replacement of naphthalene ring with thiophene. However, weak electron-withdrawing, as well as electron-donating groups at the 4′-position of the distal ring, improves the inhibitory activity against SGLT2 [64].

2.11. Quinazolinone Derivatives

2.11.1. Heterocyclic Quinazolinone Derivatives

El-Sayed et al., synthesized and tested quinazolinone-based rhodanine-3-acetic acid derivatives for inhibitory activity against aldose reductase. They reported **57a** (Figure 13) with the highest inhibitory activity (IC_{50} = 0.0497 μM) and was found to be 3-times more active than the reference drug epalrestat. *In silico* studies demonstrated the highest binding affinity (−11.05 kcal/mol) of **57a** and the polar anion binding site occupancy of the enzyme. The presence of H bonding with Tyr48 residue and hydrophobic interaction with Leu300 residue was reported. The reduction in potency was reported with bulky groups at the 3-phenyl ring of quinazolinone moiety, but the presence of $-OCH_3$ at the central benzene ring enhanced the activity [65].

2.11.2. Alkoxy Quinazolinone Derivatives

Javaid et al. developed and evaluated 2-arylquinazolin-4(3H)-one derivatives as yeast α-glucosidase inhibitors. Four derivatives of **58** (Figure 13) showed several hundred-fold higher activities than the standard drug acarbose, (IC_{50} = 0.3 ± 0.01 to 117.9 ± 1.76 μM) and **58a** (Figure 13) displayed the highest activity (IC_{50} = 0.3 ± 0.1 μM). The nature of inhibition was revealed by the kinetic study as competitive inhibition (K_i = 0.43 ± 0.0067 μM). The $-OCH_2CH_3$, -OH and -Ph groups on **58a** were found responsible for the highest activity due to interactions with residues at the enzyme binding site. *In silico* studies showed π-π stacking interactions of aromatic rings of **58a** with Trp376, Trp481, and Trp516 residues, responsible for its greater stability and binding affinity [66].

2.11.3. Non-Heterocyclic Quinazolinone Derivatives

Wei et al., also developed and examined quinazolinone derivatives for their α-glucosidase inhibition. They reported analogues, **59a** and **59b** (Figure 13) with the highest inhibitory activity (IC_{50} = 12.5 ± 0.1 and 15.6 ± 0.2 μM, respectively). The inhibition was found to be enhanced with -Cl and -Br and lost with the presence of -F, $-NO_2$, or $-N(CH_3)_2$ at C-4′ position of the phenyl ring. H bonding (O atom of quinazoline, -Cl groups with Ala451 and Ser44 residues), electrostatic along with hydrophobic interactions were found between **59a** and the α-glucosidase enzyme. But **59b** interacts weakly through hydrophobic interactions with residues His348, Ala444 and Ala454 of the enzyme [67].

Zhang et al., designed quinazoline-1-deoxynojirimycin hybrid and checked α-glucosidase inhibition activity. They reported **60** (Figure13) as the most potent α-glucosidase inhibitor (IC_{50} = 0.09 μM) compared to the standard drug miglitol due to the presence of 1-DNJ moiety at the C-7 position, linked by -$OCH_2CH_2CH_3$ chain. Thus, **60a** can lead to the future development of α-glucosidase inhibitors [68].

Ibrahim et al., synthesized and assessed quinazoline-4(3H)-one derivative as PPAR-γ and SUR agonist. They found compounds **61a** and **61b** (Figure 13) with the highest PPAR-γ agonistic potency (IC_{50} = 0.350 and 0.369 μM, respectively) along with potent insulin-secreting activities (EC_{50} values of 0.97 and 1.01 μM, respectively). *In silico* studies revealed their high affinity towards PPAR-γ and SUR, suggesting their further development as a new drug [69].

2.12. Quinazoline and Quinoxaline Derivatives

2.12.1. Heterocyclic Quinazoline-Triazole Hybrids

Saeedi et al., synthesized quinazolinone-1,2,3-triazole derivatives and checked their inhibition potential on α-glucosidase. They found analogues **62a** and **62b** (Figure 13) with the highest potency (IC_{50} = 181.0 ± 1.4 and 192.3 ± 1.8 μM, respectively). *In silico* studies revealed the presence of H-bonding and pi-pi stacking interactions between the quinazolinone moiety of **62a** with the His279 residues of the α-glucosidase enzyme. The molecules possessing substituents at 4th position of benzyl moiety were found with enhanced activity, particularly with 4-Br group (highest inhibition). In case of **62b**, several hydrophobic and H bonding interactions, specifically with 3-OCH_3 group at the phenyl ring of **62b** with the Arg312 residue of the α-glucosidase enzyme were reported [70].

2.12.2. Heterocyclic Quinazoline Derivatives

Ali et al., developed and evaluated quinazoline-thiazoline derivatives against the DPP-4 enzyme. They found analogue **63a** (Figure 13) the most active (IC_{50} = 0.76 nM). The presence of -NO_2 at the R2 position of phenyl ring was observed to increase the inhibition activity. *In silico* studies demonstrated many non-covalent interactions such as H-bonding, π-π stacking and hydrophobic interactions between **63a**, and residues Arg125, Arg699, residues Arg125, Phe357, Tyr547, and residues Glu205, Try662, Try631, Asn710, Trp659, Ser630, Gly632, Val546, His740, Lys544 of the protein respectively.

Hence, **63a** can be used for the future development of novel antidiabetic drugs [71].

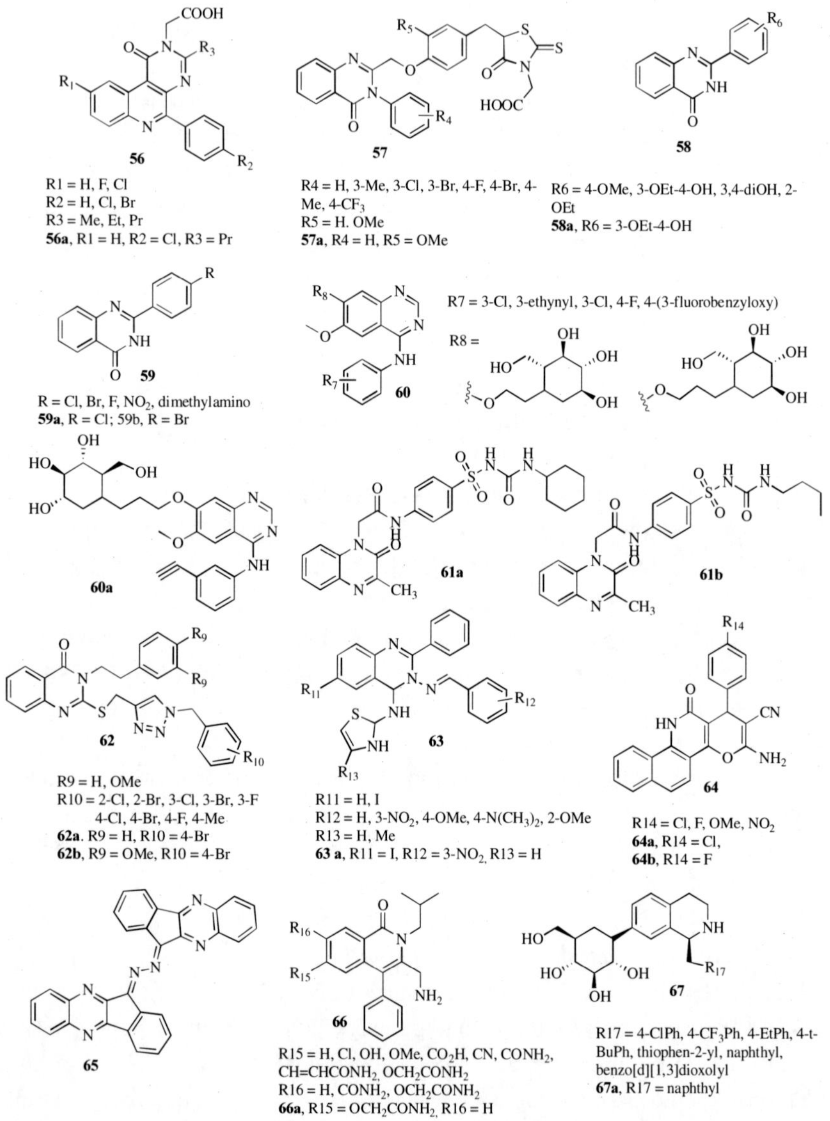

Figure 13. Quinolines, isoquinoline, quinazoline and quinoxaline analogues as antidiabetic agents.

2.12.3. Heterocyclic Quinoline Hybrids

Nikookar et al. reported and evaluated dihydropyrano[3,2-c]quinoline derivatives for α-glucosidase inhibition. Analogues **64a** and **64b** (Figure 13) displayed the highest enzyme inhibition (IC_{50} = 10.3 ± 0.3 and 15.7 ± 0.5 μM, respectively). The substitution of phenyl ring at 4th position enhanced the activity. The compound **64a** was found as un-competitive (K_i = 11 μM) and **64b** as a non-competitive inhibitor (K_i = 28 μM) as per kinetic studies. These compounds were found safe during cytotoxicity studies on breast cancer cell lines [72].

2.12.4. Heterocyclic Quinoxaline Hybrids

Khan et al., reported and assessed Indeno-quinoxaline hybrids against α-glucosidase. Amongst the series, **65** (Figure 13) exhibited the highest enzyme inhibition (IC_{50} = 18.23 ± 0.37 μM), in comparison to standard drug acarbose (IC_{50} = 38.25 ± 0.12 μM) due to the presence of ylidene type structure [73].

2.13. Miscellaneous Derivatives

2.13.1. Substituted Pyrrole Acetate Derivatives

Xiu et al., designed and checked 1-Acetyl-5-phenyl-1H-pyrrol-3-ylacetate (**68**) (Figure 14) for aldose reductase inhibition. They found **68** as potent aldose reductase inhibitor (IC_{50} = 0.0223 μM) and prevented HG-induced HBZY-1 cell to death at 0.9 μM, compared to standard drug epalrestat. It was also found to decrease the blood sugar levels of STZ-induced DN rats implying its potential as a clinical candidate for type 2 diabetes [74].

2.13.2. N-Substituted Pyrroles and Pyrrolidines

Winters et al., designed and examined N-arylpyrroles as GPR120 agonists. Authors reported compound **69a** (Figure 14) with 2,6-difluoropropionic acid moiety as a potent GPR120 agonist (EC_{50} = 80 nM). The substitution at 4th position of aryl group was found to improve the activity. Compound **69a** showed a good PK profile, a positive effect in the oral glucose tolerance test on mice, noteworthy decreased blood glucose (dose of 30 mg/kg) and body weight by 4.6% in the DIO mouse model. It also displayed good selectivity and potency for related receptor GPR40 [75].

2.13.3. Halogenated Cyanopyrrolidine Analogues as DPP-4 Inhibitors

Fukushima et al., designed a potent DPP-IV inhibitor **70** (IC_{50} = 4.6 nM) (Figure 14) from the 4-fluoro-2-cyanopyrrolidine derivatives. X-ray crystallography evaluations displayed the fitting of 2-hydroxy-1,1-dimethylethyl moiety of analogue **70** in the core pocket of the enzyme formed by Arg358, His126, Ser201, Arg358 and Phe357 to achieve high affinity. It was found to reduce the plasma glucose in an oral glucose tolerance test in rats (dose = 0.3 mg/kg) and inhibits DPP-IV after glucose loading at 0.1 and 0.3 mg/kg at 15min. The benzenesulphonic acid salt of **70** (**TS-021**), is a potent and long-duration DPP-IV inhibitor selected as a clinical candidate [76].

Fukushima et al., also synthesized and evaluated 3- or 4-substituted 2-cyanopyrrolidines derivatives as DPP-IV inhibitors. Authors reported 4-F derivatives more potent and gave positive results for the glucose tolerance test than 3-substituted ones in rats. Analogue **70a** (Figure 14) was found to be most potent (IC_{50} = 0.6 nM) and lowered the blood glucose level in an oral glucose tolerance test, in Zucker fatty rats suggesting the future utility of these compounds as antidiabetic drugs [77].

Haffner et al., also synthesized and evaluated 2-cyano-4-fluoro-thiovalyl-pyrrolidines against DPP-IV. They found analogue **71a** (Figure 14) as the most potent among series, with longest duration of activity in both dogs and rats. It caused inhibition of DPP-4 to 84% (dose =1 mpk) in rat with a 6h duration and >12h above the IC_{50} = 0.2 mpk in the dog. The pharmacokinetic profile of **71a** was observed better amongst the series (K_i = 53 nM) [78].

Wang et al., designed and assessed imidazoline-2-cyanopyrrolidine analogues for their DPP-IV inhibition. Authors found compound **72a** (Figure 14) with the highest inhibitory activity (IC_{50} = 2.0 nM) due to two $-OCH_3$ groups in the phenyl ring [79].

Tsai et al., also developed and evaluated arylcyclopropylamine-2-cyanopyrrolidine based hybrids against DPP-4. Compound **73a** (Figure 14) was found with the highest inhibition potency (IC_{50} = 0.15 μM) and selectivity due to the presence of -F group on 2-cyanopyrrolidine (S form). It also showed a moderate bioavailability (42%), exceptional pharmacokinetic profiles ($t_{1/2}$ = 4.8 h) in rats, and lowered plasma glucose levels to 73% (dose = 10 mg/kg) [80].

Liu et al., developed and checked (S)-phenylalanine analogues with a 2-cyanopyrrolidine moiety, as DPP-4 inhibitors. Almost all the derivatives showed potent inhibitory activity along with selectivity and compound **74a** (Figure 14) showed the highest potency (IC_{50} = 0.247 μM) as well as better selectivity. The phenylalanine analogues were found with better activity than alanine derivatives. The ring expansion from cyclopropyl to cyclobutyl, caused a loss of activity. In silico studies showed the occupancy of 2-cyanopyrrolidine ring of **74a** into the hydrophobic S1 pocket of the enzyme. The NH_2 and -C=O groups showed H-bond interactions with residues Glu205, Glu206, and Asn710, respectively. The N-1 nitrogen atom of the triazole moiety of **74a** also showed H-bonding interactions with the enzyme residue Arg358, for better fit and higher DPP-4 inhibition potency [81].

Liu et al., also developed and examined benzyl-phenylalanine derivatives with a 2-cyanopyrrolidine moiety, as DPP-4 inhibitors. All analogues displayed potent inhibitory activity and selectivity but analogue **75a** (Figure 14) showed the most potent activity (IC_{50} = 3.79 nM) as well as better selectivity against DPP-4. The molecules with substitution at p-position of benzyl group displayed better activity than at -o/-m-position. **75a** also reported to reduce the blood glucose levels in the oral glucose tolerance test of normal Sprague Dawley rats and inhibit the glucose-induced blood glucose increase by 28% (dose =10 mg/kg) [82].

Wang et al., also developed, and tested carbonitrile-pyrrolidine-2 and 4-fluoropyrrolidine derivatives against DPP-4 inhibitors. They reported compound **76a** (Figure 14) the most active (IC_{50} = 0.017 μM), with moderate selectivity and reduce plasma glucose levels to 27.57% (dose = 30 mg/kg) in ICR mice in oral glucose resistance tests due to its high binding affinity with the enzyme where the 4-fluoropyrrolidine moiety occupied the S1 pocket of the enzyme, and the -F forms H bond with various enzyme residues [83].

Ji et al., synthesized and investigated α-amino pyrrole-2-carbonitrile analogues with hetero-aromatic moieties against DPP-4. They found 77**a** and **77b** (Figure 14) as the most potent (IC_{50} = 0.004 μM and IC_{50} = 0.01 μM, respectively) due to the presence of p-fluoropyrrolidine-2-carbonitrile moeity, which occupy the hydrophobic pocket. In contrast, the -C=O and α-NH_2 groups formed H-bond interactions with the amino acid residues. The -F atom in the pyrrole-2-carbonitrile enhances the activity owing to H bonding with the enzyme residue [84].

2.13.4. Heterocyclic Pyrrolidine Analogues

Kondo et al., also designed and examined L-prolylpyrrolidine derivatives as DPP-IV inhibitors. From the series, analogue **78a** (Figure 14) was found to be most potent (IC_{50} = 14 nM for human DPP- IV) due to its S-containing hetero-aromatic moiety and 95% plasma DPP-IV inhibition in normal rats (dose =3mg/kg) with a 30 min duration. It was found active in both human as well as rat plasma (IC_{50} = 41 and 60 nM, respectively) [85].

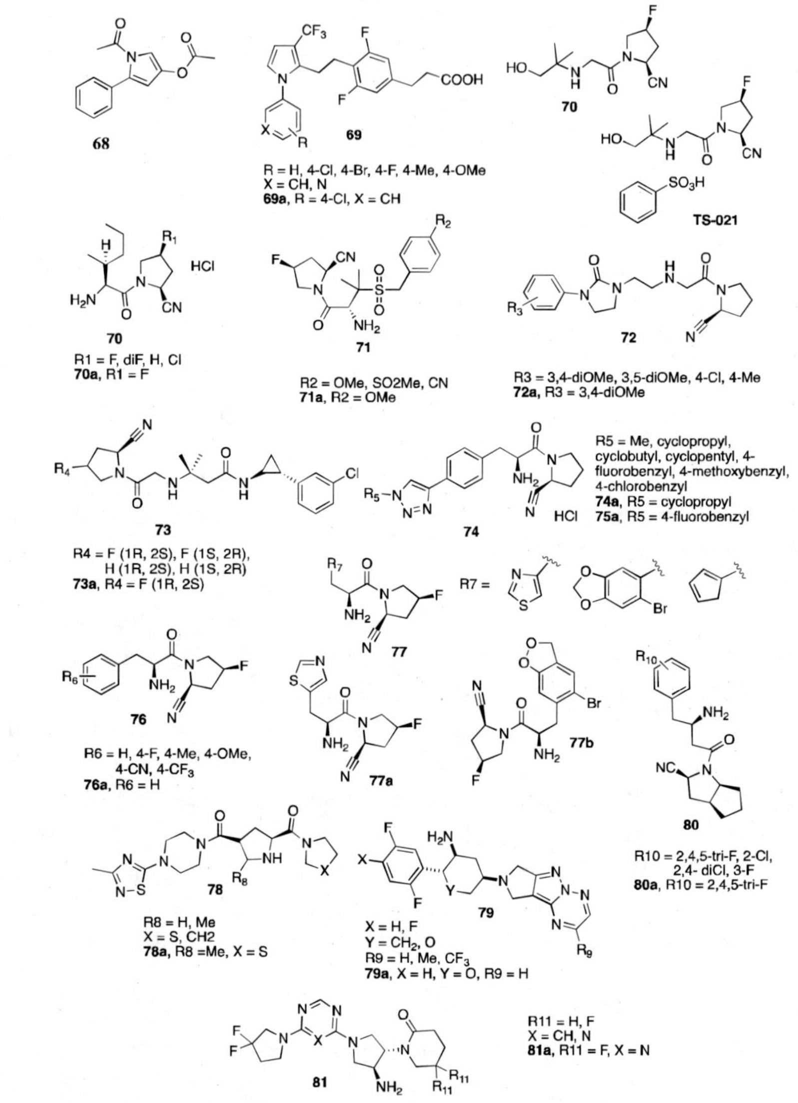

Figure 14. Pyrrole analogues as antidiabetic agents.

Cox et al., developed 5,6,5- and 5,5,6- tricyclic pyrrolidines analogues against the DPP-4. They reported analogue **79a** (Figure 14), from the 5,5,6-tricyclic pyrrolidine series, as the most potent (IC_{50} = 0.12 nM). The replacement of X=H to -F caused a rise in DDP-8 inhibition potency. Analogue **79a** showed excellent DPP-8 and FAP selectivity (>250000 fold).

But, its pharmacokinetics profile (PK) was not satisfactory compared to standard omarigliptin [86].

Ji et al., synthesized and evaluated β-amino pyrrole-2-carbonitrile analogues against DPP-4. Compound **80a** (Figure 14) with 2,4,5-trifluoro group was found to have the highest potency (IC_{50} = 0.01 μM). In silico studies revealed the presence of H bonding interactions between -F atom and the enzyme residues Ser630 along with hydrophobic interactions of octahydrocyclopenta[b]pyrrole-2-carbonitrile moiety of **80a** with the residues Phe357, Ser209, Arg125 occupying the S2 pocket of the enzyme which enhances its activity against DPP-4. The molecules with electron-donating groups at the para-position of the benzene ring were inactive [87].

Andrews et al., designed and tested 3-amino-4-substituted pyrrolidine analogues against DPP-4. They found compound **81a** (Figure 14) as the most potent (IC_{50} = 23 ± 9 nM) due to gem-difluoro group on the lactam moiety and inhibits DPP-4 up to>80% for 20 h in humans (dose = 100 mg/kg) suggesting its candidature for the further modifications to treat diabetes [88].

2.13.5. Imidazole-Chromene Hybrids

Gopinath et al., investigated and synthesized chiral-2H-chromene-N-imidazole-amino acid conjugates against aldose reductase enzyme. Analogue **82a** (Figure 15) displayed the highest enzyme inhibition (IC_{50} = 0.031 ± 0.082 μM) in comparison to standard compound sorbinil (IC_{50} = 0.43 ± 0.014 μM) and reduced the blood sugar levels of STZ-induced rats depending upon dose. The presence of 4-Cl group on the phenyl ring attached to imidazole was found mandatory for activity [89].

2.13.6. Imidazole-Triazole Hybrids

Wang et al., designed and checked imidazole-triazole hybrids as α-glucosidase inhibitors. They found analogue **83a** (Figure 15) with the highest potency (IC_{50} = 15.16 ± 0.18 μM). The presence of 3-BrPh group was reported as essential, and -Cl, -F groups reduced the activity. The shifting of ethoxy group from 2nd to 4th position at phenylacetamide showed a reduction in activity. Analogue **83a** was reported as a non-competitive inhibitor (K_i = 14.78 μM) as per kinetics studies. The molecular docking studies demonstrated the involvement of van der Waals interaction between its ethoxy phenyl group and the bottom pocket of the enzyme, along with a CH–π and an arene-cation interaction with the Tyr71 and Arg439 residue, respectively. -PhBr group interacts with enzyme through hydrophobic and CH–π interaction with residue His239.

Amide group and triazole ring interact through H bond with enzyme residues (Glu276, Asp214 and Thr215, respectively) [90].

2.13.7. Imidazole Pyrazole Hybrids

Chaudhry et al. evaluated imidazole-pyrazole hybrids against α-glucosidase and reported analogues **84a** and **84b** (Figure 15) with the highest potency (IC_{50} = 25.19 ± 0.004 and 33.62 ± 0.03 μM, respectively) due to H bonding interactions of N atom of pyrazole ring with Asn241 as well as of O atom of NO_2 group with Arg312 amino acid residue. The presence of electron-donating groups like -OCH_3 at R7 and R8 positions were found to reduce the activity [91].

2.13.8. Imidazole-Quinolinone Hybrids

Ikuma et al., reported and evaluated imidazo-quinolin-4(5H)-one analogues as DPP-4 inhibitors. Authors reported analogue **85a** (Figure 15) as the most potent and selective inhibitor (IC_{50} = 6.0 nM) compound with 5-methyl-2-oxo-1,3-dioxol-4-yl methyl ester group as R displayed maximum inhibitory potential. **85a** showed 87% and 64% DPP-4 inhibition in SD rats at the (dose =3 mg/ kg) at 1 and 10h, respectively, compared to the standard sitagliptin as per *in vivo* analysis suggesting its potential for diabetes [92].

2.13.9. Benzimidazole Analogues

Ozil et al., reported bis-benzimidazole derivatives and examined their potential against α-glucosidase. Analogue **86a** (Figure 15) possessed the maximum potency (IC_{50} = 0.44 ± 0.04 μM) in comparison to standard acarbose (IC_{50} = 13.34 ± 1.26 μM). The activity was found to enhance with the attachment of electron-withdrawing groups such as NO_2 on the benzimidazole. H bonding interactions were found between -NH_2 and -C=O of **86a** and Asp1526, Asp1157, Trp1369 and Try1251 of the α-glucosidase. Van der Waal interactions were also observed for **86a** with the Tyr1251, Phe1559, Asp1279 and Trp1355 of the α-glucosidase as per in silico studies, suggesting it as lead for further modifications and development as an antidiabetic drug [93].

2.13.10. Benzimidazole-Thiourea Hybrids

Zawawi et al., synthesized and screened benzimidazole-thiourea hybrids against α-glucosidase. Analogues **87a** and **87b** (Figure 15) presented the highest potency (IC_{50} = 50.57 ± 0.81 and 35.83 ± 0.66 μM, respectively). They found enhanced inhibition activity with the substitution of electron-withdrawing groups at 4th position of phenyl ring, while electron-donating groups reduced the activity.

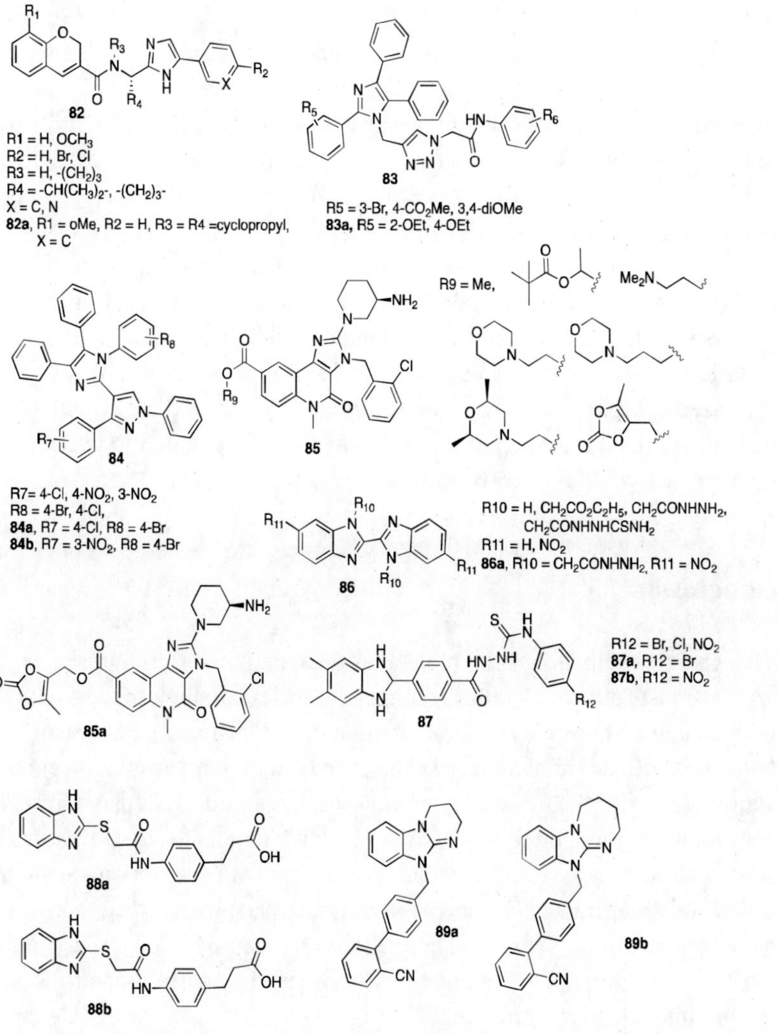

Figure 15. Imidazole analogues as antidiabetic agents.

In silico studies showed the presence of H bonding and arene-arene interactions between **87a** with Glu276 and Phe157 of the enzyme. The -C=O oxygen of the benzamide moiety and imidazole moiety of **87b** forms two H-bonds with His245 and Glu276, respectively. Hydrophobic and arene-arene interactions were also reported for **87b** with the binding site of the enzyme [94].

Hidalgo-Figueroa et al., designed carboxylic acids derivatives of benzimidazole as dual PPAR-γ/GPR40 agonist. Analogues **88a** and **88b** (Figure 15) exhibited the maximum agonistic activity in both receptors. **88a** enhanced the mRNA expression of PPAR-γ and GPR40 by 7- and 2-fold, respectively. In silico studies demonstrated the significant affinity of **88a** towards both targets. In vivo studies in a diabetic mice model revealed a good anti-hyperglycaemic effect by **88b** (dose = 50 mg/kg), suggesting their potential as dual PPAR-γ/GPR40 agonist [95].

Babkov et al., synthesized biphenyl-benzimidazole analogues and reported their potency as allosteric AMPK activators and AT1 receptor antagonists. (Figure 15) Compounds **89a** and **89b** were found with significant AMPK activity (EC_{50} = 0.34 μM and 0.44 μM, respectively) along with Cu^{2+} catalyzed inhibition of ascorbate oxidation (IC_{50} = 5.32 μM and 4.96 μM, respectively). At the concentration of 100 μM, compound **89b** was reported as the most active AMPK activator [96].

Conclusion

This chapter summarizes the molecules designed by different research groups and the most active molecules amongst the series, along with their interactions with the various proteins depending upon the agonistic or antagonistic actions. Numerous drugs are available in the market with the variable mechanism of action but still the, diabetes could not be cured. Extensive research is continuously going on to unleash the effective molecule for its treatment. The strategy based on the interaction of structural moieties present in the molecules found active during *in vitro* and *in vivo* studies can prove effective in designing new antidiabetic molecules. These molecules can be designed by analyzing the type and number of interactions between the scaffolds and the protein, paving the way to a future clinical drug.

References

[1] Kaul K, Tarr JM, Ahmad SI, Kohner EM, Chibber R. Introduction to diabetes mellitus. *Diabetes.* 2013:1-11.

[2] Rom S, Zuluaga-Ramirez V, Gajghate S, Seliga A, Winfield M, Heldt NA, Kolpakov MA, Bashkirova YV, Sabri AK, Persidsky Y. Hyperglycemia-driven neuroinflammation compromises BBB leading to memory loss in both diabetes mellitus (DM) type 1 and type 2 mouse models. *Molecular neurobiology.* 2019;56(3):1883-96.

[3] McQuaid K. *Current medical diagnosis and treatment.* New York: Lange Medical Books; 2001.

[4] Kerru N, Singh-Pillay A, Awolade P, Singh P. Current anti-diabetic agents and their molecular targets: A review. European Journal of Medicinal Chemistry. 2018;152:436-88.

[5] Ali F, Khan KM, Salar U, Taha M, Ismail NH, Wadood A, Riaz M, Perveen S. Hydrazinyl arylthiazole based pyridine scaffolds: Synthesis, structural characterization, in vitro α-glucosidase inhibitory activity, and in silico studies. *European Journal of Medicinal Chemistry.* 2017;138:255-72.

[6] Shah S, Javaid K, Zafar H, Khan KM, Khalil R, Ul-Haq Z, Perveen S, Choudhary MI. Synthesis, and In vitro and in silico α-glucosidase inhibitory studies of 5-chloro-2-aryl benzo [d] thiazoles. *Bioorganic Chemistry.* 2018;78:269-79.

[7] Kim KS. & Joon S. Rhee Effect of Acetylation on EmulSifying Properties of Glycinin. *J. Agr. Food Chem.* 1990;38.

[8] Yki JH. Drug Therapy: Thiazolidinediones. *N Engl J Med.* 2004;351:1106-18.

[9] Parks D. Tommkinson NCO. Villeneuve MS. Blanchard SG. Willson TM Bioorg *Med Chem Lett.* 1998;8:3657.

[10] Madhavan GR, Chakrabarti R, Kumar SK, Misra P, Mamidi RN, Balraju V, Kasiram K, Babu RK, Suresh J, Lohray BB. Novel phthalazinone and benzoxazinone containing thiazolidinediones as antidiabetic and hypolipidemic agents. *European journal of medicinal chemistry.* 2001;36(7-8):627-37.

[11] Nazreen S, Alam MS, Hamid H, Yar MS, Shafi S, Dhulap A, Alam P, Pasha M, Bano S, Alam MM. Design, synthesis, in silico molecular docking and biological evaluation of novel oxadiazole based thiazolidine-2, 4-diones bis-heterocycles as PPAR-γ agonists. *European Journal of Medicinal Chemistry.* 2014;87:175-85.

[12] Yanagisawa H, Takamura M, Yamada E, Fujita S, Fujiwara T, Yachi M, Isobe A, Hagisawa Y. Novel oximes having 5-benzyl-2, 4-thiazolidinedione as antihyperglycemic agents: synthesis and structure–activity relationship. *Bioorganic & medicinal chemistry letters.* 2000;10(4):373-5.

[13] Nazreen S, Alam MS, Hamid H, Yar MS, Dhulap A, Alam P, Pasha M, Bano S, Alam MM, Haider S. Thiazolidine-2, 4-diones derivatives as PPAR-γ agonists: Synthesis, molecular docking, in vitro and in vivo antidiabetic activity with hepatotoxicity risk evaluation and effect on PPAR-γ gene expression. *Bioorganic & medicinal chemistry letters.* 2014;24(14):3034-42.

[14] Bansal G, Singh S, Monga V, Thanikachalam PV, Chawla P. Synthesis and biological evaluation of thiazolidine-2, 4-dione-pyrazole conjugates as antidiabetic, anti-inflammatory and antioxidant agents. *Bioorganic chemistry.* 2019;92:103271.

[15] Bhattarai BR, Kafle B, Hwang J-S, Ham SW, Lee K-H, Park H, Han I-O, Cho H. Novel thiazolidinedione derivatives with anti-obesity effects: dual action as PTP1B

inhibitors and PPAR-γ activators. *Bioorganic & medicinal chemistry letters.* 2010;20(22):6758-63.

[16] Ha YM, Park YJ, Kim J-A, Park D, Park JY, Lee HJ, Lee JY, Moon HR, Chung HY. Design and synthesis of 5-(substituted benzylidene) thiazolidine-2, 4-dione derivatives as novel tyrosinase inhibitors. *European journal of medicinal chemistry.* 2012;49:245-52.

[17] Wang Z, Liu Z, Lee W, Kim S-N, Yoon G, Cheon SH. Design, synthesis and docking study of 5-(substituted benzylidene) thiazolidine-2, 4-dione derivatives as inhibitors of protein tyrosine phosphatase 1B. *Bioorganic & Medicinal Chemistry Letters.* 2014;24(15):3337-40.

[18] Mahapatra MK, Kumar R, Kumar M. Synthesis, biological evaluation and in silico studies of 5-(3-methoxybenzylidene) thiazolidine-2, 4-dione analogues as PTP1B inhibitors. *Bioorganic Chemistry.* 2017;71:1-9.

[19] Maccari R, Ottanà R, Curinga C, Vigorita MG, Rakowitz D, Steindl T, Langer T. Structure–activity relationships and molecular modelling of 5-arylidene-2, 4-thiazolidinediones active as aldose reductase inhibitors. *Bioorganic & medicinal chemistry.* 2005;13(8):2809-23.

[20] Maccari R, Ottanà R, Ciurleo R, Rakowitz D, Matuszczak B, Laggner C, Langer T. Synthesis, induced-fit docking investigations, and in vitro aldose reductase inhibitory activity of non-carboxylic acid containing 2, 4-thiazolidinedione derivatives. *Bioorganic & medicinal chemistry.* 2008;16(11):5840-52.

[21] Maccari R, Vitale RM, Ottanà R, Rocchiccioli M, Marrazzo A, Cardile V, Graziano ACE, Amodeo P, Mura U, Del Corso A. Structure–activity relationships and molecular modelling of new 5-arylidene-4-thiazolidinone derivatives as aldose reductase inhibitors and potential anti-inflammatory agents. *European journal of medicinal chemistry.* 2014;81:1-14.

[22] Yoshida T, Sakashita H, Akahoshi F, Hayashi Y. [(S)-γ-(4-Aryl-1-piperazinyl)-l-prolyl] thiazolidines as a novel series of highly potent and long-lasting DPP-IV inhibitors. *Bioorganic & medicinal chemistry letters.* 2007;17(9):2618-21.

[23] Yoshida T, Akahoshi F, Sakashita H, Sonda S, Takeuchi M, Tanaka Y, Nabeno M, Kishida H, Miyaguchi I, Hayashi Y. Fused bicyclic heteroarylpiperazine-substituted L-prolylthiazolidines as highly potent DPP-4 inhibitors lacking the electrophilic nitrile group. *Bioorganic & medicinal chemistry.* 2012;20(16):5033-41.

[24] Javid M, Rahim F, Taha M, Rehman H, Nawaz M. A. wadood, S. Imran, I. Uddin, A. Mosaddik, KM Khan. *Bioorganic Chemistry.* 2018.

[25] Khanna S, Bahal R, Bharatam PV. In silico studies on PPARγ agonistic heterocyclic systems. *QSAR and Molecular Modeling Studies in Heterocyclic Drugs I.* 2006:149-80.

[26] Kharbanda C, Alam MS, Hamid H, Javed K, Shafi S, Ali Y, Alam P, Pasha M, Dhulap A, Bano S. Novel benzenesulfonylureas containing thiophenylpyrazoline moiety as potential antidiabetic and anticancer agents. *Bioorganic & medicinal chemistry letters.* 2014;24(22):5298-303.

[27] Kharbanda C, Alam MS, Hamid H, Javed K, Dhulap A, Bano S, Ali Y. Antidiabetic effect of novel benzenesulfonylureas as PPAR-γ agonists and their anticancer effect. *Bioorganic & Medicinal Chemistry Letters.* 2015;25(20):4601-5.

[28] Ovais S, Pushpalatha H, Reddy GB, Rathore P, Bashir R, Yaseen S, Dheyaa A, Yaseen R, Tanwar O, Akthar M. Synthesis and biological evaluation of some new pyrazoline substituted benzenesulfonylurea/thiourea derivatives as anti-hyperglycaemic agents and aldose reductase inhibitors. European Journal of Medicinal Chemistry. 2014;80:209-17.

[29] Deka N, Uravane M, Anthony J, Bhumra SK, Nair A, B-Rao C, Patel D, Sivaramakrishnan H. Design and synthesis of non-TZD peroxisome proliferator-activated receptor γ (PPARγ) modulator. *Medicinal Chemistry Research.* 2014;23(4):2150-9.

[30] Taygerly JP, McGee LR, Rubenstein SM, Houze JB, Cushing TD, Li Y, Motani A, Chen J-L, Frankmoelle W, Ye G. Discovery of INT131: a selective PPARγ modulator that enhances insulin sensitivity. *Bioorganic & medicinal chemistry.* 2013;21(4):979-92.

[31] Du Y, Ling H, Shen J, Li Q. Discovery of novel, potent, selective and cellular active ADC type PTP1B inhibitors via fragment-docking-oriented de novel design. *Bioorganic & Medicinal Chemistry*. 2015;23(15):4891-8.

[32] Liu P, Du Y, Song L, Shen J, Li Q. Novel, potent, selective and cellular active ABC type PTP1B inhibitors containing (methanesulfonyl-phenyl-amino)-acetic acid methyl ester phosphotyrosine mimetic. *Bioorganic & Medicinal Chemistry.* 2015;23(21):7079-88.

[33] Liu P, Du Y, Song L, Shen J, Li Q. Discovery of novel, high potent, ABC type PTP1B inhibitors with TCPTP selectivity and cellular activity. *European Journal of Medicinal Chemistry.* 2016;118:27-33.

[34] Ghareb N, El-Sayed NM, Abdelhameed R, Yamada K, Elgawish MS. Toward a treatment of diabesity: Rational design, synthesis and biological evaluation of benzene-sulfonamide derivatives as a new class of PTP-1B inhibitors. *Bioorganic Chemistry.* 2019;86:322-38.

[35] Ji Y, Chen X, Chen H, Zhang X, Fan Z, Xie L, Ma B, Zhu C. Designing of acyl sulphonamide based quinoxalinones as multifunctional aldose reductase inhibitors. *Bioorganic & Medicinal Chemistry.* 2019;27(8):1658-69.

[36] Sharma R, Soman SS. Design and synthesis of sulfonamide derivatives of pyrrolidine *and piperidine as anti-diabetic agents. European Journal of Medicinal Chemistry.* 2015;90:342-50.

[37] Abd El-Karim SS, Anwar MM, Syam YM, Nael MA, Ali HF, Motaleb MA. Rational design and synthesis of new tetralin-sulfonamide derivatives as potent anti-diabetics and DPP-4 inhibitors: 2D & 3D QSAR, in vivo radiolabeling and bio distribution studies. *Bioorganic chemistry.* 2018;81:481-93.

[38] Eeda V, Wu D, Lim H-Y, Wang W. Design, synthesis, and evaluation of potent novel peroxisome proliferator-activated receptor γ indole partial agonists. *Bioorganic & medicinal chemistry letters.* 2019;29(22):126664.

[39] Islam MS, Barakat A, Al-Majid AM, Ali M, Yousuf S, Choudhary MI, Khalil R, Ul-Haq Z. Catalytic asymmetric synthesis of indole derivatives as novel α-glucosidase inhibitors in vitro. *Bioorganic Chemistry.* 2018;79:350-4.

[40] Wang G, Wang J, Xie Z, Chen M, Li L, Peng Y, Chen S, Li W, Deng B. Discovery of 3, 3-di (indolyl) indolin-2-one as a novel scaffold for α-glucosidase inhibitors: In silico studies and SAR predictions. *Bioorganic chemistry.* 2017;72:228-33.

[41] Gollapalli M, Taha M, Ullah H, Nawaz M, AlMuqarrabun LMR, Rahim F, Qureshi F, Mosaddik A, Ahmat N, Khan KM. Synthesis of Bis-indolylmethane sulfonohydrazides derivatives as potent α-Glucosidase inhibitors. *Bioorganic chemistry.* 2018;80:112-20.

[42] Nazir M, Abbasi MA, Siddiqui SZ, Khan KM, Salar U, Shahid M, Ashraf M, Lodhi MA, Khan FA. New indole based hybrid oxadiazole scaffolds with N-substituted acetamides: As potent anti-diabetic agents. Bioorganic chemistry. 2018;81:253-63.

[43] Taha M, Rahim F, Imran S, Ismail NH, Ullah H, Selvaraj M, Javid MT, Salar U, Ali M, Khan KM. Synthesis, α-glucosidase inhibitory activity and in silico study of tris-indole hybrid scaffold with oxadiazole ring: As potential leads for the management of type-II diabetes mellitus. *Bioorganic* chemistry. 2017;74:30-40.

[44] Tavani C, Bianchi L, De Palma A, Passeri GI, Punzi G, Pierri CL, Lovece A, Cavalluzzi MM, Franchini C, Lentini G. Nitro-substituted tetrahydroindolizines and homologs: Design, kinetics, and mechanism of α-glucosidase inhibition. *Bioorganic & Medicinal Chemistry Letters.* 2017;27(17):3980-6.

[45] Naureen S, Chaudhry F, Munawar MA, Ashraf M, Hamid S, Khan MA. Biological evaluation of new imidazole derivatives tethered with indole moiety as potent α-glucosidase inhibitors. *Bioorganic Chemistry.* 2018;76:365-9.

[46] Chu K-F, Song J-S, Chen C-T, Yeh T-K, Hsieh T-C, Huang C-Y, Wang M-H, Wu S-H, Yao C-H, Chao Y-S. Synthesis and biological evaluation of N-glucosyl indole derivatives as sodium-dependent glucose co-transporter 2 inhibitors. *Bioorganic chemistry.* 2019;83:520-5.

[47] Nomura S, Yamamoto Y, Matsumura Y, Ohba K, Sakamaki S, Kimata H, Nakayama K, Kuriyama C, Matsushita Y, Ueta K. Novel indole-N-glucoside, TA-1887 as a sodium glucose cotransporter 2 inhibitor for treatment of type 2 diabetes. *ACS medicinal chemistry letters.* 2014;5(1):51-5.

[48] Darwish KM, Salama I, Mostafa S, Gomaa MS, Khafagy E-S, Helal MA. Synthesis, biological evaluation, and molecular docking investigation of benzhydrol-and indole-based dual PPAR-γ/FFAR1 agonists. *Bioorganic & Medicinal Chemistry Letters.* 2018;28(9):1595-602.

[49] Khan M, Yousaf M, Wadood A, Junaid M, Ashraf M, Alam U, Ali M, Arshad M, Hussain Z, Khan KM. Discovery of novel oxindole derivatives as potent α-glucosidase inhibitors. *Bioorganic & Medicinal Chemistry.* 2014;22(13):3441-8.

[50] Luthra T, Lalitha KN, Agarwal R, Uma A, Sen S. Design, synthesis and in vitro study of densely functionalized oxindoles as potent α-glucosidase inhibitors. *Bioorganic & Medicinal Chemistry.* 2018;26(18):4996-5005.

[51] Taha M, Imran S, Rahim F, Wadood A, Khan KM. Oxindole based oxadiazole hybrid analogs: Novel α-glucosidase inhibitors. *Bioorganic chemistry.* 2018;76:273-80.

[52] Sun Y, Su K, Valentine J, Rosa-Bauza Y, Ellman J, Elboudwarej O, Mukherjee B, Craik C, Shuman M, Chen F. Zhang. X Time-Resolved Single-Step Protease Activity Quantification Using Nanoplasmonic Resonator Sensors. *ACS Nano.* 2010;4:978-84.

[53] Han K, Li Y, Zhang Y, Teng Y, Ma Y, Wang M, Wang R, Xu W, Yao Q, Zhang Y. Design, synthesis and docking study of novel tetracyclic oxindole derivatives as α-glucosidase inhibitors. *Bioorganic & Medicinal Chemistry Letters.* 2015;25(7):1471-5.

[54] Iqbal Z, Hameed S, Ali S, Tehseen Y, Shahid M, Iqbal J. Synthesis, characterization, hypoglycemic and aldose reductase inhibition activity of arylsulfonylspiro [fluorene-9, 5′-imidazolidine]-2′, 4′-diones. *European Journal of Medicinal Chemistry.* 2015;98:127-38.

[55] Iqbal Z, Morahan G, Arooj M, Sobolev AN, Hameed S. Synthesis of new arylsulfonylspiroimidazolidine-2, 4-diones and study of their effect on stimulation of insulin release from MIN6 cell line, inhibition of human aldose reductase, sorbitol accumulations in various tissues and oxidative stress. *European Journal of Medicinal Chemistry.* 2019;168:154-75.

[56] Chen T, Ning M, Ye Y, Wang K, Leng Y, Shen J. Design, synthesis and structure-activity relationship studies of GPR40 agonists containing amide linker. *European Journal of Medicinal Chemistry.* 2018;152:175-94.

[57] Xie F, Liang Y, Xia Y, Luo S, Jiang F, Fu L. Discovery of 2-ethoxy-4-(methoxymethyl) benzamide derivatives as potent and selective PTP1B inhibitors. *Bioorganic Chemistry.* 2019;92:103273.

[58] Mohammadi-Khanaposhtani M, Rezaei S, Khalifeh R, Imanparast S, Faramarzi MA, Bahadorikhalili S, Safavi M, Bandarian F, Esfahani EN, Mahdavi M. Design, synthesis, docking study, α-glucosidase inhibition, and cytotoxic activities of acridine linked to thioacetamides as novel agents in treatment of type 2 diabetes. *Bioorganic Chemistry.* 2018;80:288-95.

[59] Maheshwari N, Karthikeyan C, Bhadada SV, Verma AK, Sahi C, Moorthy NHN, Trivedi P. Design, synthesis and biological evaluation of some tetrazole acetamide derivatives as novel non-carboxylic PTP1B inhibitors. *Bioorganic Chemistry.* 2019;92:103221.

[60] Li X, Xu Q, Li C, Luo J, Li X, Wang L, Jiang B, Shi D. Toward a treatment of diabesity: In vitro and in vivo evaluation of uncharged bromophenol derivatives as a new series of PTP1B inhibitors. *European Journal of Medicinal Chemistry.* 2019;166:178-85.

[61] Chatzopoulou M, Patsilinakos A, Vallianatou T, Prnova MS, Žakelj S, Ragno R, Stefek M, Kristl A, Tsantili-Kakoulidou A, Demopoulos VJ. Decreasing acidity in a series of aldose reductase inhibitors: 2-Fluoro-4-(1H-pyrrol-1-yl) phenol as a scaffold for improved membrane permeation. *Bioorganic & Medicinal Chemistry.* 2014;22(7):2194-207.

[62] Crespo I, Giménez-Dejoz J, Porte S, Cousido-Siah A, Mitschler A, Podjarny A, Pratsinis H, Kletsas D, Pares X, Ruiz FX. Design, synthesis, structure-activity relationships and X-ray structural studies of novel 1-oxopyrimido [4, 5-c]

quinoline-2-acetic acid derivatives as selective and potent inhibitors of human aldose reductase. *European Journal of Medicinal Chemistry.* 2018;152:160-74.

[63] Banno Y, Miyamoto Y, Sasaki M, Oi S, Asakawa T, Kataoka O, Takeuchi K, Suzuki N, Ikedo K, Kosaka T. Identification of 3-aminomethyl-1, 2-dihydro-4-phenyl-1-isoquinolones: a new class of potent, selective, and orally active non-peptide dipeptidyl peptidase IV inhibitors that form a unique interaction with Lys554. *Bioorganic & medicinal chemistry.* 2011;19(16):4953-70.

[64] Pan X, Huan Y, Shen Z, Liu Z. Synthesis and biological evaluation of novel tetrahydroisoquinoline-C-aryl glucosides as SGLT2 inhibitors for the treatment of type 2 diabetes. *European Journal of Medicinal Chemistry.* 2016;114:89-100.

[65] El-Sayed S, Metwally K, El-Shanawani AA, Abdel-Aziz LM, El-Rashedy AA, Soliman ME, Quattrini L, Coviello V, la Motta C. Quinazolinone-based rhodanine-3-acetic acids as potent aldose reductase inhibitors: Synthesis, functional evaluation and molecular modeling study. *Bioorganic & Medicinal Chemistry Letters.* 2017;27(20):4760-4.

[66] Javaid K, Saad SM, Rasheed S, Moin ST, Syed N, Fatima I, Salar U, Khan KM, Perveen S, Choudhary MI. 2-Arylquinazolin-4 (3H)-ones: A new class of α-glucosidase inhibitors. *Bioorganic & Medicinal Chemistry.* 2015;23(23):7417-21.

[67] Wei M, Chai W-M, Wang R, Yang Q, Deng Z, Peng Y. Quinazolinone derivatives: Synthesis and comparison of inhibitory mechanisms on α-glucosidase. *Bioorganic & Medicinal Chemistry.* 2017;25(4):1303-8.

[68] Zhang Y, Gao H, Liu R, Liu J, Chen L, Li X, Zhao L, Wang W, Li B. Quinazoline-1-deoxynojirimycin hybrids as high active dual inhibitors of EGFR and α-glucosidase. *Bioorganic & Medicinal Chemistry Letters.* 2017;27(18):4309-13.

[69] Ibrahim MK, Eissa IH, Alesawy MS, Metwaly AM, Radwan MM, ElSohly MA. Design, synthesis, molecular modeling and anti-hyperglycemic evaluation of quinazolin-4 (3H)-one derivatives as potential PPARγ and SUR agonists. *Bioorganic & medicinal chemistry.* 2017;25(17):4723-44.

[70] Saeedi M, Mohammadi-Khanaposhtani M, Pourrabia P, Razzaghi N, Ghadimi R, Imanparast S, Faramarzi MA, Bandarian F, Esfahani EN, Safavi M. Design and synthesis of novel quinazolinone-1, 2, 3-triazole hybrids as new anti-diabetic agents: In vitro α-glucosidase inhibition, kinetic, and docking study. *Bioorganic chemistry.* 2019;83:161-9.

[71] Ali Z, Akhtar MJ, Haider MR, Khan AA, Siddiqui AA, Yar MS. Design and synthesis of quinazoline-3, 4-(4H)-diamine endowed with thiazoline moiety as new class for DPP-4 and DPPH inhibitor. *Bioorganic chemistry.* 2017;71:181-91.

[72] Nikookar H, Mohammadi-Khanaposhtani M, Imanparast S, Faramarzi MA, Ranjbar PR, Mahdavi M, Larijani B. Design, synthesis and in vitro α-glucosidase inhibition of novel dihydropyrano [3, 2-c] quinoline derivatives as potential anti-diabetic agents. *Bioorganic chemistry.* 2018;77:280-6.

[73] Khan MS, Munawar MA, Ashraf M, Alam U, Ata A, Asiri AM, Kousar S, Khan MA. Synthesis of novel indenoquinoxaline derivatives as potent α-glucosidase inhibitors. *Bioorganic & medicinal chemistry.* 2014;22(3):1195-200.

[74] Xiu Z-M, Wang L-P, Fu J, Xu J, Liu L. 1-Acetyl-5-phenyl-1H-pyrrol-3-ylacetate: An aldose reductase inhibitor for the treatment of diabetic nephropathy. *Bioorganic & Medicinal Chemistry Letters.* 2017;27(18):4482-7.

[75] Winters MP, Sui Z, Wall M, Wang Y, Gunnet J, Leonard J, Hua H, Yan W, Suckow A, Bell A. Discovery of N-arylpyrroles as agonists of GPR120 for the treatment of type II diabetes. *Bioorganic & Medicinal Chemistry Letters.* 2018;28(5):841-6.

[76] Fukushima H, Hiratate A, Takahashi M, Mikami A, Saito-Hori M, Munetomo E, Kitano K, Chonan S, Saito H, Suzuki A. Synthesis and structure–activity relationships of potent 4-fluoro-2-cyanopyrrolidine dipeptidyl peptidase IV inhibitors. *Bioorganic & medicinal chemistry.* 2008;16(7):4093-106.

[77] Fukushima H, Hiratate A, Takahashi M, Saito M, Munetomo E, Kitano K, Saito H, Takaoka Y, Yamamoto K. Synthesis and structure–activity relationships of potent 3-or 4-substituted-2-cyanopyrrolidine dipeptidyl peptidase IV inhibitors. *Bioorganic & medicinal chemistry.* 2004;12(23):6053-61.

[78] Haffner CD, McDougald DL, Reister SM, Thompson BD, Conlee C, Fang J, Bass J, Lenhard JM, Croom D, Secosky-Chang MB. 2-Cyano-4-fluoro-1-thiovalylpyrrolidine analogues as potent inhibitors of DPP-IV. *Bioorganic & medicinal chemistry letters.* 2005;15(23):5257-61.

[79] Wang L, Zhang B, Ji J, Li B, Yan J, Zhang W, Wu Y, Wang X. Synthesis and evaluation of structurally constrained imidazolidin derivatives as potent dipeptidyl peptidase IV inhibitors. *European journal of medicinal chemistry.* 2009;44(8):3318-22.

[80] Tsai T-Y, Hsu T, Chen C-T, Cheng J-H, Yeh T-K, Chen X, Huang C-Y, Chang C-N, Yeh K-C, Hsieh S-H. Novel trans-2-aryl-cyclopropylamine analogues as potent and selective dipeptidyl peptidase IV inhibitors. *Bioorganic & medicinal chemistry.* 2009;17(6):2388-99.

[81] Liu Y, Wu Y, Wu H, Tang L, Wu P, Liu T, Hu Y. Design, Synthesis, Biological Evaluation, and Docking Studies of (S)-Phenylalanine Derivatives with a 2-Cyanopyrrolidine Moiety as Potent Dipeptidyl Peptidase 4 Inhibitors. *Chemical Biology & Drug Design.* 2013;82(2):140-6.

[82] Liu Y, Si M, Tang L, Shangguan S, Wu H, Li J, Wu P, Ma X, Liu T, Hu Y. Synthesis and biological evaluation of novel benzyl-substituted (S)-phenylalanine derivatives as potent dipeptidyl peptidase 4 inhibitors. *Bioorganic & medicinal chemistry.* 2013;21(18):5679-87.

[83] Wang J, Feng Y, Ji X, Deng G, Leng Y, Liu H. Synthesis and biological evaluation of pyrrolidine-2-carbonitrile and 4-fluoropyrrolidine-2-carbonitrile derivatives as dipeptidyl peptidase-4 inhibitors for the treatment of type 2 diabetes. *Bioorganic & medicinal chemistry.* 2013;21(23):7418-29.

[84] Ji X, Su M, Wang J, Deng G, Deng S, Li Z, Tang C, Li J, Li J, Zhao L. Design, synthesis and biological evaluation of hetero-aromatic moieties substituted pyrrole-2-carbonitrile derivatives as dipeptidyl peptidase IV inhibitors. *European journal of medicinal chemistry.* 2014;75:111-22.

[85] Kondo T, Nekado T, Sugimoto I, Ochi K, Takai S, Kinoshita A, Hatayama A, Yamamoto S, Kishikawa K, Nakai H. Design and synthesis of DPP-IV inhibitors lacking the electrophilic nitrile group. *Bioorganic & medicinal chemistry.* 2008;16(4):1613-31.

[86] Cox JM, Chu HD, Kuethe JT, Gao Y-D, Scapin G, Eiermann G, He H, Li X, Lyons KA, Metzger J. The discovery of novel 5, 6, 5-and 5, 5, 6-tricyclic pyrrolidines as potent and selective DPP-4 inhibitors. *Bioorganic & Medicinal Chemistry Letters.* 2016;26(11):2622-6.

[87] Ji X, Xia C, Wang J, Su M, Zhang L, Dong T, Li Z, Wan X, Li J, Li J. Design, synthesis and biological evaluation of 4-fluoropyrrolidine-2-carbonitrile and octahydrocyclopenta [b] pyrrole-2-carbonitrile derivatives as dipeptidyl peptidase IV inhibitors. *European Journal of Medicinal Chemistry.* 2014;86:242-56.

[88] Andrews KM, Beebe DA, Benbow JW, Boyer DA, Doran SD, Hui Y, Liu S, McPherson RK, Neagu C, Parker JC. 1-((3S, 4S)-4-amino-1-(4-substituted-1, 3, 5-triazin-2-yl) pyrrolidin-3-yl)-5, 5-difluoropiperidin-2-one inhibitors of DPP-4 for the treatment of type 2 diabetes. *Bioorganic & medicinal chemistry letters.* 2011;21(6):1810-4.

[89] Gopinath G, Sankeshi V, Alaparthi MD, Bandaru S, Pasala VK, Chittineni PR, Krupadanam GD, Sagurthi SR. Design and synthesis of chiral 2H-chromene-N-imidazolo-amino acid conjugates as aldose reductase inhibitors. *European Journal of Medicinal Chemistry.* 2016;124:750-62.

[90] Wang G, Peng Z, Wang J, Li J, Li X. Synthesis and biological evaluation of novel 2, 4, 5-triarylimidazole–1, 2, 3-triazole derivatives via click chemistry as α-glucosidase inhibitors. *Bioorganic & medicinal chemistry letters.* 2016;26(23):5719-23.

[91] Chaudhry F, Naureen S, Ashraf M, Al-Rashida M, Jahan B, Munawar MA, Khan MA. Imidazole-pyrazole hybrids: Synthesis, characterization and in-vitro bioevaluation against α-glucosidase enzyme with molecular docking studies. *Bioorganic Chemistry.* 2019;82:267-73.

[92] Ikuma Y, Hochigai H, Kimura H, Nunami N, Kobayashi T, Uchiyama K, Umezome T, Sakurai Y, Sawada N, Tadano J. Discovery of 3H-imidazo [4, 5-c] quinolin-4 (5H)-ones as potent and selective dipeptidyl peptidase IV (DPP-4) inhibitors: use of a carboxylate prodrug to improve bioavailability. *Bioorganic & Medicinal Chemistry.* 2015;23(4):779-90.

[93] Ozil M, Emirik M, Beldüz A, Ülker S. Molecular docking studies and synthesis of novel bisbenzimidazole derivatives as inhibitors of α-glucosidase. *Bioorganic & Medicinal Chemistry.* 2016;24(21):5103-14.

[94] Zawawi NKNA, Taha M, Ahmat N, Ismail NH, Wadood A, Rahim F. Synthesis, molecular docking studies of hybrid benzimidazole as α-glucosidase inhibitor. *Bioorganic chemistry. 2017;70:184-91.*

[95] Hidalgo-Figueroa S, Navarrete-Vázquez G, Estrada-Soto S, Giles-Rivas D, Alarcón-Aguilar FJ, León-Rivera I, Giacoman-Martínez A, Pérez EM, Almanza-Pérez JC. Discovery of new dual PPARγ-GPR40 agonists with robust antidiabetic activity: Design, synthesis and in combo drug evaluation. *Biomedicine & Pharmacotherapy.* 2017;90:53-61.

[96] Babkov DA, Zhukowskaya ON, Borisov AV, Babkova VA, Sokolova EV, Brigadirova AA, Litvinov RA, Kolodina AA, Morkovnik AS, Sochnev VS. Towards multi-target antidiabetic agents: Discovery of biphenyl-benzimidazole conjugates as AMPK activators. *Bioorganic & medicinal chemistry letters.* 2019;29(17):2443-7.

Chapter 10

Phytoconstituents as Antidiabetic Agents and Their Chemical Aspects

Nancy Saini
Manish Vyas
and Sanjeev Kumar Sahu*
School of Pharmaceutical Sciences, Lovely Professional University, Phagwara, (Punjab), India

Abstract

Diabetes mellitus (DM) is the world's third leading cause of death after cancer, heart disease, and stroke, and it is one of the most challenging diseases to treat today. DM and its effects are expensive to treat, not only for people with it but also for healthcare systems worldwide. The development of various antidiabetic agents has been widely studied in recent decades. Natural products (NPs) have long been an essential source of medicines, with natural resources accounting for about half of the drugs currently used. Many natural products, especially those derived from plants, have been suggested for DM treatment. This chapter mainly focuses on bioactive phytoconstituents exhibiting antidiabetic activity with their chemistry aspects.

Keywords: diabetes mellitus, natural products, antidiabetic activity, phytoconstituents

* Corresponding Author's Email: sanjeevsahu82@yahoo.co.in.

In: Management of Diabetes Mellitus Based on Natural Products
Editors: Yachana Mishra and Vijay Mishra
ISBN: 979-8-88697-853-7

1. Introduction

Since the past decade, diabetes mellitus (DM) has been a health disorder. It is the most common non-infective disease. During the pathological condition of glycemia, the cells cannot recognize the decreased insulin production by the beta cells of the pancreas or insulin. It may lead to other important disorders like angiopathy, neuropathy, diabetic retinopathy, and nephropathy [1]. For more than 50 years, the worldwide prevalence of DM has been gradually rising, and it has already at pandemic proportions [2]. Most DM was about 150 million in 2000 and 220 million in 2010 [3, 4]. In 2003, the WHO estimated that 194 million people had diabetes, nearly two-thirds living in developing countries [5]. These data are increasing year-wise [5] and rising to 578 million (10.2%) by 2030 and 700 million (10.9%) by 2045, as per projections [6]. Increased thirst (polydipsia), increased appetite (polyphagia), increased urination (polyuria), reduced weight, and exhaustion are some of the signs and symptoms of severe insulin deficiency and hyperglycemia [7]. Diabetic retinopathy, which may result in blurring of vision due to the reduced VEGF levels and may eventually result in vision loss; nephropathy may result in kidney failure; peripheral neuropathy, which may cause foot ulcers, amputations and articulations of Charcot; and autonomous neuropathy, which may cause gastrointestinal, genitourinary, and cardiovascular symptoms as well as dysfunction of sexual activities. Cardiovascular atherosclerosis and cerebrovascular diseases are more prevalent in diabetic patients. Diabetes people are more likely to have high blood pressure and altered lipoprotein metabolism [8].

The great majority of diabetes cases fall into two primary etiopathogenetic groups: (i) type 1 diabetes (T1DM), which is caused by an absolute lack of insulin secretion, (ii) type 2 diabetes (T2DM) [9-12], and (iii) gestational diabetes (GD) [13]. T1DM is an autoimmune disease in which pancreatic beta-cells are destroyed. T2DM is a disease of increasingly impaired glucose regulation caused by a combination of malfunctioning pancreatic beta cells and insulin resistance [12]. As the obesity and T2DM epidemics continue, GD, defined as diabetes diagnosed during pregnancy but not overt diabetes, is becoming more common [10]. Furthermore, some studies have classified diabetes based on factors including Steroid-induced diabetes mellitus (SIDM), double diabetes, brittle diabetes, and maturity-onset diabetes of the young (MODY). SIDM is an abnormal rise in blood glucose in a patient with or without a history of DM related to glucocorticoid use [13]. The combination of symptoms of T1DM and T2DM has recently been referred to as "double diabetes," for example, when a person with T1DM becomes overweight/obese and insulin resistance worsens [14].

The term "brittle diabetes" refers to cases in which the instability, for whatever reason, causes significant life disruption and frequent and/or lengthy hospitalization. It affects about 3/1000 insulin-dependent diabetes individuals, primarily young women [15]. MODY is a type of diabetes caused by a mutation in a single gene involved in the development and function of -cells, which is inherited in an autosomal dominant way [16]. Neonatal diabetes mellitus (NDM) can be classified into three types based on phenotypic characteristics: temporary, persistent, and syndromic. In babies with insulin-dependent hyperglycemia, with blood glucose levels consistently greater than 250 mg/dL and no other cause, NDM should be explored. In a large multinational cohort study of 1020 patients diagnosed with diabetes before the age of six months, 80% had a genetic diagnosis [17].

2. Naturally Occurring Heterocyclic Compounds as Antidiabetic Agents

Heterocyclic compounds are cyclic compounds with oxygen, nitrogen, and sulfur components in the ring around the carbon atom [18]. The phytochemical constituents of the heterocyclic compounds with medical and dietary properties are essential to the pharmaceutical industry [19]. The amalgamation, properties, and applications of heterocyclic mixtures, particularly important in improving medicine, are the only focus of heterocyclic chemistry. A carbocyclic compound is a naturally occurring cyclic particle in which all carbon molecules are arranged in rings. When the ring structure of a chemical contains at least one element other than carbon, the compound is said to be heterocyclic. Nitrogen, oxygen, and sulfur are the most common hetero molecules; however, heterocyclic rings with additional hetero components are also well-known [20]. Alkaloids, antimicrobials, essential amino acids, nutrition, hemoglobin, chemicals, and many produced medicines and colors are just a few examples of the wide range of mixes that contain heterocyclic ring structures [19]. Saturated and unsaturated compounds are the two main categories of heterocyclic compounds. With altered steric characteristics, saturated heterocyclic molecules behave like their acyclic derivatives. Some novel heterocyclic compounds have developed in the past few years with their significant antidiabetic effects. These heterocyclic rings are displayed in Table 1.

Table 1. Rings with heteroatoms

Ring with Heteroatoms	Saturated			Unsaturated		
	Nitrogen	**Oxygen**	**Sulphur**	**Nitrogen**	**Oxygen**	**Sulphur**
Three	Aziridine	Oxirane	Thiirane	Azirine	Oxirene	Thiirene
	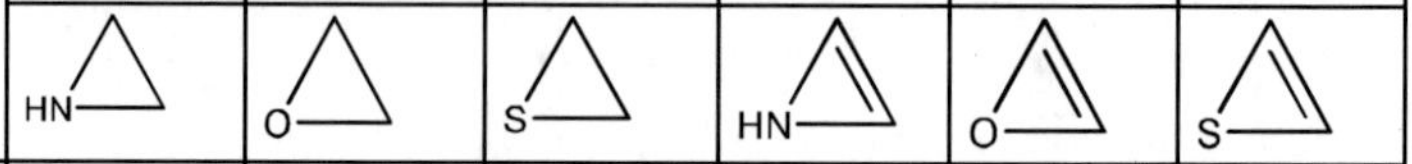					
Four	Azetidine	Oxetane	thietane	Azete	Oxete	Thiete
	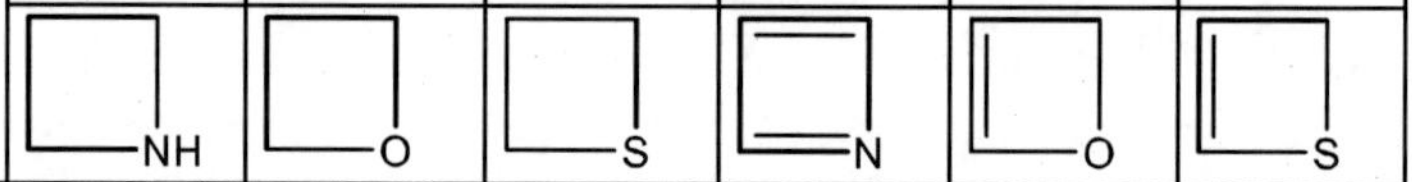					
Five	Pyrrolidine	Oxolane	Thiolane	Pyrrole	Furan	Thiophene
	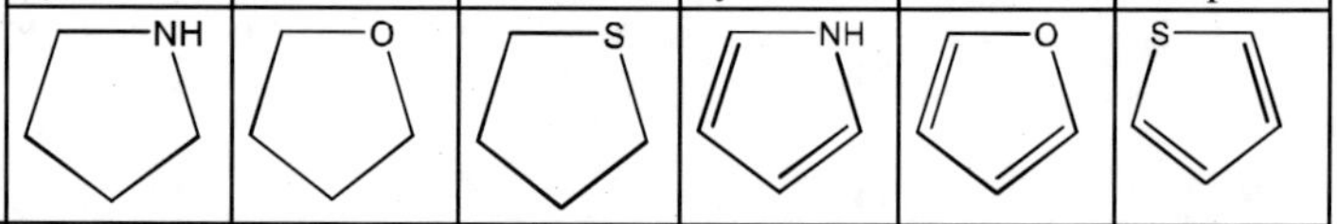					
Six	Piperidine	Oxane	Thiane	Pyridine	Pyran	Thiopyran
	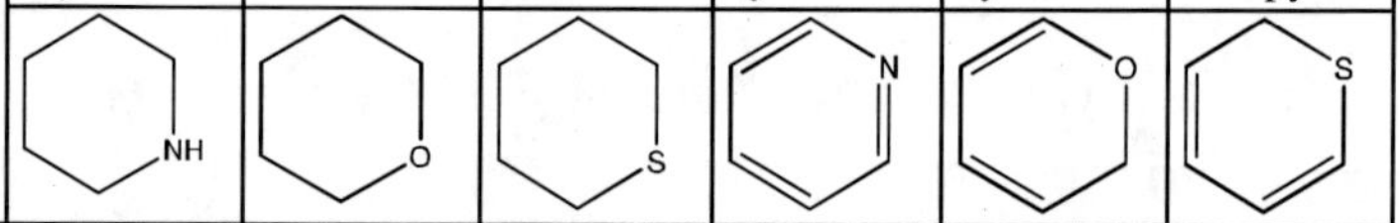					
Seven	Azepane	Oxepane	Thiepane	Azepine	Oxepine	Thiepine
	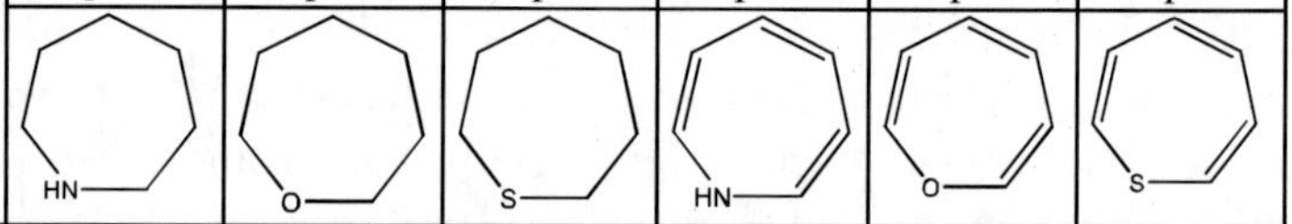					
Eight	Azocane	Oxocane	Thiocane	Azocine	Oxocine	Thiocine
	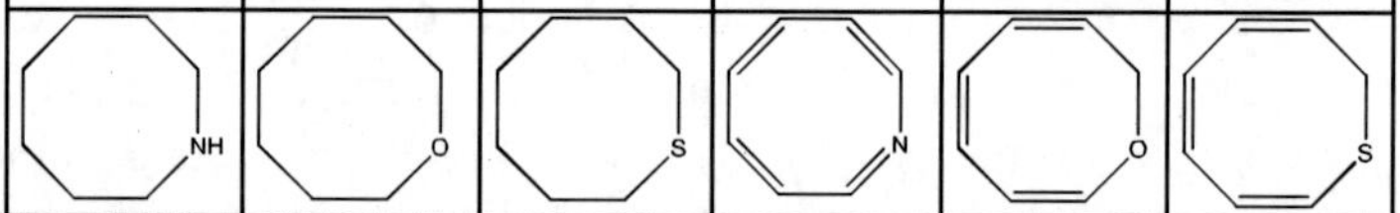					
Nine	Azonane	Oxonane	Thionane	Azonine	Oxonine	Thionine
	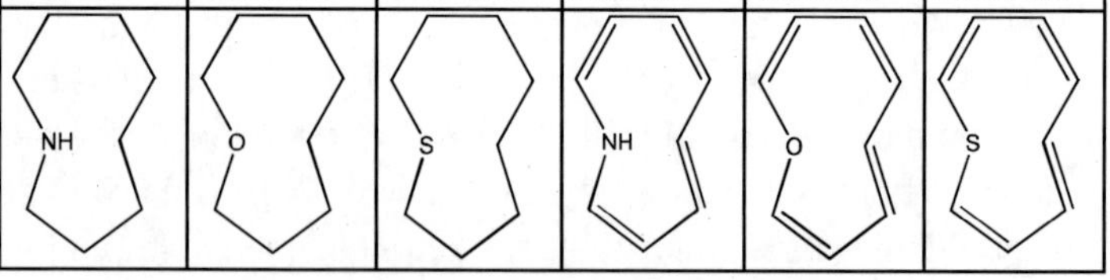					

Because of advances in chemical and pharmaceutical research, several bioactive compounds have been obtained from NPs, particularly in DM medicinal plants, and have been isolated, purified, and studied. These chemicals are divided into several categories based on their qualities, including saponins, flavonoids, anthraquinones, terpenes, coumarins, phenolics, and other substances.

2.1. Saponins

A group of secondary metabolites known as saponins is present in various plant species and some marine organisms. They are categorized as steroidal and nonsteroidal and comprise non-aglycones sugar and sugar chain units. The types of triterpene groups depend on the aglycone type. Attaching aglycone to one, two, or three sugars is possible. Three side chains would also work. Different alternatives are available for steroidal aglycones and aglycones made of triterpenes (-H, -COOH, -CH3) (Table 2) [21-26]. It has been demonstrated that several saponins, which are primarily found in medicinal plants, have anti-diabetic characteristics and can lower blood sugar, change blood sugar levels, and enhance insulin sensitivity and sugar tolerance.

The bitter melon (*Momordica charantia*), a popular herb, determines the total composition of the five novels' momordicosides Q (1), R (2), S (3) cucurbitane glycosides. These substances and their aglycones have demonstrated considerable insulin (100 nM) equivalent conversion of glucose transporter 4 (GLUT4) into cell membranes in the L6 myotubes and the 3T3-L1 adipocyte. According to one study, these substances activate AMP-activated protein kinase (AMPK), an enzyme that controls fat metabolism and permits glucose absorption [21].

A new dammarane-saponin, phanoside (4), discovered in the plant *Gynostemma pentaphyllum* Thunb has been reported to stimulate insulin secretion in the independent islands of rat pancreas. Phenoside increases insulin secretion in vitro by around four times at 16.7 mM glucose and ten times at 3.3 mM glucose. These sugar levels are supplemented by a factor of two by 2 M glibenclamide. When administered orally to rats with hyperglycemia, phenoside (40 and 80 mg/mL) enhanced glucose tolerance and raised plasma insulin levels. K-ATP and L-Ca^{2+} type channels, which impact the exocytotic machinery of beta cells, appear to be remote from the action [22, 27].

New steroid 28-Nor-22 (R) Witha 2,6,23-trienolide is produced by *Elephantopus scaber* acetone extract (5). This substance has been demonstrated to lower blood sugar levels and restore insulin levels in diabetic rats created by streptozotocin (STZ) by pancreatic cell activation and subsequent insulin release [23].

Table 2. Heterocyclic saponins

Compound No.	Structure	Mechanism
1.	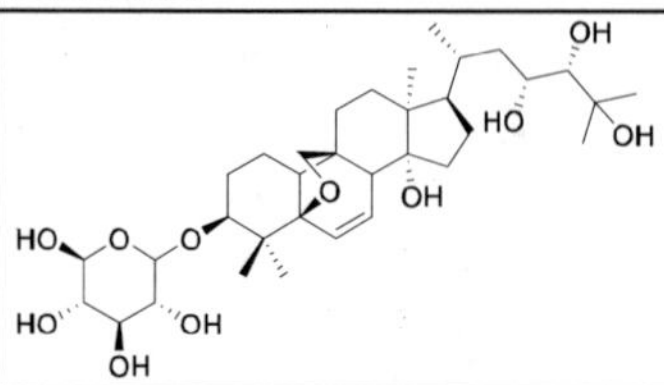	Enhance fatty acid oxidation [21]
2.	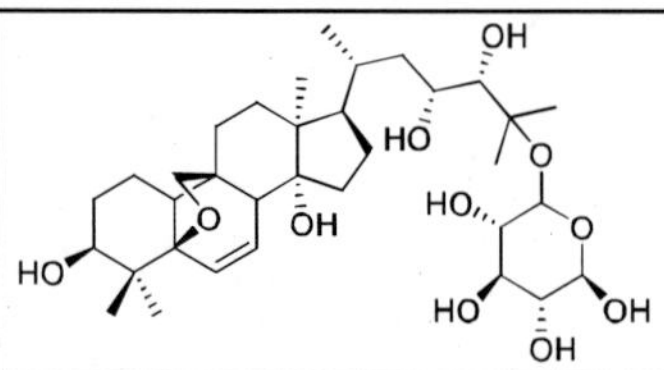	Enhance fatty acid oxidation [21]
3.	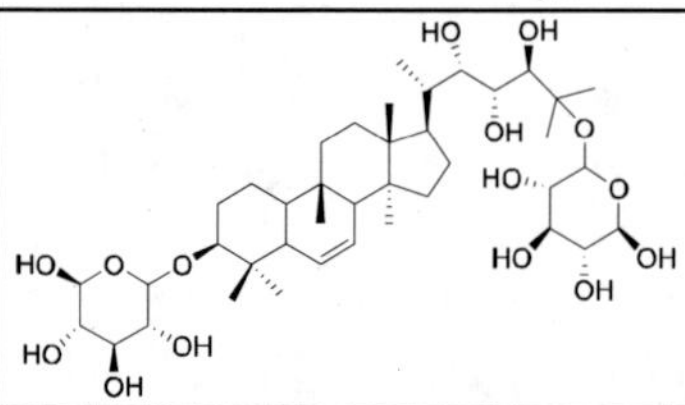	Enhance fatty acid oxidation [21]
4.	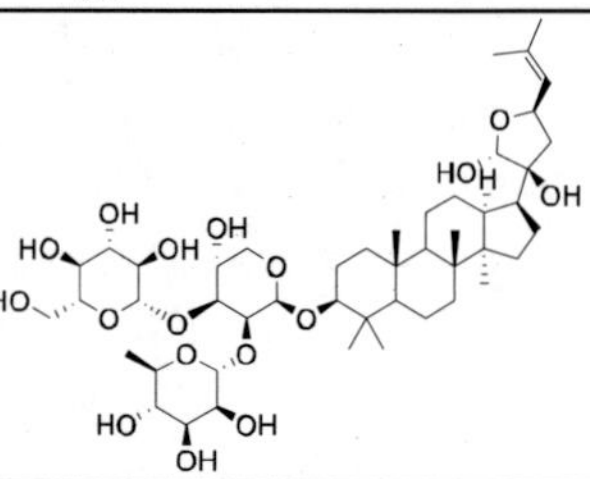	Stimulate insulin secretion [22]
5.	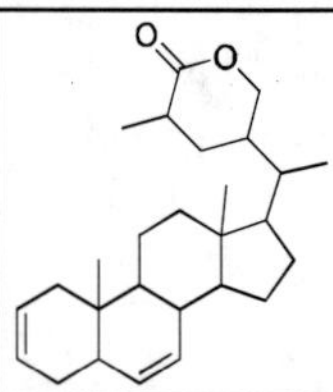	Pancreatic cell activation [23]
6.	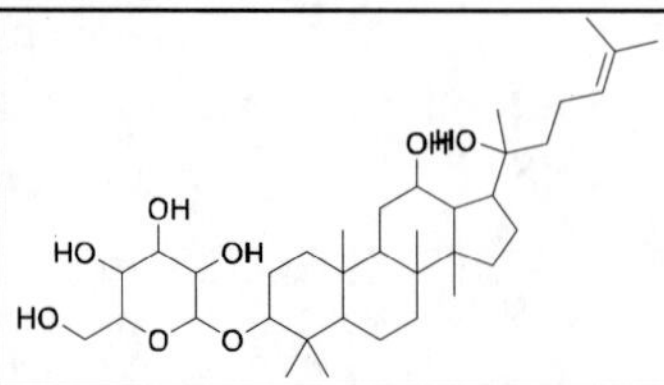	Decrease blood sugar level [24]

Compound No.	Structure	Mechanism
7.	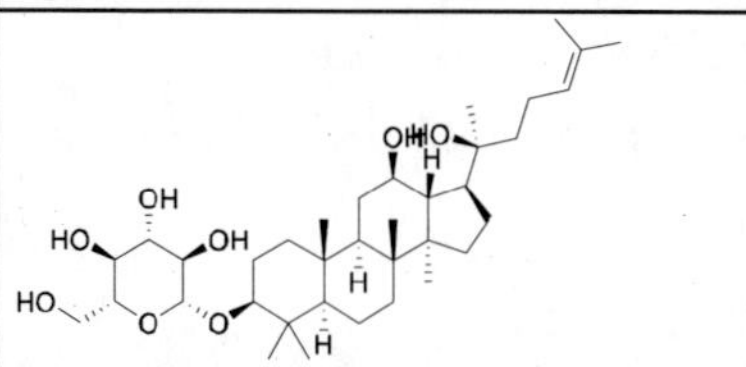	Reduce blood sugar level [24]
8.	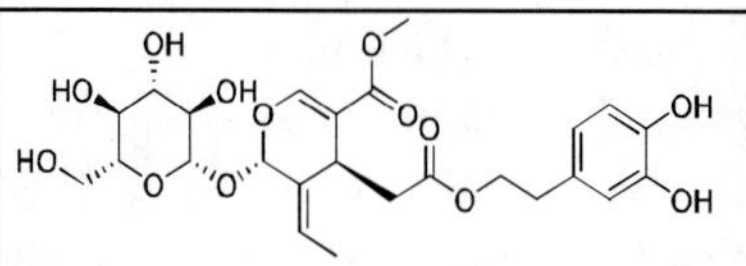	Raises insulin sensitivity, accelerates pancreatic β-cells' ability to secrete insulin, and enhances glucose transfer [25]
9.	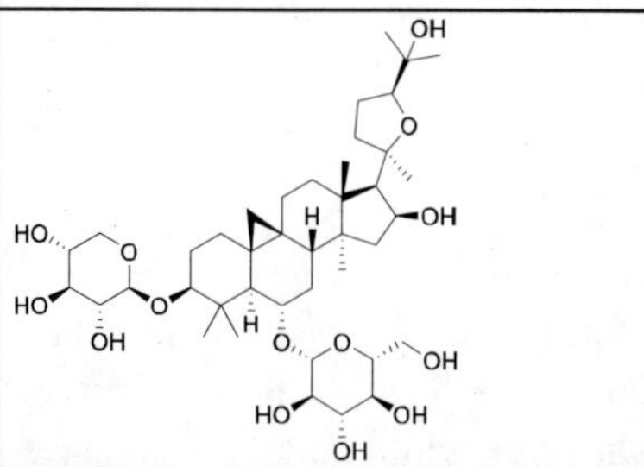	Promoted gastrointestinal absorption effects [26]
10.	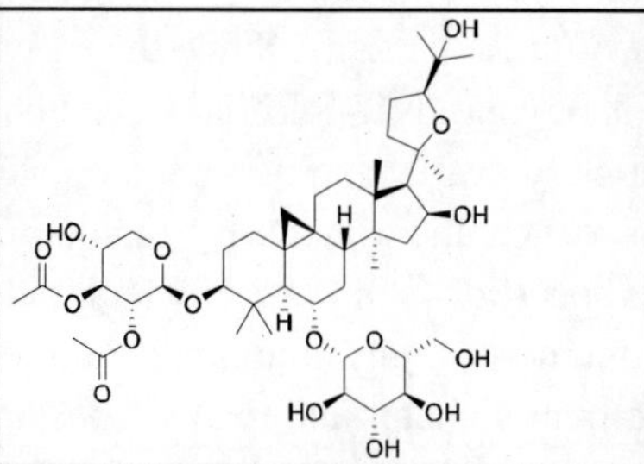	Promoted gastrointestinal absorption effects [26]

The active saponins ginsenoside Re (6) and ginsenoside Rh2 (7) are present in *Panax ginseng*. They significantly affect the levels of cholesterol and blood sugar. According to Zhang et al., phosphatidylinositol 3-kinase and cascade signals are sent after stimulation of insulin signaling on the IR substrate-1 by ginsenoside Re. Additionally, ginsenoside Re inhibits the activity of cJun and NF-kappaB and stops NF-kappaB from degrading [28]. According to Lai et al., the ginsenoside Rh2 route that decreases plasma glucose is based on elevated endorphin synthesis, which stimulates opioid receptors and results in better expression of glucose transporter subtype 4 [29].

The traditional antidiabetic and antihypertensive medicines, *Olea europea* and *Ligustrum japonicum* produce oleanolic acid and oleuropein (8). According to studies, oleanolic acid improved sugar tolerance in rats on a high-fat diet by lowering serum glucose and insulin levels. Oleanolic acid is an agonist of TGR5, a synthetic G-protein receptor antagonist that mediates some of its many cellular and physiological effects. Hence TGR5 agonists may be used to treat metabolic disorders [30].

Astragalus membranaceus (Fisch.) Bge. var. mongholicus (Bge.) Hsiao or *Astragalus membranaceus* (Fisch.) Bge. produces astragalosides IV (9) and I (10), active cycloartane saponins with a high triterpenoid type. According to studies, they were discovered to have protective benefits in mice during the early stages of diabetic nephropathy. By lowering carbohydrate absorption in the small intestine and colon, these substances are well known for inhibiting amylase, an enzyme necessary for treating T2DM [31-33].

2.2. Flavonoids

Flavonoids are naturally occurring phenolic substances. Flavonoids include aromatic hydroxyl groups, which give them their antioxidant effects. Biochemical flavonoids have a wide range of impacts, and their potent antioxidant activity is one of those benefits. Since the early 1980s, studies on the therapeutic potential of flavonoids in DM have been conducted. The auto poly ADP-ribosylation of poly synthetase polymerase, which promotes cell regeneration and protects pancreatic islands by maintaining the Reg gene transcriptional complex, is specifically inhibited by antioxidant flavonoids and free radical scavengers. Numerous physiologically active flavonoids have recently been identified to treat diabetes and related consequences.

Quercetin (11), (-) - epicatechin (12), and rutin (13), the three most prevalent flavonoids in plants, can boost antioxidant levels, lessen hyperglycemia and cell death in rat mice, and inhibit NO, insulin production and insulin release in remote islands [34-36].

The rat microsomal rat liver glucose-6-phosphatase bioassay was used to assess the antidiabetic effects of two flavonoids, quercetin 3-O- (2-galloyl) rhamnoside (14) and kaempferol 3-O-(2-galloyl) rhamnoside (15). The findings demonstrated that compounds 14 and 15 considerably reduced the neo glucogenic potential of liver fragments and had a considerable inhibitory effect on microsomal glucose-6-phosphatase disruption, with an IC_{50} of about 30 M [37].

The methanolic extract of Pueraria lobata roots produced novel 2-aryl benzofuran puerariafuran (16) and coumestrol (17). With IC_{50} values of 0.53 and 0.19 M, respectively, they demonstrated a strong inhibitory effect on increased glycation products (AGEPs) in vitro [38]. The release of ethyl acetate from *Erigeron annuus* flowers yielded the novel 2,3-dioxygenated flavanone erigeroflavanone (18), which inhibited the formation of AGEPs and rat lens aldose reductase (AR) [39].

Sulfuretin (19) was examined for its effects on AR and AGEP compounds using targeted bioactivity and isolation. It was produced from the ethyl acetate component of *Rhus verniciflua.* Both AR and AGEP were inhibited significantly. Sulfuretin inhibited the AGEP (IC_{50} = 124.7 M) nearly ten times more than aminoguanidine (value IC_{50} = 1231.0 M) [40].

Two dihydro flavonol glycosides, engletin (20) and astilbin (21), were produced from acetic ether extract of *Stelechocarpus cauliflorus* leaves. They merely differ regarding the number of hydroxyl groups in their aglycone, yet they exhibit various anti-aldose and anti-AGEP properties. Compared to human combined AR, engeletin demonstrated 23 times greater inhibitory activity than astilbin (26.7M; IC_{50} = 1.16 M). Astilbin and quercetin together effectively controlled AGEP growth [41].

Myricetin (22), an active component of *Abelmoschus moschatus* (Malvaceae), has been tested to ameliorate insulin resistance in Zucker-obese rats. By enhancing post-receptor insulin signaling in the muscles, which is connected to improved PI3-kinase activity associated with IRS-1 and GLUT 4 activity, myricetin increases insulin sensitivity [42].

The effect of prolonged genistein (23) therapy on aorta reactivation was examined in STZ-deficient mice. The findings demonstrated that genistein effectively prevented aberrant vascular remodeling in diabetic rats by lowering oxidative stress on the aortic tissue wall and vascular remodeling in diabetic rats through NO- and prostaglandin-based pathways [43]. Furthermore, in C57BL / KsJ-db / db mice, genistein's hypoglycemic effects were discovered, along with those of hesperidin (24), naringin (25), and daidzein (26). They were partially mediated by liver enzymes controlling glucose [44]. Flavonoids with a typical benzo-pyrone structure are a component of the major phases of secondary metabolites (Table 3) [45-63].

Many other flavonoids demonstrated antidiabetic properties through anti-oxidation techniques, inhibiting glucosidase, including scutellarin (27) from *Erigeron multiradiatus*, eupatilin (28) from *Artemisia princeps* Pampanini, isoginkgetin (29) from *Gingko biloba* L., and saponarin (30) from *Tinospora cordifolia* [64-66].

Table 3. Heterocyclic flavonoids

Compound No.	Structure	Mechanism
11.	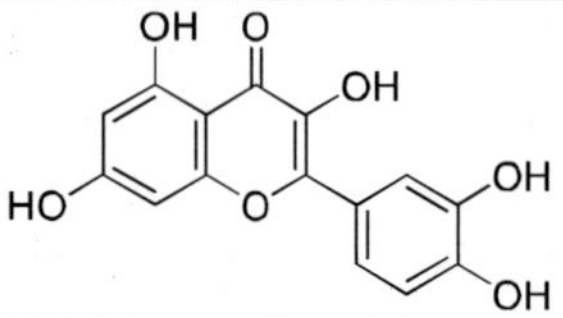	Insulin secretory and insulin-sensitizing actions are inhibited, and peripheral tissues use glucose more effectively as a result [45]
12.	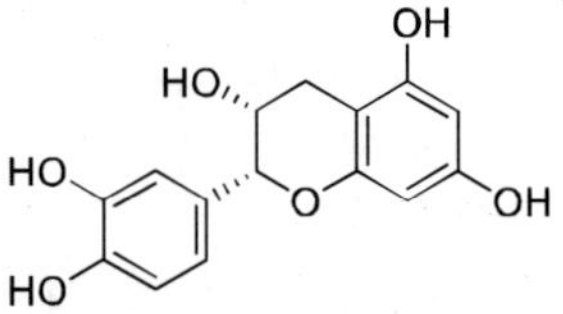	It exhibited a protective effect and restored blood glucose levels via -cell regeneration [46, 47]
13.	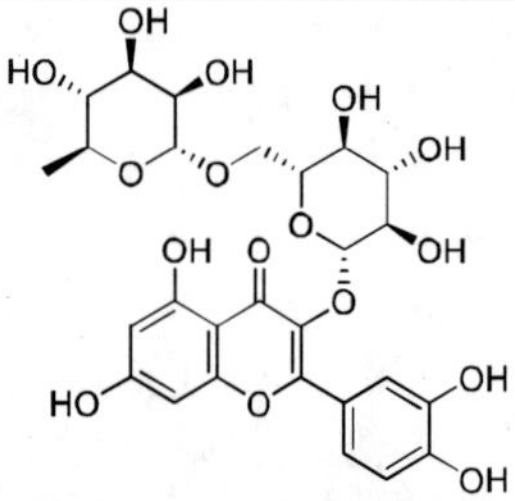	Reduction in the absorption of carbohydrates from the small intestine, a suppression of tissue gluconeogenesis, an increase in tissue glucose uptake, stimulation of beta cell insulin secretion, and defense against Langerhans islet degeneration [48]
14.	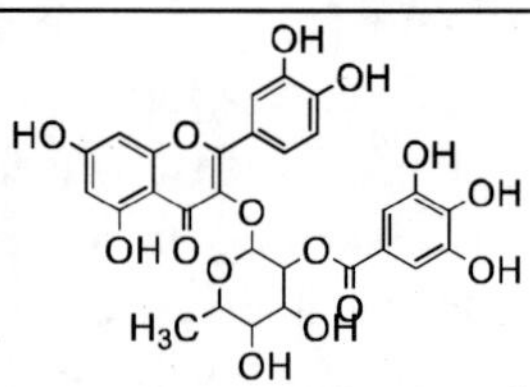	Without altering the catalytic subunit or the phosphate/pyrophosphate transporter (T2) of the G-6-Pase system, it inhibits the glucose-6-phosphate (G-6-P) transporter (T1) [49]
15.	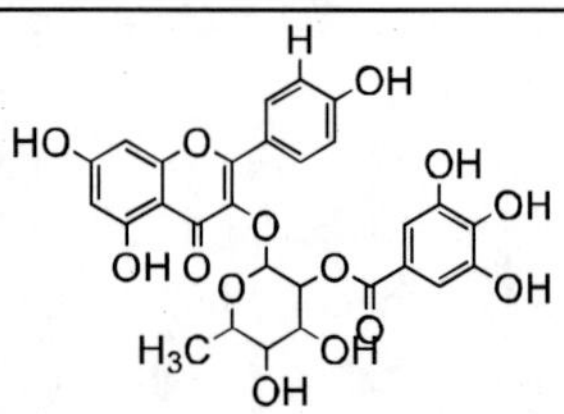	Without altering the catalytic subunit or the phosphate/pyrophosphate transporter (T2) of the G-6-Pase system, it inhibits the glucose-6-phosphate (G-6-P) transporter (T1) [49]
16.	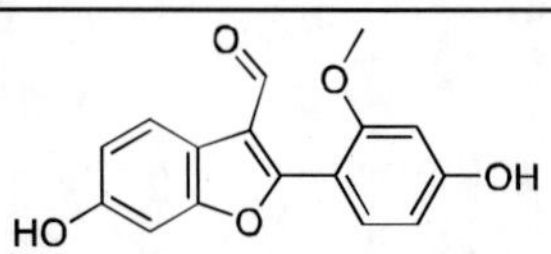	Inhibition of AGEs formation [38]

Compound No.	Structure	Mechanism
17.	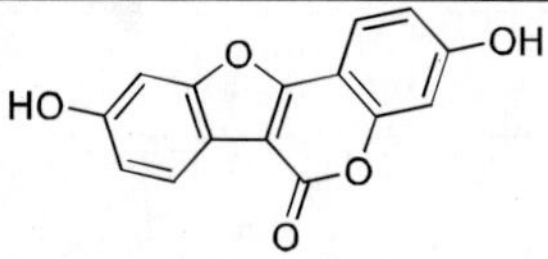	Inhibition of AGEs formation [50]
18.	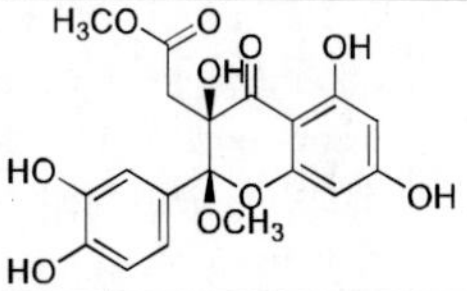	AGEs inhibitor [51]
19.	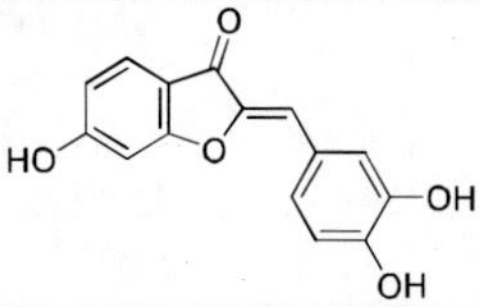	AGEs inhibitor [52]
20.	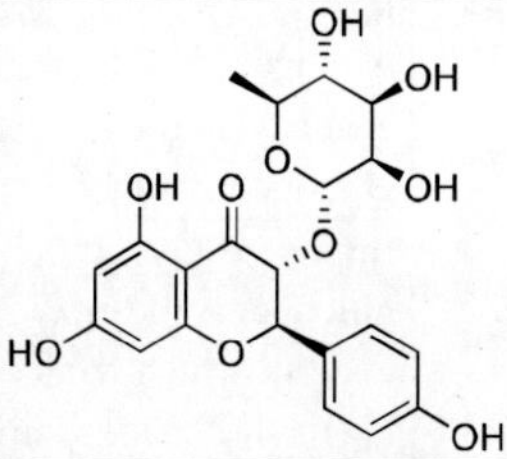	Inhibition of AGEs [53]
21.	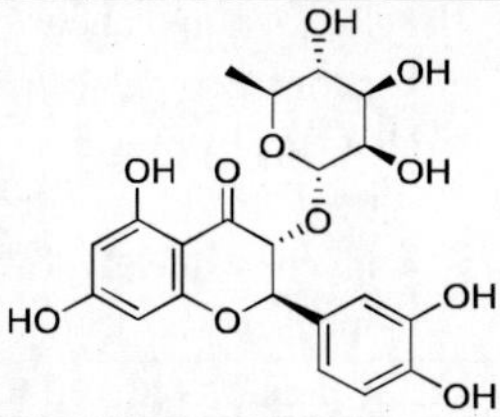	Alpha glucosidase inhibitor [54]
22.	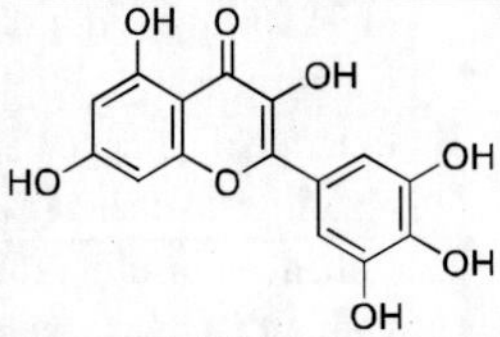	Increases insulin sensitivity [55]
23.	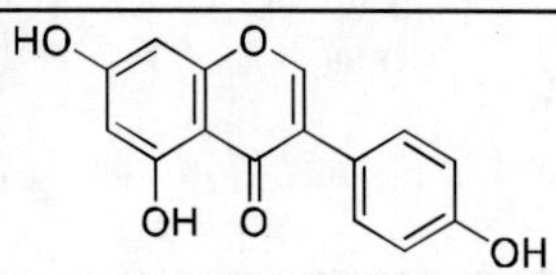	Direct effects on beta-cell proliferation, insulin production driven by glucose, and prevention of apoptosis [56]

Table 3. (Continued)

Compound No.	Structure	Mechanism
24.	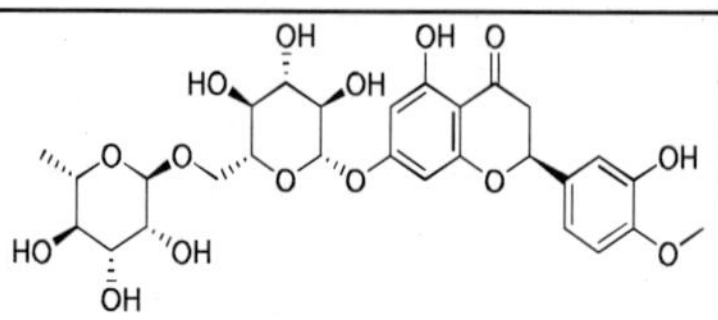	Hesperidin treatment may boost insulin and hence decrease glucose levels as well as change the amount of glycogen in diabetic tissues due to improved glycolytic and gluconeogenic enzymes, which may block pancreatic islet damage through its antioxidative activity [57]
24.	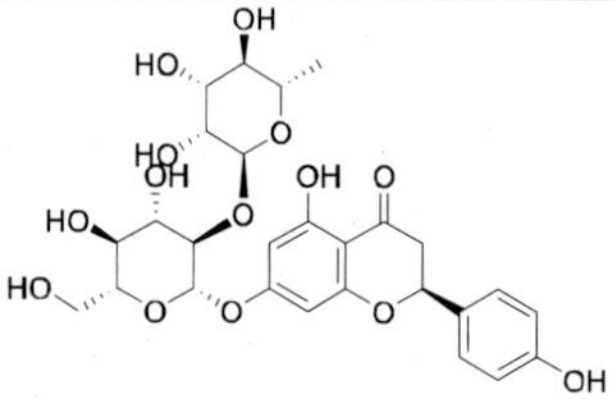	Improved glycolytic and gluconeogenetic enzymes boost insulin and hence lower glucose levels, reduce pancreatic islet damage through antioxidative efficacy, and change the amount of glycogen in diabetic tissues [58]
25.	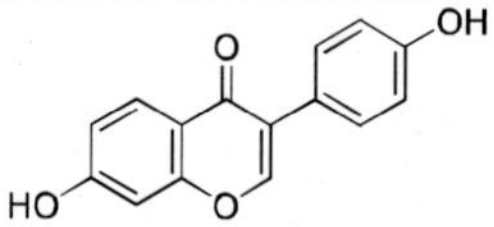	Improved glycolytic and gluconeogenic enzymes increase insulin, which reduces glucose levels. It changes the amount of glycogen in diabetic tissues. These actions also reduce pancreatic islet damage by preventing oxidative stress, and they increase insulin and consequently lower blood glucose levels [59]
26.	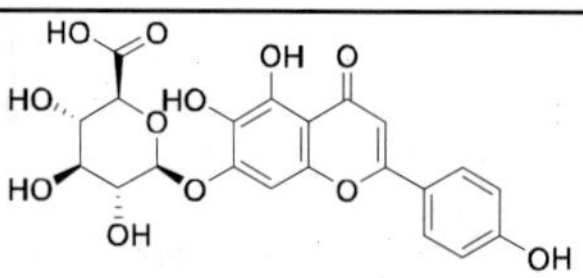	Scutellarin reduced the symptoms of T2DM, including fibrosis, body weight loss, hyperlipidemia, and functional damage to the heart with histological changes [60]
27.	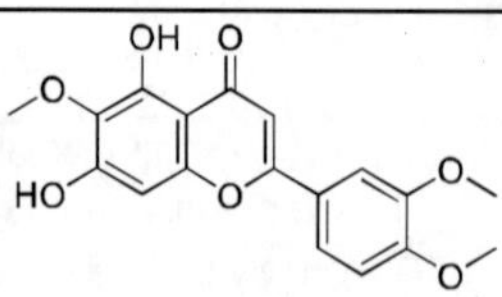	Enhanced insulin production without a precise mechanism; nonetheless, K+-ATP sensitive and Ca^{2+} voltage-dependent channels, which are crucial for insulin secretion, are involved [61]

Compound No.	Structure	Mechanism
28.	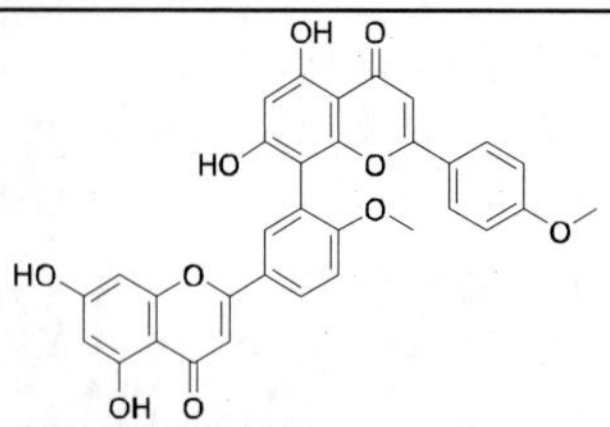	Adipogenesis [62]
29.	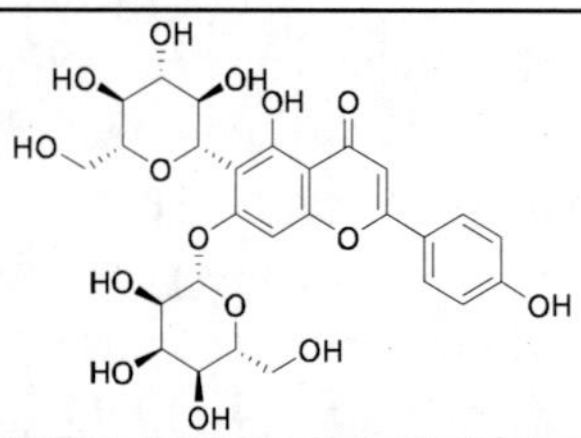	α-glucosidase inhibitor [63]

2.3. Anthraquinones

The inhibitory action of chryso-obtusin-2-O-D-glucoside (31) derived from acetic ether extract of *Cassia tora* seeds was examined using in vitro bioassays (Table 4). It also suppresses AGEPsBSA production using indirect AGEP-ELISA more effectively than the AGEPs inhibitor aminoguanidine. Compound 31 strongly blocked the AR mouse lens with IC_{50} values of 8.8 M [67, 68].

Table 4. Heterocyclic anthraquinones

Compound No.	Structure	Mechanism
1.	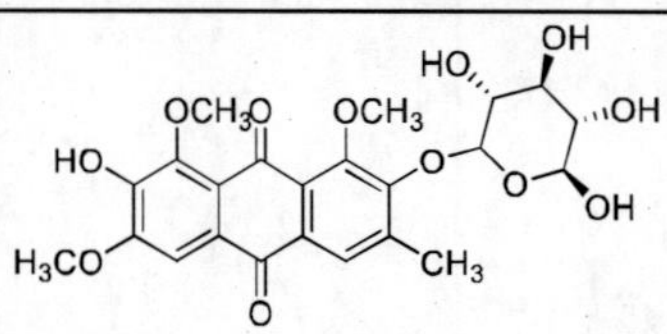	inhibiting effects on both PTP1B and -glucosidase [68]

2.4. Terpenes

New sesquiterpene glycoside nerolidol-3-O-l-rhamnopyranosyl-(1-->4) - alpha-l-rhamnopyranosyl – (1-->2)-[alpha-l- rhamnopyranosyl(1-->6)-beta-d-glucopyranoside (32) was isolated from dried leaves of loquat, *Eriobotrya japonica* (Thunb.) Lindl. Compound 32 at doses of 25 and 75 mg/kg demonstrated a significant ($p < 0.05$) hypoglycemic activity in alloxan-induced diabetic rats [69].

A useful compound called costunolide (33) is present in the Costusspeciosus plant. It reduces plasma glucose considerably and dose-dependently ($p < 0.05$). Additionally, an oral dose of costunolide (20 mg/kg) increases plasma insulin, muscle glycogen, high-density lipoprotein (HDL) cholesterol, and serum protein while dramatically decreasing glycosylated haemoglobin, total serum cholesterol, triglycerides, and LDL cholesterol. By reducing NO on the islands, costunolide may promote the synthesis of insulin [70].

Table 5. Heterocyclic terpenes

Compound No.	Structure	Mechanism
1.	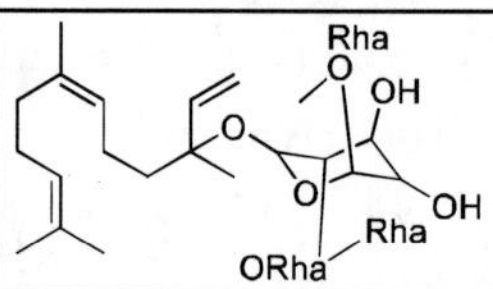	Inhibition of glucocidase [72]
2.	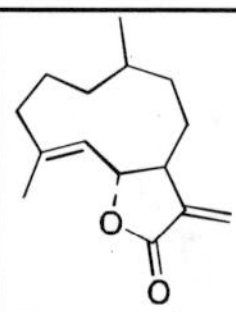	Block CTL-mediated cytotoxicity [73]
3.	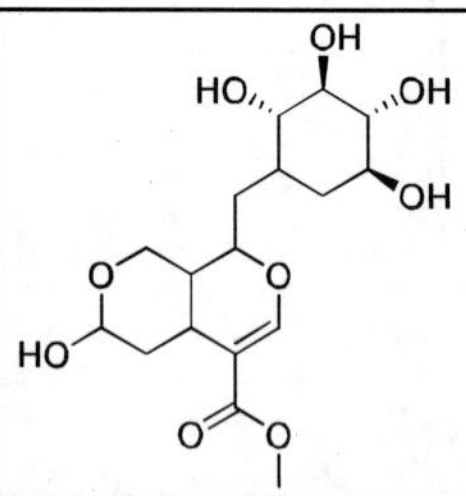	Alpha glucosidase inhibitor [74]

An active substance extracted from *Cornus officinalis* is called morroniside (34). Yokozawa et al. investigated the effects of morroniside on kidney injury in diabetic rats treated with STZ. Morroniside significantly reduced serum glucose and urine protein levels in diabetic mice when administered orally for 20 days at 20 mg/kg [71]. It also prevented oxidative stress. Table 5 shows heterocyclic terpenes and antidiabetic actions [72-74].

2.5. Coumarins and Lignans

Peucedanol 7-O-D-glucopyranoside (35), a coumarin, was found in 80% of the ethanol extracted from *Peucedani radix* (*Peucedanum japonicum*, Umbelliferae) (Table 6). At a dosage of 5.8 mg/kg, compound 35 lowered postprandial hyperglycemia by 39%. It has been demonstrated that plasma glucose uptake increases insulin resistance and triggers an overproduction of glucose transporter-4 in skeletal muscle [75, 76].

Eighty percent of the ethanol extracts of *Peucedani radix* (*Peucedanum japonicum*, Umbelliferae) contained the coumarin peucedanol 7-O-D-glucopyranoside (35). Compound 35 decreased postprandial hyperglycemia by 39% at 5.8 mg/kg. Plasma glucose drop was observed to be promoted by increased insulin resistance and overexpression of glucose transporter-4 in skeletal muscle.

Table 6. Heterocyclic coumarins

Compound No.	Structure	Mechanism
1.	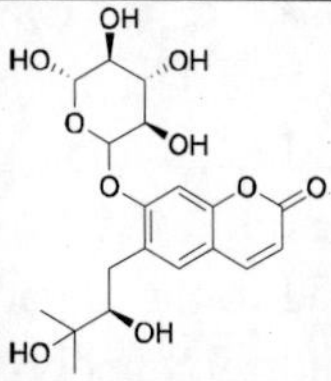	Alpha glucosidase inhibitor [72]
2.	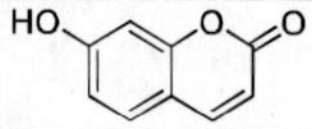	Decreased insulin resistance and high blood sugar levels and increased hepatic glycogen [76]

The bitter orange (*Citrus aurantium*) and golden apple (*Aegle marmelos* Correa) contain umbelliferone (7-hydroxycoumarin) (36). According to research by Pugalendi and colleagues, umbelliferone may protect the liver and kidneys against the creation of fatty acids, lower blood sugar and cholesterol levels, reduce lipid peroxidation, and improve antioxidant levels. These results demonstrate the antidiabetic and anti-hyperlipidemic effects of umbelliferone [77].

2.6. Phenolics

A new compound, 2,5-dihydroxy-4,3-di-(-D-glucopyranosyloxy)-trans-stilbene, was produced by *Morus bombycis* Koidzumi (37). At doses ranging from 200 to 800 mg/kg, this medication reduced hyperglycemia in STZ-induced diabetic rats, and its effect on blood sugar levels was comparable to that of tolbutamide (Table 7) [78].

Table 7. Heterocyclic phenolics

Compound No.	Structure	Mechanism
1.	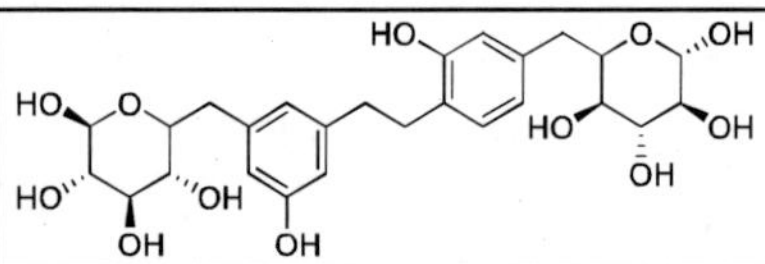	Alpha glucosidase inhibitor [78]

2.7. Other Compounds

Bidens pilosa has a novel polyacetylenic glucoside called cytopiloyne (38), which prevents T1DM via controlling T cells, and decreases CD4+ T cell proliferation and type 1 differentiation. In addition, lymph nodes and the pancreatic spleen had fewer CD4+ T cells after long-term cytopiloyne treatment. The new carbohydrate (39) discovered in the aqueous extracts of the roots and rhizomes of *Psacalium peltatum* showed hypoglycemic activity at dose of 100 mg/kg, compared to tolbutamide and insulin in alloxan-treated diabetic rats [79].

According to studies on rats and mice, the brucines E (40) and D (41) present in *Brucea javanica* (L.) seeds reduce blood sugar levels. When normoglycemic mice were administered 1 mg/kg of compounds 40 and 41, their blood glucose levels decreased by 40.07 ± 11.45% and 48.82 ± 13.34%, respectively. Compounds 40 and 41 significantly reduced blood glucose levels in STZ-treated animals by 73.57 ± 13.64% and 87.99 ± 2.91% [80], respectively. These two substances may function as insulin secretagogues (Table 8) [81-85].

Table 8. Other heterocyclic compounds

Compound No.	Structure	Mechanism
3.	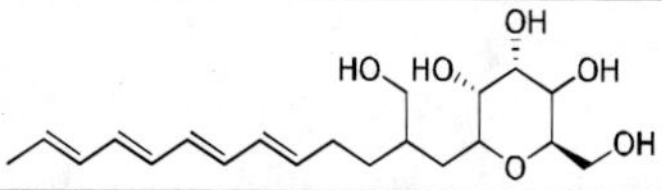	decreased postprandial glycemia and elevated blood insulin levels [81]
4.	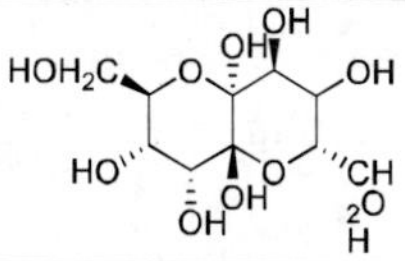	Lower blood sugar level [82]
5.	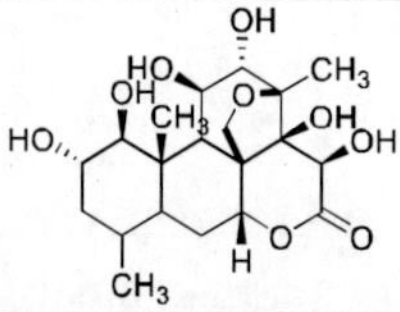	Reduce blood sugar level [83]
6.	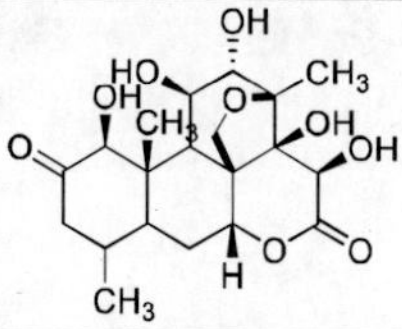	Reduce blood sugar level [83]
7.	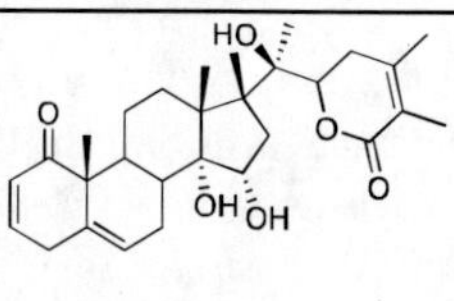	By controlling hepatic glucose production, coagulanolide is effective in the management of fasting hyperglycemia in T2DM [84]
8.	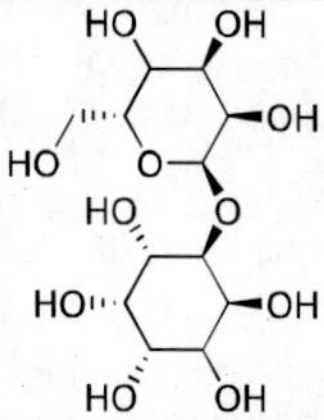	Improve insulin resistance and the progression of T2DM [85]
9.	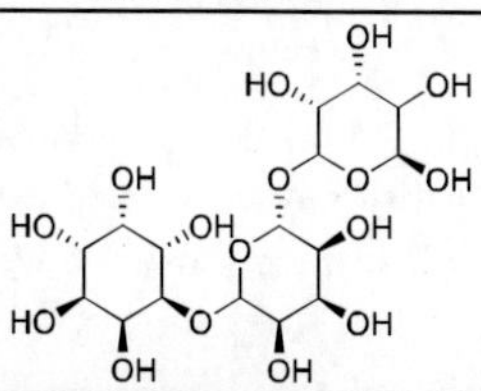	Improve insulin resistance and the progression of T2DM [85]

Both mice with normoglycemic diabetes and those with STZ were protected from post-hyperglycemia after succulent load by coagulanolide, which can be found in the fruit of *Withania coagulans*. Additionally, it increased the db/db mice's ability to tolerate glucose and significantly reduced their FBG profile. Comparing coagulanolide to the standard antidiabetic medicine metformin, it was observed that the average effective dose of coagulanolide was around 25 mg/kg in patients with STZ-induced diabetes in mice [86].

The traditional Indian herb *Mucuna pruriens* has been investigated for its hypoglycemic and anti-hyperglycemic benefits. It has created three novel cyclitols, including D-chiro-inositol and its two galacto-derivatives (43 and 44). This remedy significantly impacts hypoglycemia [87].

Conclusion

Medicine derived from natural resources has significant value in treating health disorders. Most phytochemicals with antidiabetic bioactivity manage diabetes by lowering hyperglycemia and hyperlipidemia, inhibiting amylase, and regulating insulin secretion.

References

[1] Agarwal P, Gupta R. Alpha-amylase inhibition can treat diabetes mellitus. *Research and Reviews Journal of Medical and Health Sciences*. 2016;5(4):1-8.

[2] Aschner P, Karuranga S, James S, Simmons D, Basit A, Shaw JE, Wild SH, Ogurtsova K, Saeedi P. The International Diabetes Federation's guide for diabetes epidemiological studies. *Diabetes Research and Clinical Practice*. 2021;172.

[3] Atlas D. International diabetes federation. *IDF Diabetes Atlas, 7th edn* Brussels, Belgium: International Diabetes Federation. 2015;33.

[4] Skyler JS. Diabetes mellitus: pathogenesis and treatment strategies. *Journal of medicinal chemistry*. 2004;47(17):4113-7.

[5] Whiting DR, Guariguata L, Weil C, Shaw J. IDF diabetes atlas: global estimates of the prevalence of diabetes for 2011 and 2030. *Diabetes research and clinical practice*. 2011;94(3):311-21.

[6] Ogurtsova K, da Rocha Fernandes J, Huang Y, Linnenkamp U, Guariguata L, Cho NH, Cavan D, Shaw J, Makaroff L. IDF Diabetes Atlas: Global estimates for the prevalence of diabetes for 2015 and 2040. *Diabetes research and clinical practice*. 2017;128:40-50.

[7] Kahanovitz L, Sluss PM, Russell SJ. Type 1 diabetes–a clinical perspective. *Point of care.* 2017;16(1):37.
[8] Association AD. Diagnosis and classification of diabetes mellitus. *Diabetes care.* 2010;33(Supplement_1):S62-S9.
[9] Association AD. Diagnosis and classification of diabetes mellitus. *Diabetes care.* 2014;37(Supplement_1):S81-S90.
[10] Blair M. Diabetes mellitus review. *Urologic nursing*. 2016;36(1).
[11] Coustan DR. Gestational diabetes mellitus. *Clinical chemistry*. 2013;59(9):1310-21.
[12] Maraschin JdF. Classification of diabetes. *Diabetes*. 2013:12-9.
[13] Hwang JL, Weiss RE. Steroid-induced diabetes: a clinical and molecular approach to understanding and treatment. *Diabetes/metabolism research and reviews*. 2014;30(2):96-102.
[14] Merger SR, Kerner W, Stadler M, Zeyfang A, Jehle P, Mueller-Korbsch M, Holl R, Initiative D, mellitus GBCND. Prevalence and comorbidities of double diabetes. Diabetes research and clinical practice. 2016;119:48-56.
[15] Vantyghem M-C, Press M, editors. Management strategies for brittle diabetes. *Annales d'endocrinologie*; 2006: Elsevier.
[16] Urbanová J, Brunerová L, Brož J. Hidden MODY—Looking for a Needle in a Haystack. *Frontiers in Endocrinology*. 2018;9:355.
[17] Lemelman MB, Letourneau L, Greeley SAW. Neonatal diabetes mellitus: an update on diagnosis and management. *Clinics in perinatology*. 2018;45(1):41-59.
[18] Hemming K. 1, 2, 4-Oxadiazoles. *Comprehensive heterocyclic chemistry III*: Elsevier Ltd; 2008. p. 243-314.
[19] Singh LP. A Review of Heterocyclic Compounds for Antidiabetic Activity. *Systematic Reviews in Pharmacy*. 2022;13(4):410-3.
[20] Vitaku E, Smith DT, Njardarson JT. Analysis of the structural diversity, substitution patterns, and frequency of nitrogen heterocycles among US FDA approved pharmaceuticals: miniperspective. *Journal of medicinal chemistry.* 2014;57(24):10257-74.
[21] Tan M-J, Ye J-M, Turner N, Hohnen-Behrens C, Ke C-Q, Tang C-P, Chen T, Weiss H-C, Gesing E-R, Rowland A. Antidiabetic activities of triterpenoids isolated from bitter melon associated with activation of the AMPK pathway. *Chemistry & biology.* 2008;15(3):263-73.
[22] Hoa NK, Norberg A, Sillard R, Van Phan D, Thuan ND, Dzung DTN, Jörnvall H, Östenson C-Gr. The possible mechanisms by which phanoside stimulates insulin secretion from rat islets. *Journal of Endocrinology*. 2007;192(2):389-94.
[23] Daisy P, Jasmine R, Ignacimuthu S, Murugan E. A novel steroid from Elephantopus scaber L. an ethnomedicinal plant with antidiabetic activity. *Phytomedicine*. 2009;16(2-3):252-7.
[24] Cho WC, Chung W-S, Lee SK, Leung AW, Cheng CH, Yue KK. Ginsenoside Re of Panax ginseng possesses significant antioxidant and anti-hyperlipidemic efficacies in streptozotocin-induced diabetic rats. *European journal of pharmacology*. 2006;550(1-3):173-9.

[25] Da Porto A, Brosolo G, Casarsa V, Bulfone L, Scandolin L, Catena C, Sechi LA. The pivotal role of oleuropein in the antidiabetic action of the Mediterranean diet: A concise review. *Pharmaceutics*. 2021;14(1):40.

[26] Wang N, Siu F, Zhang Y. Effect of astragaloside IV on diabetic gastric mucosa in vivo and in vitro. *American Journal of Translational Research*. 2017;9(11):4902.

[27] Norberg A, Hoa NK, Liepinsh E, Van Phan D, Thuan ND, Jörnvall H, Sillard R, Östenson C-Gr. A novel insulin-releasing substance, phanoside, from the plant Gynostemma pentaphyllum. *Journal of Biological Chemistry*. 2004;279(40): 41361-7.

[28] Zhang Z, Li X, Lv W, Yang Y, Gao H, Yang J, Shen Y, Ning G. Ginsenoside Re reduces insulin resistance through inhibition of c-Jun NH2-terminal kinase and nuclear factor-κB. *Molecular endocrinology*. 2008;22(1):186-95.

[29] Lai D-M, Tu Y-K, Liu I-M, Chen P-F, Cheng J-T. Mediation of β-endorphin by ginsenoside Rh2 to lower plasma glucose in streptozotocin-induced diabetic rats. *Planta medica*. 2006;72(01):9-13.

[30] Gao D, Li Q, Li Y, Liu Z, Liu Z, Fan Y, Han Z, Li J, Li K. Antidiabetic potential of oleanolic acid from Ligustrum lucidum Ait. *Canadian Journal of Physiology and Pharmacology*. 2007;85(11):1076-83.

[31] Sato H, Genet C, Strehle A, Thomas C, Lobstein A, Wagner A, Mioskowski C, Auwerx J, Saladin R. Anti-hyperglycemic activity of a TGR5 agonist isolated from Olea europaea. *Biochemical and biophysical research communications*. 2007;362(4):793-8.

[32] Qi L-W, Yu Q-T, Li P, Li S-L, Wang Y-X, Sheng L-H, Yi L. Quality evaluation of Radix Astragali through a simultaneous determination of six major active isoflavonoids and four main saponins by high-performance liquid chromatography coupled with diode array and evaporative light scattering detectors. *Journal of Chromatography A*. 2006;1134(1-2):162-9.

[33] Xiaoxing Y, Yindi Z, Junxian Y, Pei Z, Jianping S, Jun Q, Haiwei W, Xiang Z. The antioxidative effects of astragalus saponin I protect against development of early diabetic nephropathy. *Journal of pharmacological sciences*. 2006;101(2):166-73.

[34] Coskun O, Kanter M, Korkmaz A, Oter S. Quercetin, a flavonoid antioxidant, prevents and protects streptozotocin-induced oxidative stress and β-cell damage in rat pancreas. *Pharmacological research*. 2005;51(2):117-23.

[35] Quine SD, Raghu PS. Effects of (-)-epicatechin, a flavonoid on lipid peroxidation and antioxidants in streptozotocin-induced diabetic liver, kidney and heart. *Pharmacol Rep*. 2005;57(5):610-5.

[36] Kamalakkannan N, Prince P. Rutin improves the antioxidant status in streptozotocin-induced diabetic rat tissues. *Molecular and cellular biochemistry*. 2006;293(1):211-9.

[37] Estrada O, Hasegawa M, Gonzalez-Mujíca F, Motta N, Perdomo E, Solorzano A, Méndez J, Méndez B, Zea EG. Evaluation of flavonoids from Bauhinia megalandra leaves as inhibitors of glucose-6-phosphatase system. *Phytotherapy Research: An International Journal Devoted to Pharmacological and Toxicological Evaluation of Natural Product Derivatives*. 2005;19(10):859-63.

[38] Jang DS, Kim JM, Lee YM, Kim YS, Kim J-H, Kim JS. Puerariafuran, a new inhibitor of advanced glycation end products (AGEs) isolated from the roots of Pueraria lobata. *Chemical and pharmaceutical bulletin*. 2006;54(9):1315-7.

[39] Yoo NH, Jang DS, Yoo JL, Lee YM, Kim YS, Cho J-H, Kim JS. Erigeroflavanone, a flavanone derivative from the flowers of Erigeron annuus with protein glycation and aldose reductase inhibitory activity. *Journal of Natural Products*. 2008;71(4):713-5.

[40] Lee EH, Song D-G, Lee JY, Pan C-H, Um BH, Jung SH. Inhibitory effect of the compounds isolated from Rhus verniciflua on aldose reductase and advanced glycation endproducts. *Biological and Pharmaceutical Bulletin*. 2008;31(8):1626-30.

[41] Wirasathien L, Pengsuparp T, Suttisri R, Ueda H, Moriyasu M, Kawanishi K. Inhibitors of aldose reductase and advanced glycation end-products formation from the leaves of Stelechocarpus cauliflorus RE Fr. *Phytomedicine*. 2007;14(7-8):546-50.

[42] Liu I-M, Tzeng T-F, Liou S-S, Lan T-W. Improvement of insulin sensitivity in obese Zucker rats by myricetin extracted from Abelmoschus moschatus. *Planta Medica*. 2007;73(10):1054-60.

[43] Baluchnejadmojarad T, Roghani M. Chronic administration of genistein improves aortic reactivity of streptozotocin-diabetic rats: mode of action. *Vascular pharmacology*. 2008;49(1):1-5.

[44] Jung UJ, Lee M-K, Jeong K-S, Choi M-S. The hypoglycemic effects of hesperidin and naringin are partly mediated by hepatic glucose-regulating enzymes in C57BL/KsJ-db/db mice. *The Journal of nutrition*. 2004;134(10):2499-503.

[45] M Eid H, S Haddad P. The antidiabetic potential of quercetin: underlying mechanisms. *Current medicinal chemistry*. 2017;24(4):355-64.

[46] Iftikhar A, Aslam B, Iftikhar M, Majeed W, Batool M, Zahoor B, Amna N, Gohar H, Latif I. Effect of Caesalpinia bonduc polyphenol extract on alloxan-induced diabetic rats in attenuating hyperglycemia by upregulating insulin secretion and inhibiting JNK signaling pathway. *Oxidative Medicine and Cellular Longevity*. 2020;2020.

[47] Nie T, Cooper GJ. Mechanisms underlying the antidiabetic activities of polyphenolic compounds: A review. *Frontiers in Pharmacology*. 2021;12.

[48] Joseph B, Jini D. Antidiabetic effects of Momordica charantia (bitter melon) and its medicinal potency. *Asian pacific journal of tropical disease*. 2013;3(2):93-102.

[49] Gonzalez-Mujica F, Motta N, Estrada O, Perdomo E, Méndez J, Hasegawa M. Inhibition of hepatic neoglucogenesis and glucose-6-phosphatase by quercetin 3-O-α (2 ″-galloyl) rhamnoside isolated from Bauhinia megalandra leaves. *Phytotherapy Research: An International Journal Devoted to Pharmacological and Toxicological Evaluation of Natural Product Derivatives*. 2005;19(7):624-7.

[50] Zywno H, Bzdega W, Kolakowski A, Kurzyna P, Harasim-Symbor E, Sztolsztener K, Chabowski A, Konstantynowicz-Nowicka K. The influence of coumestrol on sphingolipid signaling pathway and insulin resistance development in primary rat hepatocytes. *Biomolecules*. 2021;11(2):268.

[51] Brahmachari G. Bio-flavonoids with promising antidiabetic potentials: A critical survey. *Research signpost*. 2011;661(2):187-212.

[52] Kwon Y, Cho S, Kim J, Lee Y, Lee S, Lee M, editors. Hypoglycemic effect of Cordyceps militaris Polymolecules in Streptozotocin-Induced Diabetic Rats. *Proceedings of the PSK Conference; 2001: The Pharmaceutical Society of Korea*.

[53] Irmisch S, Ruebsam H, Jancsik S, Man Saint Yuen M, Madilao LL, Bohlmann J. Flavonol biosynthesis genes and their use in engineering the plant antidiabetic metabolite montbretin A. Pla*nt Physiology*. 2019;180(3):1277-90.

[54] Irawan C, Rochaeni H, Sulistiawaty L, Roziafanto AN. Phytochemical Screening, LC-MS Studies and Antidiabetic Potential of Methanol Extracts of Seed Shells of Archidendron bubalinum (Jack) IC Nielson (Julang Jaling) from Lampung, Indonesia. *Pharmacognosy Journal*. 2018;10(6s).

[55] Taheri Y, Suleria HAR, Martins N, Sytar O, Beyatli A, Yeskaliyeva B, Seitimova G, Salehi B, Semwal P, Painuli S. Myricetin bioactive effects: Moving from preclinical evidence to potential clinical applications. *BMC complementary medicine and therapies*. 2020;20(1):1-14.

[56] Patel IC, Hakim M, Prajapati R, Solanki A, Panigrahi J. In *Vitro Approach and Quantification of "Puerarin and Genistein": Valuable Antidiabetic Compounds from Pueraria tuberosa.* Biotechnology of Anti-diabetic Medicinal Plants: Springer; 2021. p. 1-24.

[57] Sundaram R, Nandhakumar E, Haseena Banu H. Hesperidin, a citrus flavonoid ameliorates hyperglycemia by regulating key enzymes of carbohydrate metabolism in streptozotocin-induced diabetic rats. *Toxicology Mechanisms and Methods*. 2019;29(9):644-53.

[58] Den Hartogh DJ, Tsiani E. Antidiabetic properties of naringenin: A citrus fruit polyphenol. *Biomolecules*. 2019;9(3):99.

[59] Das D, Sarkar S, Bordoloi J, Wann SB, Kalita J, Manna P. Daidzein, its effects on impaired glucose and lipid metabolism and vascular inflammation associated with type 2 diabetes. *Biofactors*. 2018;44(5):407-17.

[60] Huo Y, Mijiti A, Cai R, Gao Z, Aini M, Mijiti A, Wang Z, Qie R. Scutellarin alleviates type 2 diabetes (HFD/low dose STZ)-induced cardiac injury through modulation of oxidative stress, inflammation, apoptosis and fibrosis in mice. *Human & Experimental Toxicology*. 2021;40(12_suppl):S460-S74.

[61] Escandón-Rivera SM, Mata R, Andrade-Cetto A. Molecules isolated from Mexican hypoglycemic plants: A Review. *Molecules*. 2020;25(18):4145.

[62] Shao N, Feng Z, Li N. Isoginkgetin inhibits inflammatory response in the fibroblast-like synoviocytes of rheumatoid arthritis by suppressing matrix metallopeptidase 9 expression. *Chemical Biology & Drug Design*. 2022;99(6):923-9.

[63] Jain A, Dasgupta N, Ranjan S, Singh V, Singh H, Purohit SD, Mishra NC, Yadav NP, Haque S, Mishra BN. Whey protein based electrosprayed nanospheres for encapsulation and controlled release of bioactive compounds from Tinospora cordifolia extract. *Innovative Food Science & Emerging Technologies*. 2021;69:102671.

[64] Luo P, Tan Z-H, Zhang Z-F, Zhang H, Liu X-F, Mo Z-J. Scutellarin isolated from Erigeron multiradiatus inhibits high glucose-mediated vascular inflammation. *Yakugaku Zasshi*. 2008;128(9):1293-9.

[65] Kang Y-J, Jung UJ, Lee M-K, Kim H-J, Jeon S-M, Park YB, Chung H-G, Baek N-I, Lee KT, Jeong T-S. Eupatilin, isolated from Artemisia princeps Pampanini, enhances hepatic glucose metabolism and pancreatic β-cell function in type 2 diabetic mice. *Diabetes Research and Clinical Practice*. 2008;82(1):25-32.

[66] Liu G, Grifman M, Macdonald J, Moller P, Wong-Staal F, Li Q-X. Isoginkgetin enhances adiponectin secretion from differentiated adiposarcoma cells via a novel pathway involving AMP-activated protein kinase. *Journal of Endocrinology*. 2007;194(3):569-78.

[67] Jang DS, Lee GY, Kim YS, Lee YM, Kim C-S, Yoo JL, Kim JS. Anthraquinones from the seeds of Cassia tora with inhibitory activity on protein glycation and aldose reductase. *Biological and Pharmaceutical Bulletin*. 2007;30(11):2207-10.

[68] Ali MY, Park S, Chang M. Phytochemistry, Ethnopharmacological Uses, Biological Activities, and Therapeutic Applications of Cassia obtusifolia L.: A Comprehensive Review. *Molecules*. 2021;26(20):6252.

[69] Chen J, Li W, Wu J, Ren B, Zhang H. Hypoglycemic effects of a sesquiterpene glycoside isolated from leaves of loquat (Eriobotrya japonica (Thunb.) Lindl.). *Phytomedicine*. 2008;15(1-2):98-102.

[70] Eliza J, Daisy P, Ignacimuthu S, Duraipandiyan V. Normo-glycemic and hypolipidemic effect of costunolide isolated from Costus speciosus (Koen ex. Retz.) Sm. in streptozotocin-induced diabetic rats. *Chemico-biological interactions*. 2009;179(2-3):329-34.

[71] Yokozawa T, Yamabe N, Kim HY, Kang KS, Hur JM, Park CH, Tanaka T. Protective effects of morroniside isolated from Corni Fructus against renal damage in streptozotocin-induced diabetic rats. *Biological and Pharmaceutical Bulletin*. 2008;31(7):1422-8.

[72] El Ridhasya F, Rahim N, Almurdani M, Hendra R, Teruna HY. Antidiabetic Constituents from Helminthostachys zeylanica (L) Hook (Ophioglossaceae). *Pharmacognosy Journal*. 2020;12(2).

[73] Rashwan AS, El-Beltagy MA, Saleh SY, Ibrahim IA. Potential role of cinnamaldehyde and costunolide to counteract metabolic syndrome induced by excessive fructose consumption. *beni-suef university journal of basic and applied sciences*. 2019;8(1):1-8.

[74] He K, Song S, Zou Z, Feng M, Wang D, Wang Y, Li X, Ye X. *The hypoglycemic and synergistic effect of loganin, morroniside, and ursolic acid isolated from the fruits of Cornus officinalis. Phytotherapy Research*. 2016;30(2):283-91.

[75] Lee SO, Choi SZ, Lee JH, Chung SH, Park SH, Kang HC, Yang EY, Cho HJ, Lee KR. Antidiabetic coumarin and cyclitol compounds fromPeucedanum japonicum. *Archives of pharmacal research*. 2004;27(12):1207-10.

[76] Ranđelović S, Bipat R. A Review of Coumarins and Coumarin-Related Compounds for Their Potential Antidiabetic Effect. *Clinical Medicine Insights: Endocrinology and Diabetes*. 2021;14:11795514211042023.

[77] Ramesh B, Viswanathan P, Pugalendi KV. Protective effect of umbelliferone on membranous fatty acid composition in streptozotocin-induced diabetic rats. *European journal of pharmacology*. 2007;566(1-3):231-9.

[78] Pereira AC, Arruda MS, da Silva EA, da Silva MN, Lemos VS, Cortes SF. Inhibition of α-glucosidase and hypoglycemic effect of stilbenes from the Amazonian plant Deguelia rufescens var. urucu (Ducke) AMG Azevedo (Leguminosae). *Planta medica*. 2012;78(01):36-8.

[79] Contreras C, Roman R, Perez C, Alarcón F, Zavala M, Pérez S. Hypoglycemic activity of a new carbohydrate isolated from the roots of Psacalium peltatum. *Chemical and pharmaceutical bulletin*. 2005;53(11):1408-10.

[80] NoorShahida A, Wong TW, Choo CY. Hypoglycemic effect of quassinoids from Brucea javanica (L.) Merr (Simaroubaceae) seeds. *Journal of ethnopharmacology*. 2009;124(3):586-91.

[81] Chang CL-T, Liu H-Y, Kuo T-F, Hsu Y-J, Shen M-Y, Pan C-Y, Yang W-C. Antidiabetic effect and mode of action of cytopiloyne. *Evidence-Based Complementary and Alternative Medicine*. 2013;2013.

[82] Vyas M. Nutritional profile of spinach and its antioxidant & antidiabetic evaluation. *International Journal of Green Pharmacy* (IJGP). 2017;11(03).

[83] Patle D, Vyas M, Khatik GL. A review on natural products and herbs used in the management of diabetes. *Current diabetes reviews*. 2021;17(2):186-97.

[84] Singh A, Singh N, Akanksha, Jayendra, Maurya R, Srivastava A. Coagulanolide modulates hepatic glucose metabolism in C57BL/KsJ-db/db mice. *Human & experimental toxicology*. 2012;31(10):1056-65.

[85] Sánchez-Hidalgo M, León-González AJ, Gálvez-Peralta M, González-Mauraza NH, Martin-Cordero C. D-Pinitol: A cyclitol with versatile biological and pharmacological activities. *Phytochemistry Reviews*. 2021;20(1):211-24.

[86] Maurya R, Singh AB, Srivastava AK. Coagulanolide, a withanolide from Withania coagulans fruits and anti-hyperglycemic activity. *Bioorganic & Medicinal Chemistry Letters*. 2008;18(24):6534-7.

[87] Donati D, Lampariello LR, Pagani R, Guerranti R, Cinci G, Marinello E. Antidiabetic oligocyclitols in seeds of Mucuna pruriens. *Phytotherapy Research: An International Journal Devoted to Pharmacological and Toxicological Evaluation of Natural Product Derivatives*. 2005;19(12):1057-60.

Chapter 11

Natural Products in the Treatment of Diabetes: An Insight into the Mechanism of Action

Pranav Kumar Prabhakar[1,*]
and Yachana Mishra[2]
[1]Division of Research and Development, Lovely Professional University, Phagwara, (Punjab), India
[2]School of Bioengineering and Biosciences, Lovely Professional University, Phagwara, (Punjab), India

Abstract

Elevated blood glucose levels are a hallmark of diabetes mellitus (DM), a metabolic condition brought on by inadequate or inefficient insulin secretor response (hyperglycemia). A variety of syndromes make up the DM category. The body uses glucose primarily for energy, and when someone has DM, their body manages glucose inconsistently. Three defects primarily cause the start of hyperglycemia in DM: increased hepatic glucose synthesis, decreased insulin secretion, and reduced insulin action. Conventional medications for diabetes work to improve insulin sensitivity, boost insulin production, and/or lower blood glucose levels. The most well-known hypoglycemic herbs, including fenugreek, ginseng, gymnema, bitter melon, *Coptis chinensis*, and banaba, boost insulin secretion and promote skeletal muscle and adipose tissue glucose uptake, blocking intestinal glucose absorption, and reducing hepatic glucose synthesis. Although the therapeutic effect of these phytomedicines has been consistently demonstrated in humans and animals, multi-centric large-scale clinical trials have not been conducted to assess the efficacy and safety of these herbal medicines and their

---

* Corresponding Author's Email: prabhakar.iitm@gmail.com.

In: Management of Diabetes Mellitus Based on Natural Products
Editors: Yachana Mishra and Vijay Mishra
ISBN: 979-8-88697-853-7

interactions with conventional medications when both are administered at the same time.

Keywords: diabetes mellitus, blood glucose level, herbal medicines, hyperglycemia

1. Introduction

Diabetes mellitus (DM) is a chronic disease caused by inherited and/or acquired deficiency in insulin production by the pancreas or by the ineffectiveness of the insulin produced. Such a deficiency results in increased glucose concentrations in the blood, which damages many of the body's systems, particularly the blood vessels and nerves. DM is a metabolic disorder and abnormally high blood glucose levels (hyperglycemia) [1]. DM can be divided into two major categories insulin-dependent diabetes mellitus (IDDM) or type 1 (an autoimmune disease of younger patients with a lack of insulin production causing hyperglycemia and a tendency towards ketosis) and noninsulin-dependent diabetes mellitus (NIDDM) or type 2 (a metabolic disorder resulting from the body's inability to produce enough or properly utilize insulin hence patients have hyperglycemia but are ketosis resistant). Over 90% of patients with diabetes have type 2. Currently, an estimated 170 million people worldwide suffer from diabetes mellitus, which is predicted to double by 2030 [2-4]. The reason for this global rise is the growth of the aged population, increasing trends towards obesity, unhealthy diet, and sedentary lifestyle [5, 6]. This condition requires medical treatment and several lifestyle changes.

Apart from currently available therapeutic options, many herbal medicines have been recommended to treat diabetes. Plants have been used traditionally throughout the world because of their effectiveness, fewer side effects, and relatively low cost [7,8]. Therefore, the investigation on such agents from traditional medicinal plants has become more important. Today, managing diabetes without any side effects is still a challenge to the medical fraternity. A wide array of plant-derived active principles have demonstrated antidiabetic activity. The main active constituents of these plants include alkaloids, glycosides, galactomannan gum, polysaccharides, peptidoglycan, hypoglycans, guanidine, steroids, carbohydrates, glycopeptides, terpenoids, amino acids and inorganic ions [9]. These affect various metabolic cascades, which directly or indirectly affect the level of glucose in the human body.

2. Synthetic Antidiabetic Drugs

The currently available antidiabetic drugs manage the blood glucose levels under normal range by supplementing insulin, improving insulin sensitivity, increasing insulin secretion from the pancreas, decreasing glucose absorption from the intestinal tract and/or glucose uptake by tissue cells. There are several types of glucose-lowering drugs, including insulin secretagogues (sulfonylureas, meglitinides), insulin sensitizers (biguanides, metformin, thiazolidinediones) and α-glucosidase inhibitors (miglitol, acarbose) [10-12]. The mechanism of insulin release from β-cells in response to changes in blood glucose concentration is a complex process [13]. The insulin stimulation followed by cascade signaling enhances glucose intake, utilization and storage in various tissues. In diabetic patients, the body loses insulin production capacity due to pancreatic β-cell apoptosis or insulin insensitivity [14].

3. Natural Products in Diabetes Treatment

Management of diabetes without any side effects is still a challenge to the medical fraternity [15]. Traditional medicinal plants with various active principles and properties have been used since ancient times [16, 17]. Medicinal plants have multiple beneficial activities, including manipulating carbohydrate metabolism by various mechanisms, preventing and restoring integrity and functioning of β-cells, insulin-releasing activity, improving glucose uptake and utilization, and antioxidant properties. However, a few herbal medicines have been well characterized, and their efficacy has been demonstrated in systematic clinical trials [18], similar to commercially available synthetic drugs [19]. Adverse effects from herbal remedies are not rare, but their frequency and severity are unknown [20].

4. Mechanism of Action of Commonly Used Medicinal Plants

There are different natural medicines used for combating diabetes also, and thousands of dietary supplements are commercially marketed for people with diabetes. However, only a fraction of these products have reliable clinical evidence of effectiveness. The phytochemicals work through various metabolic pathways involving glucose or its derivatives as substrate or product. They affect glucose metabolism (glycolysis, Kreb's cycle), pentose phosphate pathways, glycogenesis, glycogenolysis, gluconeogenesis, absorption of glucose via the alimentary canal, and increase insulin release, its production, and its efficacy [13]. Many of these natural medicines modulate blood sugar levels through various mechanisms. Each herb consists of various components, only a few of which may be therapeutically effective [21,22].

4.1. Ginseng

This is the most studied medicinal plant for its hypoglycemic activities. *Panax ginseng,* also known as Chinese or Korean, has the highest therapeutic potency. *Panax quinquefolius,* i.e., American ginseng has medium potency, while *Panax japonicus* (Japanese ginseng) is considered to have low potency. The most commonly used therapeutic ginseng is *Panax ginseng*. Ginseng can decrease blood glucose by affecting various pathways.

Korean red ginseng (0.1-1.0 g/mL) significantly stimulates insulin release from isolated rat pancreatic islets at a glucose concentration of 3.3 mM [23]. The treatment with oral administration of H-AG (heat-processed American ginseng) at a dose of 100 mg/kg of body weight for 20 days decreased serum levels of glucose, glycosylated proteins and hemoglobin A1C in streptozotocin (STZ)-induced diabetic rats. The treatment also improved the decreased creatinine clearance levels and decreased the accumulation of N (ε)-(carboxymethyl) lysine and its receptors in the kidney [24]. *Radix Ginseng Alba* improved hyperglycemia in KKAy mice, possibly by blocking intestinal glucose absorption and inhibiting the hepatic glucose-6-phosphatase. *Radix Ginseng Palva* has a similar effect through the up-regulation of adipocytic PPAR-y protein expression and inhibiting intestinal glucose absorption [25].

Panax ginseng and American ginseng contain ginsenosides, which are thought to decrease insulin resistance and improve insulin sensitivity [26-28]. *Panax quinquefolius* increases body weight and reduces cholesterol levels, PPAR actions and triglyceride metabolism in male Zucker diabetic fatty (ZDF) rats with T2DM [29]. *P. quinquefolius* improves postprandial glycemia in patients with T2DM [30]. Ginsenoside Rh2 decreases plasma glucose concentrations within 60 minutes in a dose-dependent manner in rats fed with fructose-rich chow and after a single intravenous injection in STZ-induced insulin-resistant rats [31]. The ginsenoside Rh2 might be acting through the release of ACh from nerve terminals, stimulating muscarinic M(3) receptors in pancreatic cells to increase insulin secretion [32-34].

4.2. Bitter Gourd (*Momordica charantia*)

The antidiabetic components in bitter melon include charantin, vicine, polypeptide-p, alkaloids, and other non-specific bioactive antioxidants [35, 36]. A hypoglycemic peptide, Polypeptide-p, has been isolated from fruits, seeds, and tissue of *Momordica charantia* Linn (bitter gourd) [37]. Oleanolic acid glycosides, isolated from bitter melon, improved glucose tolerance in T2DM by preventing sugar from being absorbed in the intestines. In STZ-induced diabetic mice, bitter melon decreased the blood glucose via suppression of STZ-induced peroxidation and apoptosis in β-cells by increasing the glycogen content in the liver and muscle and activating hepatic glucokinase, hexokinase, and phosphofructokinase [38-42].

Reported adverse effects of bitter melon include hypoglycemic coma, convulsions in children, reduced fertility in mice, a favism-like syndrome, increased activities of γ-glutamyl transferase and alkaline phosphatase in animals, and headaches in humans. The mechanism of action remains to be fully established. Bitter melon can be used as a dietary supplement in herbal medicine to manage diabetes and/or metabolic syndromes [43-45].

4.3. Coptis Chinensis (Huanglian)

Berberine is an isoquinoline alkaloid and the active ingredient present in Coptis chinensis. It is found in plant roots, rhizomes, stems, and barks. Intragastric administration of berberine in diabetic rats decreased fasting blood glucose levels and total cholesterol, triglyceride and LDL-C in the serum, whereas it increased HDL-C and NO level, and blocked the increment of SOD and GSH-px levels [46]. It increases GLUT4 translocation in adipocytes and myotubes [47], increases AMPK activity and decreases glucose-stimulated insulin secretion (GSIS) and palmitate-potential insulin secretion in MIN6 cells and rat islets [48]. It also increases the expressions of PPAR α/δ/γ proteins in the liver [49], increases the expressions of the insulin receptor in the liver and skeletal muscle cells, and improves cellular glucose consumption in the presence of insulin [50]. Berberine also significantly decreases the activity of intestinal disaccharidases and β-glucuronidase in STZ-induced diabetic rats [51, 52]. Studies showed that berberine restored damaged pancreas tissues in diabetic rats induced by alloxan. Berberine is found to lower fasting and postprandial blood glucose in 48 adult patients with T2DM [53, 54].

4.4. Banaba (*Lagerstroemia Speciosa*)

Diabetes patients in North America commonly use Banaba, which contains two important constituents and has two crucial effects on diabetic patients. Banaba extracts containing corosolic acid and ellagitannins seem to have an insulin-like effect and activate insulin receptors [55]. The latter activity is thought to be secondary to the activation of the insulin receptor tyrosine kinase or the inhibition of tyrosine phosphatase.

4.5. Fenugreek (*Trigonella Foenum-Graecum*)

Fenugreek is an herbal remedy sourced from the dried seeds of a plant native to India, China, and North Africa. Studies with mice indicate that 4-hydroxyisoleucine (an amino acid derived from fenugreek) may help to stimulate the secretion of insulin, reduce insulin resistance, and decrease blood sugar levels [56]. Preliminary research shows that T2DM patients who mix 15 g of ground, powdered fenugreek seeds with a meal have lower postprandial glucose levels when compared to the control [57]. This might be due to a bulk laxative effect and slow carbohydrate absorption from the gastrointestinal tract. But fenugreek also seems to enhance insulin release due to the presence of 4-isoleucine [58]. Studies show that the adjunct use of fenugreek seeds improves glycemic control and decreases insulin resistance in mild T2DM patients. There is also a favorable effect on hypertriglyceridemia and improvement in HDL-cholesterol levels [59].

Fenugreek and Sodium orthovanadate alone or in low-dose combination have effectively controlled ocular histopathological and biochemical abnormalities associated with diabetic retinopathy [60]. Low doses of Vanadate and fenugreek in combination normalize altered membrane-linked functions and GLU4 distribution without any side effects [61, 62]. Fenugreek seeds are rich in protein and contain the unique free amino acid 4-hydoxyisoleucine (4-OH-Ile), which has been characterized as one of the active ingredients for blood glucose control [63, 64].

4.6. *Gymnema*

Gymnema has been tested as a hypoglycemic agent in combination with insulin, and the results are encouraging [65, 66]. The plant extract works by increasing endogenous insulin production or serum C-peptide levels. Therefore, C-peptide is used as a marker to monitor endogenous insulin release. Gymnema also decreases total cholesterol levels, triglycerides and LDL cholesterol; instead, it enhances HDL cholesterol levels.

Conclusion

Diabetes is a metabolic disorder arising mainly due to a fault in insulin production or mounting resistance to its action. In the case of DM, the most severe problem is the side effect that occurs due to the accumulation of glucose. This excess glucose is converted into various compounds and free radicals, damaging the vital organs and organelles. There are no specific medicines in the market to treat these complications.

Several plants can reduce glucose production, induce glucose utilization, and combat secondary complications. Herbal treatments have been used in patients with insulin-dependent and non-insulin-dependent diabetes, diabetic retinopathy, diabetic peripheral neuropathy, etc. However, less than 1% of plants have been screened pharmacologically, and only a fraction for DM. This needs further exploration before drugs and nutraceuticals can be developed from these natural resources. Many herbal therapies have not undergone proper scientific assessment, and some potentially cause serious toxic effects and major drug-to-drug interaction. Continued research is necessary to elucidate the pharmacological activities of herbal remedies.

References

[1] Lin Y, Sun Z. Current Views on Type II Diabetes. *J. Endocrinol.* 2010;204(1):1-11.

[2] King H, Aubert R E, Herman W H. Global burden of diabetes, 1995-2025: prevalence, numerical estimates, and projections. *Diabetes Care* 1998;21(9):1414-1431.

[3] Marx J. Unraveling the causes of diabetes. *Science* 2002;296(5568):686-689.

[4] Mohler M L, He Y, Wu Z, Dong J H, Miller D D. Recent and emerging anti-diabetes targets. *Med. Res. Rev.* 2009;29(1):125-195.

[5] Bagust A, Hopkinson P K, Maier W, Currie C J. An economic model of the long-term health care burden of Type II diabetes. *Diabetologia* 2001;44(12):2140-2155.

[6] Harris M I, Flegal K M, Cowie C C, Eberhardt M S, Goldstein D E, Little R R, Wiedmeyer H M, Byrd-Holt D D. Prevalence of diabetes, impaired fasting glucose,

and impaired glucose tolerance in U.S. adults. The Third National Health and Nutrition Examination Survey, 1988-1994. *Diabetes Care* 1998;21(4):518-524.

[7] Gupta RK, Kesari AN, Murthy PS, Chandra R, Tandon V, Watal G. Hypoglycemic and antidiabetic effect of ethanolic extract of leaves of *Annona squamosa* L. in experimental animals. *J. Ethnopharmacol.* 2005;99(1):75-81.

[8] Alarcon-Aguilara F J, Roman-Ramos R, Perez-Gutierrez S, Aguilar-Contreras A, Contreras-Weber C C, Flores-Saenz J L. Study of the anti-hyperglycemic effect of plants used as antidiabetics. *J. Ethnopharmacol.* 1998;61(2):101-110.

[9] Prabhakar P K, Doble M. A target based therapeutic approach towards diabetes mellitus using medicinal plants. *Curr. Diabetes Rev.* 2008;4(4): 291-308.

[10] Modi P. Diabetes beyond insulin: Review of new drugs for treatment of diabetes mellitus. *Curr. Drug Discov. Technol.* 2007;4(1):39-47.

[11] Hui H, Zhao X, Perfetti R. Structure and function studies of glucagon-like peptide-1 (GLP-1): The designing of a novel pharmacological agent for the treatment of diabetes. *Diabetes Metab. Res. Rev.* 2005;21(4):313-331.

[12] Garber A J, Spann S J. An overview of incretin clinical trials. *J. Fam. Pract.* 2008; 57(9Suppl):S10-S18.

[13] Prabhakar P K, Doble M. Mechanism of action of medicinal plants towards diabetes mellitus-a review., in: J. N. Govil, V.K. Singh, R. Bhardwaj (Eds.) Recent Progress in Medicinal Plants, Vol 22, Studium Press, LLC, USA, 2008, pp. 187-210.

[14] Hui H, Dotta F, Di Mario U, Perfetti R. Role of caspases in the regulation of apoptotic pancreatic islet beta-cells death. *J. Cell Physiol.* 2004;200 (2):177-200.

[15] Kameswararao B, Kesavulu MM, Apparao C. Evaluation of antidiabetic effect of Momordica cymbalaria fruit in alloxan-diabetic rats. *Fitoterapia* 2003;74(1-2):7-13.

[16] Middleton E, Kandaswami C, Theoharides T C. The Effects of Plant Flavonoids on Mammalian Cells:Implications for Inflammation, Heart Disease, and Cancer. *Pharmacol. Rev.* 2000;52 (4):673-751.

[17] Grover J K, Vats V. Shifting the Paradigm From Conventional to Alternative Medicines :An Introduction on Traditional Indian Medicines. *Asia Pacific Biotech. News* 2001;5(1): 28-32.

[18] Ernst E. Herbal medicines: where is the evidence? BMJ 2000; 321(7258):395-396.

[19] Wood A J J, De Smet PAGM. Herbal Remedies. *N. Engl. J. Med.* 2002;347(25): 2046-2056.

[20] Inamdar N, Edalat S, Kotwal V, Pawar S. *Care with nature's cure: Herbal drugs. Pharmacognosy Review* 2007; 1(2):361-368.

[21] Liu R H. Potential synergy of phytochemicals in cancer prevention: Mechanism of action. *J. Nutr.* 2004;**134**(12 Suppl)**:**3479S-3485S.

[22] Kawase M, Wang R, Shiomi T, Saijo R, Yagi K. Antioxidative activity of (-)-epigallocatechin-3-(3"-O-methyl) gallate isolated from fresh tea leaf and preliminary results on its biological activity. *Biosci. Biotechnol. Biochem.* 2000;**64**(10)**:**2218-2220.

[23] Kim K, Kim H Y. Korean red ginseng stimulates insulin release from isolated rat pancreatic islets, *J. Ethnopharmacol.* 2008;**120**(2)**:**190-195.

[24] Kim E K, Kwon K B, Lee J H, Park B H, Park J W, Lee H K, Jhee E C, Yang J Y. Inhibition of cytokine-mediated nitric oxide synthase expression in rat insulinoma cells by scoparone. *Biol. Pharm. Bull.* 2007;**30**(2)**:**242-246.

[25] Chung S H, Choi C G, Park S H. Comparisons between white ginseng radix and rootlet for antidiabetic activity and mechanism in KKAy mice. *Arch. Pharm. Res.* 2001;**24**(3)**:**214-218.

[26] Vuksan V, Sievenpiper J L, Koo V Y, Francis T, Beljan-Zdravkovic U, Xu Z, Vidgen E. American ginseng (*Panax quinquefolius* L) reduces postprandial glycemia in nondiabetic subjects and subjects with type 2 diabetes mellitus. *Arch. Intern. Med.* 2000;**160**(7)**:**1009-1013.

[27] Kimura M, Kimura I, Chem F J. Combined potentiating effects of Byakko-ka-ninjin-to, its constituents, rhizomes of Anemarrhena asphodeloides, timosaponin A-III, and calcium on pilocarpine-induced saliva secretion in streptozocin-diabetic mice. *Biol. Pharm. Bull.* 1996;**19**(7)**:**926-931.

[28] Sievenpiper J L, Arnason J T, Leiter L A, Vuksan V. Variable effects of American ginseng: a batch of American ginseng (*Panax quinquefolius* L.) with a depressed ginsenoside profile does not affect postprandial glycemia. *Eur. J. Clin. Nutr.* 2003;57(2):243-248.

[29] Banz W J, Iqbal M J, Bollaert M, Chickris N, James B, Higginbotham D A, Peterson R, Murphy L. Ginseng modifies the diabetic phenotype and genes associated with diabetes in the male ZDF rat. *Phytomedicine* 2007;**14**(10)**:**681-689.

[30] Wu Z, Luo J Z, Luo L. American ginseng modulates pancreatic beta cell activities. *Chin. Med.* 2007;**2:**11.

[31] Hwang J T, Lee M S, Kim H J, Sung M J, Kim H Y, Kim M S, Kwon D Y. Antiobesity effect of ginsenoside Rg3 involves the AMPK and PPAR-gamma signal pathways. *Phytother. Res.* 2009;**23**(2)**:**262-266.

[32] Lee W K, Kao S T, Liu I M, Cheng J T. Increase of insulin secretion by ginsenoside Rh2 to lower plasma glucose in Wistar rats. *Clin. Exp. Pharmacol. Physiol.* 2006;**33**(1–2)**:**27-32.

[33] Xiang Y Z, Shang H C, Gao X M, Zhang B L. A comparison of the ancient use of ginseng in traditional Chinese medicine with modern pharmacological experiments and clinical trials, *Phytother. Res.* 2008;**22**(7)**:**851-858.

[34] Kiefer D, Pantuso T. Panax ginseng. *Am. Fam. Physician.* 2003;**68**(8)**:**1539-1542.

[35] McCarty MF. Does bitter melon contain an activator of AMP-activated kinase? *Med. Hypotheses* 2004;**63**(2)**:**340-343.

[36] Krawinkel M B, Keding G B. Bitter gourd (*Momordica charantia*): A dietary approach to hyperglycemia. *Nutr. Rev.* 2006;**64:**331-337.

[37] Harinantenaina L, Tanaka M, Takaoka S, Oda M, Mogami O, Uchida M, Asakawa Y. *Momordica charantia* constituents and antidiabetic screening of the isolated major compounds. *Chem. Pharm. Bull. (Tokyo)* 2006;**54**(7)**:**1017-1021.

[38] Rathi S S, Grover J K, Vikrant V, Biswas N R. Prevention of experimental diabetic cataract by Indian Ayurvedic plant extracts. *Phytother. Res.* 2002;16(8):774-777.

[39] Shibib B A, Khan L A, Rahman R. Hypoglycaemic activity of *Coccinia indica* and *Momordica charantia* in diabetic rats: Depression of the hepatic gluconeogenic enzymes glucose-6-phosphatase and fructose-1,6-bisphosphatase and elevation of

both liver and red-cell shunt enzyme glucose-6-phosphate dehydrogenase. *Biochem. J.* 1993;292(Pt1): 267–270.

[40] Chao C Y, Huang C. Bitter gourd (*Momordica charantia*) extract activates peroxisome proliferator-activated receptors and upregulates the expression of the acyl CoA oxidase gene in H4IIEC3 hepatoma cells. *J. Biomed. Sci.* 2003;**10**(6 Pt 2)**:**782-791.

[41] Chuang C Y, Hsu C, Chao C Y, Wein Y S, Kuo Y H, Huang C J. Fractionation and identification of 9c, 11t, 13t-conjugated linolenic acid as an activator of PPAR-alpha in bitter gourd (*Momordica charantia* L.). *J. Biomed. Sci.* 2006;**13**(6)**:**763-772.

[42] Tan M J, Ye J M, Turner N, Hohnen-Behrens C, Ke C Q, Tang C P, Chen T, Weiss HC, Gesing E R, Rowland A, James D E, Ye Y. Antidiabetic Activities of Triterpenoids Isolated from Bitter Melon Associated with Activation of the AMPK Pathway. *Chem. Biol.* 2008;**15**(3)**:**263-273.

[43] Basch E, Ulbricht C, Kuo G, Szapary P, Smith M. Therapeutic applications of fenugreek. *Altern. Med. Rev.* 2003;**8**(1)**:**20-27.

[44] Chen Q, Chan L L, Li E T. Bitter melon (*Momordica charantia*) reduces adiposity, lowers serum insulin and normalizes glucose tolerance in rats fed a high fat diet. *J. Nutr.* 2003;**133**(4)**:**1088-1093.

[45] Cefalu W T, Ye J, Wang Z Q. Efficacy of dietary supplementation with botanicals on carbohydrate metabolism in humans. *Endocr. Metab. Immune Disord. Drug Targets* 2008;**8**(2)**:**76-81.

[46] Yu R, Hui H, Shlomo M. *Insulin Secretion and Action. Endocrinology (2nd).* Humana Press; 2005:311-319.

[47] Lee Y S, Kim W S, Kim K H, Yoon M J, Cho H J, Shen Y, Ye J M, Lee C H, Oh W K, Kim C T, Hohnen-Behrens C, Gosby A, Kraegen EW, James DE, Kim JB. Berberine, a natural plant product, activates AMP-activated protein kinase with beneficial metabolic effects in diabetic and insulin-resistant states. *Diabetes* 2006;**55**(8)**:**2256-2264.

[48] Zhou J Y, Zhou S W, Zhang K B, Tang J L, Guang L X, Ying Y, Xu Y, Zhang L, Li D D. Chronic effects of berberine on blood, liver glucolipid metabolism and liver PPARs expression in diabetic hyperlipidemic rats. *Biol. Pharm. Bull.* 2008;**31**(6)**:**1169-1176.

[49] Zhou L, Wang X, Shao L, Yang Y, Shang W, Yuan G, Jiang B, Li F, Tang J, Jing H, Chen M. Berberine acutely inhibits insulin secretion from beta-cells through 3', 5'-cyclic adenosine 5'-monophosphate signaling pathway. *Endocrinology* 2008;**149**(9)**:**4510-4518.

[50] Kong W J, Zhang H, Song D Q, Xue R, Zhao W, Wei J, Wang Y M, Shan N, Zhou Z X, Yang P, You X F, Li Z R, Si S Y, Zhao L X, Pan H N, Jiang J D. Berberine reduces insulin resistance through protein kinase C-dependent up-regulation of insulin receptor expression. *Metabolism* 2009;**58**(1)**:**109-119.

[51] Liu W H, Hei Z Q, Nie H, Tang F T, Huang H Q, Li X J, Deng Y H, Chen S R, Guo F F, Huang W G, Chen F Y, Liu P Q. Berberine ameliorates renal injury in streptopzotocin-induced diabetic rats by suppression of both oxidative stress and aldose reductase. *Chin. Med. J. (Engl)* 2008;**121**(8)**:**706-712.

[52] Turner N, Li J Y, Gosby A, To S W, Cheng Z, Miyoshi H, Taketo M M, Cooney G J, Kraegen E W, James D E, Hu L H, Li J, Ye J M. Berberine and its more biologically available derivative, dihydroberberine, inhibit mitochondrial respiratory complex i: A mechanism for the action of berberine to activate amp-activated protein kinase and improve insulin action. *Diabetes* 2008;**57**(5)**:**1414-1418.

[53] Yin J, Xing H, Ye J. Efficacy of berberine in patients with type 2 diabetes mellitus. *Metabolism* 2008;**57**(5)**:**712-717.

[54] Yin J, Zhang H, Ye J. Traditional Chinese medicine in treatment of metabolic syndrome. *Endocr. Metab. Immune Disord. Drug Targets* 2008;**8**(2)**:**99-111.

[55] Judy W V, Hari S P, Stogsdill W W, Judy J S, Naguib Y M, Passwater R. Antidiabetic activity of a standardized extract (Glucosol(TM)) from Lagerstroemia speciosa leaves in Type II diabetics: A dose-dependence study. *J. Ethnopharmacol.* 2003; 87(1):115-117.

[56] Sauvaire Y, Petit P, Broca C, Manteghetti M, Baissac Y, Fernandez-Alvarez J, Gross R, Roye M, Leconte A, Gomis R, Ribes G. 4-Hydroxyisoleucine: a novel amino acid potentiator of insulin secretion. *Diabetes* 1998; 47(2):206-210.

[57] Madar Z, Abel R, Samish S, Arad J. Glucose-lowering effect of fenugreek in non-insulin dependent diabetics. *Eur. J. Clin. Nutr.* 1988;42(1):51- 54.

[58] Broca C, Manteghetti M, Gross R, Baissac Y, Jacob M, Petit P, Sauvaire Y, Ribes G. 4-Hydroxyisoleucine: Effects of synthetic and natural analogues on insulin secretion. *Eur. J. Pharmacol.* 2000;390(3):339-345.

[59] Devi B A, Kamalakkannan N, Prince P S. Supplementation of Fenugreek Leaves to Diabetic Rats. Effect on Carbohydrate Metabolic Enzymes in Diabetic Liver and Kidney. *Phytother. Res.* 2003;**17**(10)**:**1231-1233.

[60] Preet A, Siddiqui M R, Taha A, Badhai J, Hussain ME, Yadava PK, Baquer NZ. Long-term effect of *Trigonella foenum graecum* and its combination with sodium orthovanadate in preventing histopathological and biochemical abnormalities in diabetic rat ocular tissues. *Mol. Cell Biochem.* 2006;289(1-2):137-147.

[61] Siddiqui M R, Moorthy K, Taha A, Hussain M E, Baquer NZ. Low doses of vanadate and Trigonella synergistically regulate Na+/K + -ATPase activity and GLUT4 translocation in alloxan-diabetic rats. *Mol. Cell Biochem.* 2006;285(1-2):17-27.

[62] Kochhar A, Nagi M. Effect of supplementation of traditional medicinal plants on blood glucose in non-insulin-dependent diabetics: A pilot study. *J. Med. Food* 2005;8(4):545-549.

[63] Annida B, Stanely Mainzen Prince P. Supplementation of fenugreek leaves reduces oxidative stress in streptozotocin-induced diabetic rats. *J. Med. Food* 2005;8(3):382-385.

[64] Flammang A M, Cifone M A, Erexson G L, Stankowski L F Jr. Genotoxicity testing of a fenugreek extract. *Food Chem. Toxicol.* 2004;42(11):1769-1775.

[65] Shanmugasundaram E R, Rajeswari G, Baskaran K, Rajesh Kumar B R, Radha Shanmugasundaram K, Kizar Ahmath B. Use of *Gymnema sylvestre* leaf extract in the control of blood glucose in insulin-dependent diabetes mellitus. *J. Ethnopharmacol.* 1990; 30(3):281-294.

[66] Baskaran K, Kizar Ahamath B, Radha Shanmugasundaram K, Shanmugasundaram ER. Antidiabetic effect of a leaf extract from Gymnema sylvestre in non-insulin-dependent diabetes mellitus patients. *J. Ethnopharmacol.* 1990;30(3):295-300.

Chapter 12

A Targeted Therapeutic Approach Based on Medicinal Plants in the Management of Diabetes Mellitus

Pranav Kumar Prabhakar[1,*]
and Yachana Mishra[2]

[1]Division of Research and Development, Lovely Professional University, Phagwara (Punjab), India
[2]School of Bioengineering and Biosciences, Lovely Professional University, Phagwara (Punjab), India

Abstract

Hyperglycemia, the defining feature of diabetes mellitus (DM), can only be explained by an insufficient or inefficient insulin secretory response. The extracts of several medicinal plants affect the Krebs cycle, gluconeogenesis, the HMP shunt pathway, cholesterol synthesis, carbohydrate absorption and metabolism, and insulin generation and release. This chapter explains medicinal plants with antidiabetic properties work.

Keywords: diabetes mellitus, antidiabetic, hyperglycemia, insulin

---

* Corresponding Author's Email: prabhakar.iitm@gmail.com.

In: Management of Diabetes Mellitus Based on Natural Products
Editors: Yachana Mishra and Vijay Mishra
ISBN: 979-8-88697-853-7

1. Introduction

The most prevalent endocrine condition, diabetes mellitus (DM), is characterized by underutilization of glucose, elevated blood sugar, and an ineffective or insufficient insulin secretory mechanism (hyperglycemia). The inability to transfer sugar from the circulation into the cells might be hereditary or acquired. DM is a severe health issue that affects 3% of the global population and 5% of the people in the US. Each year, it accounts for around 5% of all fatalities worldwide [1]. Insulin facilitates glucose uptake from the blood into the cells, liver, skeletal muscle, and adipose tissue. In diabetics, glucose builds up in the blood because these tissues cannot digest it usually. Osmotic forces start to work when blood glucose concentrations rise, increasing blood volume and urine production (polyuria). Glucose is detected in the urine when blood glucose levels exceed the renal threshold (glucosuria). An increase in thirst results from compensatory changes brought on by the body's increased water loss (polydipsia). The demand for alternative energy sources like ketone bodies rises due to some tissues' failure to absorb glucose [2]. The mechanism of action of medicinal plants in treating diabetes is covered in this chapter [3].

2. Therapeutic Strategies

Insulin sensitivity and insulin resistance are the two primary issues with insulin treatment. The oral medications are classified as hypoglycemics (also known as insulin secretagogues), and antihyperglycemics which individually target a different pathophysiological process that contributes to the development of diabetes.

Sulfonylureas have been used as hypoglycemic agents for over 50 years and continue to be a key component of type 2 DM treatment [2]. They encourage the production of more insulin by the beta cells. The pancreatic β-cells' K+ATP channel is inhibited, which allows them to carry out their role [4]. Drugs from the first generation include chlorpropamide, tolbutamide, and tolazamide. Their molecular target, the ATP-sensitive K+ channel, has a reduced binding affinity for them, requiring greater doses to be effective. Third-generation sulfonylureas (glimepiride) and second-generation sulfonylureas (glibenclamide, glipizide, and glyburide) are more powerful, have a quicker start, and typically have a shorter half-life and longer duration of action. Non-sulfonylurea insulin secretagogues include meglitinide. Similar to sulfonylurea but at a different location, they bind to an ATP-dependent K+ (KATP) channel on the cell membrane of pancreatic β-cells. They do not trigger calcium-dependent exocytosis of insulin granules [5]. Biguanides, such as metformin, have an unclear mechanism of action. However, they can reduce the plasma fasting insulin levels in hyperinsulinemia. They lower the amount of gluconeogenesis in the liver with NIDDM [6, 7], which lowers the blood glucose level. The first thiazolidinedione (TZD) with a direct insulin-sensitizing effect was troglitazone [8]. It binds to and activates the nuclear receptor known as peroxisome proliferators-activated receptor (PPAR), which controls the expression of several genes involved in metabolism [9]. The improved peripheral glucose elimination and decreased hepatic glucose production are credited with the TZD's ability to lower blood glucose levels.

Acarbose and miglitol are saccharides that inhibit glucoamylase, sucrase, maltase, and isomaltase in the small intestine brush border competitively and reversibly, delaying the breakdown of complex carbohydrates and assisting in blood pressure regulation. This significantly lessens the blood sugar rises that may occur after meals [10].

Today, the medical system still faces difficulties in managing diabetes without any adverse effects. Due to their efficiency, lack of negative side effects, and affordable price, herbal medications are frequently given. Numerous active principles produced from plants have proven to have antidiabetic properties. Alkaloids, glycosides, galactomannan gum, polysaccharides, peptidoglycans, hypoglycans, guanidine, steroids, carbohydrates, glycopeptides, terpenoids, amino acids, and inorganic ions are some of these plants' key active ingredients.

3. Medicinal Plants and Their Target Sites

Most tissues use glucose for the glucosylation of proteins and other metabolic processes, including meeting their energy needs. The sole source of energy the mammalian brain and red blood cells can utilize when not starving is glucose [11]. The significant metabolic pathways where glucose is involved-either as a substrate or a product, as well as the medicinal plants that block or stimulate one of these regulatory stages in the processes-are, are included in the following sections.

3.1. Glycolysis and Krebs Cycle

Hexokinase, phosphofructokinase, and pyruvate kinase catalyze irreversible processes in glycolysis; as a result, these enzymes should play both regulatory and catalytic functions [11]. Pyruvate is oxidized to CO_2 and H_2O via acetyl CoA with the creation of energy-equivalent NADH in the Krebs cycle, which is the primary mechanism for energy generation. The latter is oxidized in the electron transport cycle and yields ATP [11].

Numerous pharmacological plants regulate glycolysis and the Krebs cycle. Succinate dehydrogenase is activated by plants, including *Aegle marmelose* [12], *Catharanthus roseus* [13], and *Panax ginseng* [14], while malate dehydrogenase is activated by *Catharanthus roseus* [13] and *Panax ginseng* [14].

3.2. Gluconeogenesis

The process known as "gluconeogenesis" converts non-sugar carbon sources such pyruvate, lactate, glycerol, and glucogenic amino acids into glucose (primarily alanine and glutamine). Inhibitors of phosphoenol pyruvate carboxykinase include the medicinal plants *Eucommia ulmoides* [15], *Gongronema latifolium* [16], *Panax quinofolium* [17], *Syzygium aromaticum* [18, 19], and *Camellia sinensis* [20]. Inhibitors of fructose-1, 6-bisphosphatase include *Aegle marmelose* [12], *Casearia esculenta* [21]. The final regulatory enzyme in this pathway is glucose-6-phosphatase, which is inhibited by *Allium cepa* [22], *Allium sativum* [23], *Coscinium fenestratum* [24], *Eugenia jambolana* [25, 26], *Momordica charantia* [25-27], *Pterocarpus marsupium* [28], *Tinospora cordifolia* [26], and *Aconitum carmichaeli* Debeaux [29].

3.3. Hexose Monophosphate (HMP) Shunt

The HMP Shunt is a different route for glucose oxidation from the Krebs cycle and glycolysis. It produces NADPH and pentoses (ribose-5-phosphate), two crucial byproducts. The six carbons in glucose are used in an anabolic route to create five-carbon sugars. Therefore, controlling the HMP shunt in diabetic patients is crucial. In diabetics, it is crucial to regulate the enzyme glucose-6-phosphate dehydrogenase. Several plants control this enzyme. Aconitum carmichaeli Debeaux. [29], Coccinia indica [25, 30, 31], Colocassia esculenta

[32], Catharanthus roseus [13], and Dioscorea cayenensis [32] are plants that affect the enzyme glucose-6-phosphate dehydrogenase in the HMP shunt pathway.

3.4. Glycogen Synthesis

Glycogen synthase in the liver carries out a multistep process to create glycogen from wasted glucose. UDP-glucose and the non-reducing end of glycogen are two other substrates used by this enzyme. The enzyme UDP-glucose pyrophosphorylase activates glucose so that it may be utilized to synthesize glycogen. Diabetes causes a malfunction in converting glucose to glycogen, which raises blood glucose levels. *Aegle marmelose* [12], *Curcuma longa* [25, 30], *Momordica charantia* [25, 26], *Murraya koenigii* [12, 33, 34], *Ocimum sanctum* [12], *Piper betle* [35], *Coccinia indica* [30, 31], *Catharanthus roseus* [13], and *Brassica juncea* [34] are some of the plants that have an impact on the enzyme glycogen synthase function.

3.5. Glycogenolysis

The breakdown of glycogen into glucose is known as glycogenolysis, and it raises blood glucose levels [36]. Azadirachta indica leaf extract can prevent diabetic rabbits from decreasing peripheral glucose and glycogenolysis [37].

3.6. Digestion and Absorption of Carbohydrates

In a typical diet, carbohydrates account for most energy production and provide the body with more than 80% of its immediate energy needs. Starch and sucrose are two of the primary components of carbohydrates. The enzyme α-amylase found in saliva and different pancreatic secretions first breaks down starch into oligosaccharides. α-Glucisidase, a membrane-bound enzyme found in the small intestine's epithelium, catalyzes the breakdown of disaccharides and oligosaccharides into glucose [38]. Glucose is created through the digestion of starches and sugars. It then travels through the intestines and into the bloodstream before arriving to the liver. The glucose level in the blood is maintained through this mechanism. Several enzymes, such as α-glucosidase, maltase, sucrase, amylase, lactase, and isomaltase, participate in the digestion of carbohydrates. Therefore, one of the successful therapies for DM is the inhibition of α-glucosidase. Many medicinal herbs have been shown to inhibit this function, and some of these plants also reduce the absorption of carbohydrates through the brush border cell of the gut. It has been demonstrated that Bergenia ciliata's two active compounds, (-)-3-O-galloylepicatechin and (-)-3-O-galloylcatechin, inhibit rat intestinal α-glucosidase and swine pancreatic α-amylase [38]. Additionally, (-)-lyoniresinol 3-O-b-D-glucopyranoside and -xylopyranosyl (1'''2'')-b-D-galactopyranoside [39] block α-glucosidase. Despite being referred to as "diabetes pills," these inhibitors are not technically hypoglycemic agents because they do not directly affect insulin secretion or increase its sensitivity. Instead, they slow down the digestion of starch in the small intestine, allowing glucose from the starch in the meal to enter the bloodstream more gradually and be matched to a poor insulin response or low production. Such synthetic medications are sold over the counter and include miglitol and acarbose.

3.7. Insulin Secretion and Its Action

The most significant peptide hormone in the human body is insulin. Along with controlling the metabolism of carbohydrates, it also promotes lipogenesis, reduces lipolysis, and improves the transport of amino acids into cells. It is a peptide hormone that is released in response to hyperglycemia from the islets of Langerhans' β-cells. It takes a complicated procedure for β-cells to release insulin in response to variations in blood glucose levels. With the aid of GLUT 2, which is then phosphorylated by the enzyme glucokinase, some glucose initially reaches the β-cells. ATP is created by further metabolizing this changed glucose [40]. Nuclear receptor transcription factors known as peroxisome proliferator-activated receptors (PPARs) stimulate the growth of peroxisomes in living cells. They participate in the cellular metabolism of lipids, proteins, and carbohydrates [40]. The three PPAR subtypes are alpha, delta/beta, and gamma. Gamma is involved in insulin resistance, while alpha is involved in lipid metabolism and peroxisome proliferation [41]. *Aegle marmelose* (Rutaceae), *Momordica charantia*, *Glycyrrhiza glabra* (Fabaceae), *Helicteres isora* (Sterculiaceae), and *Syzyzium cumini* are examples of medicinal plants that boost PPAR gamma expression and reduce insulin resistance.

Roziglitazone, troglitazone, and piaglitazome are medications in the thiazolidinedione family that also target PPAR gamma. Significant PPARgamma ligand-binding activity is seen in dehydroglyasperin C, dehydroglyasperin D, glyasperin B, glycycoumarine, glycyrin, and glyasperin D, which were isolated from *Glycyrrhiza uralensis* and *neolgnan dehydroeugenol*, respectively [42, 43]. One of the most crucial targets for curcumin, which is produced from the root of ginger (Zingiber officinale), and 6-gingerol, a natural analog of curcumin, is PPAR gamma [44]. One of the second messengers that mediate intracellular signaling networks brought on by membrane receptor activation is cyclic AMP [45]. This process eventually results in changes to cellular functions, including metabolic processes. *Orthosiphon aristatus* [46], *Passiflora edulis* [47], *Hylocereus undatus* [48], *Luffa cylindrical* [49], *Momordica charantia* [49], and *Panax ginseng* [14] are examples of medicinal herbs that have cAMP phosphodiesterase inhibitory activity, which preserves the action of insulin.

Glucose is transported into and out of cells by glucose transporters (GLUT), which are found on vesicles in the cytoplasm. GLUT enters the membrane after being excited by glucose and performs the necessary activity. The transfer of GLUT to the plasma membrane is absent in the case of DM. Several medicinal plants, including *Aegle marmelose* [12, 50], *Allium sativum* [21], *Canna indica* [51], *Lagerstroemia speciosa* [52], *Syzyzium cumini* [50], and *Cornus officinalis* [53], aid in the efficient transport of GLUT to the plasma membrane, resulting in the transport of glucose into the cells and a reduction in blood glucose levels. By activating PI3 Kinase, insulin modifies many metabolic pathways through a series of stages [54]. However, if its response is weak, these actions are not carried out. Despite insulin's inefficiency, plants including *Aegle marmelose* [12, 50], *Helicteres isora* [55], *Vinca rosea* [25, 26], *Camellia sinensis* [19], and *Hericium erinaceus* (Fungi) [56] can activate PI3 kinase and so alter all metabolic pathways.

4. Phytoconstituents Having Hypoglycemic Potential

Several phytochemicals, including alkaloids, flavonoids, glycosides, glycolipid, polysaccharides, peptidoglycans, carbohydrates, amino acids, and saponin obtained from plant sources, have been reported to possess hypoglycemic activity.

4.1. Alkaloids

Alkaloids are amines that exist naturally and have pharmacological effects on people and animals. As part of a plant's defensive mechanism against illness, resveratrol belongs to the class of antibiotic chemicals known as phytoalexins [57]. *Tinospora cordifolia* contains berberine, a compound with strong hypoglycemia effects [58]. Blood sugar levels are lowered by alkaloids such as catharanthine, vindoline, and vindolinine isolated from *Catharanthus roseus* [59].

4.2. Polysaccharides

Aloe vera, Ocimum sanctum, and Alpinia galanga are examples of medicinal plants that contain polysaccharides, which raise insulin levels and have hypoglycemic effects. It has been demonstrated that a protein-bound polysaccharide extracted from pumpkin increases serum insulin levels, lowers blood glucose levels, and improves glucose tolerance [60].

4.3. Saponins

The glycosides of triterpinoids, steroids having a nitrogen function, and steroid alkaloids found in plants are called saponins. According to reports, *Momordica charantia*'s steroidal saponin charantin has an insulin-like action [61] by promoting the release of insulin and inhibiting glucogenesis. In animal models, the steroid β-sitosterol from *Azadirachta indica*, the diterpenoid lactone andrographolide from *Andrographis paniculata* [62], and the saponin gymnemic acid IV from *Gymnema sylvestre* all demonstrate strong hypoglycemia action [63].

4.4. Ferulic Acids

In the cell walls of many plants, including *Curcuma longa*, ferulic acid (4-hydroxy-3-methoxycinnamic acid), a flavonoid, is a highly abundant phenolic photochemical. Its antioxidant, anticancer, and blood glucose-lowering activities may offer significant health advantages [64].

4.5. Flavonoids

A naturally occurring substance known as flavonoid has both antioxidant and hypoglycemic effects. They belong to a group of secondary metabolites found in plants. Many flavonoids include flavanols, flavones, catechins, flavanones, etc. Because they ameliorate the altered glucose and oxidative metabolisms of diabetic conditions, several flavonoids have hypoglycemic effects. An essential flavonoid called quercetin is known to boost the activity of the enzyme hepatic glucokinase, most likely through improving insulin release from pancreatic islets [65]. By altering Ca^{2+} concentration, it also has a stimulatory impact on insulin secretion [66]. Hesperidin and naringin, two citrus bioflavonoids that may be added to the diet of male C57BL7KsJ-db/db mice (a T2DM model) to lower blood sugar levels, boost hepatic glucokinase activity, and increase glycogen concentration. Naringin decreases both the hepatic glucose-6-phosphatase, phosphoenolpyruvate carboxykinase, and plasma insulin C-peptide activity. When tested on obese Zucker rats (a T2DM model), genistein and soy isoflavonoids greatly improved lipid and glucose metabolism by acting as a hypoglycemic on PPAR [67]. Epigallocatechin gallate (I), a flavonoid found in green tea, lowers blood sugar levels in animals. According to reports, it works similarly to insulin in reducing hepatic glucose synthesis and increasing tyrosine phosphorylation of the insulin receptor and insulin receptor substrate-1 (IRS-1). Additionally, it increases PI3K and MAP kinase to imitate insulin and decreases phosphoenolpyruvate carboxykinase gene expression in a phosphoinositide 3-kinase-dependent manner [19]. Epicatechin, a different flavonoid, has been found to have insulin-like action [68]. This affects T2DM individuals' erythrocyte membrane-bound acetylcholinesterase [69]. Delphinidin and pelargonidin both exhibit strong hypoglycemia effects [70].

4.6. Imidazoline Compounds

Imidazoline-I binding sites are located on pancreatic beta cells, and imizoline derivatives found in some plants activate these binding sites to stimulate insulin release. In isolated human islets of Langerhans, β-carbolines from *Tribulus terrestris* were shown to boost insulin production by a factor of two to three [71].

4.6. Sulfur Containing Compounds

Hexokinase, glucose-6-phosphatase, HMG Co-A reductase, and LCAT are all activated when S-methyl cysteine sulfoxide and diallyl thiosulfinate, which were isolated from the plants *Allium sativum* [21, 72] and *Allium cepa* [22], are administered to alloxan-induced diabetic rats.

Conclusion

The American Diabetes Association (ADA) estimates that 20.8 million Americans have diabetes. Diabetes is a metabolic illness that mostly results from a problem with insulin production or increasing resistance to its effects. The most important issue is the negative effect resulting from the buildup of glucose in DM. The extra glucose is transformed into other chemicals and free radicals, which harm the organelles and essential organs. To address these issues, there are no specific medications on the market. Patients with insulin-dependent and non-insulin-dependent diabetes, diabetic retinopathy, diabetic peripheral neuropathy, etc., have employed herbal remedies for the disease. Various plants can lower glucose production, promote glucose utilization, and battle subsequent problems. Only a small portion of plants, less than 1%, have undergone pharmacological screening for DM. As a result, it is wise to consider herbal treatments for diabetes. Based on this report on the potential efficacy of medicinal plants against diabetes, it can be assumed that phytochemicals play a significant role in managing diabetes. This role requires further investigation to develop the necessary drugs and nutraceuticals from natural sources. However, some herbal treatments can potentially have substantial adverse consequences and drug-to-drug interactions since they have not all undergone the required scientific evaluation. More study is required to clarify the pharmacological actions of herbal therapies currently used to treat DM.

References

[1] WHO, Traditional medicine strategy (2002–2005). *WHO Publications*. 2002; 1–6.

[2] Ashcroft S, Ashcroft F M. The sulfonylurea receptor. *Biochim. Biophys. Acta* 1992; 1175: 45–59.

[3] Alarcon-Aguilara F J, Roman-Ramos R, Perez-Gutierrez S, Aguilar-Contreras A, Contreras-Weber C, Flores-Saenz J L. Study of the anti-hypoglycemic effect of plants used as antidiabetics. *J. Ethnopharmacol.* 1998; 61 (2): 101-10.

[4] Engler R L, Yellon D M. Sulfonylurea K A T P blockade in Type II diabetes and preconditioning in cardiovascular disease. *Circulation* 1996; 94; 2297-01.

[5] Chakraborty R, Rajagopalan R. Diabetes and insulin resistance associated disorders: Disease and therapy. *Current Science* 2002; 83**:** 1533–8.

[6] Klip A, Leiter L A. Cellular mechanism of action of metformin. *Diabetes Care* 1990; 13 (6): 696-04.

[7] Stumvoll M, Nurjhan N, Perriello G. Metabolic effects of metformin in non-insulin dependent diabetes mellitus. *N. Engl. J. Med.* 1995;333: 550–4.

[8] Day C. Thiazolidinediones: a new class of antidiabetic drugs. *Diabet Med.* 1999; 16 (3): 179–92.

[9] Schoonjans K, Auwerx J, Thiazolidinediones: an update. *Lancet* 2000; 355 (9208): 1008-1010.

[10] Puls W, Keup U, Krause H, Thomas P G, Hoffmeister F. *Glucosidase inhibition: a new approach to the treatment of diabetes, obesity and hyperlipoproteinemi*a, Naturwissenschaften 1977; 64(10): 536–537.

[11] JM Berg, JL Tymoczko, L Stryer. Biochemistry, 5th Ed. WH Freeman and Co. 644-89.

[12] Narendhirakannan R T, Subramanian S, Kandaswamy M. Biochemical evaluation of antidiabetogenic properties of some commonly used Indian plants on streptozotocin-induced diabetes in experimental rats. *Clin. Exp. Pharmacol. Physiol.* 2006; 33(12): 1150-7.

[13] Singh S N, Vats P, Suri S. Effect of an antidiabetic extract of *Catharanthus roseus* on enzymic activities in streptozotocin induced diabetic rats. *J. Ethnopharmacol.* 2001; 76: 269-77.

[14] Yeung H W, Ng T B. Hypoglycemic constituents of *Panax ginseng*. *General Pharmacolology* 1985; 16(6): 549-52.

[15] Park S A, Choi M S, Kim M J, Jung U J, Kim H J, Park K K, Noh H J, Park H M, Park Y B, Lee J S, Lee M K. Hypoglycemic and hypolipidemic action of Du-zhong (*Eucommia ulmoides* Oliver) leaves water extract in C57BL/KsJ-db/db mice. *J. Ethnopharmacol.* 2006; 107(3): 412-7.

[16] Ugochukwu N H, Babady N E. Antihyperglycemic effect of aqueous and ethanolic extracts of *Gongronema latifolium* leaves on glucose and glycogen metabolism in livers of normal and streptozotocin-induced diabetic rats. *Life Sci.* 2003; 73(15): 1925-38.

[17] Broadhurst C L, Polansky M M, Anderson R A. Insulin-like biological activity of culinary and medicinal plant aqueous extracts in-vitro. *Journal of Agricultural and Food Chemistry* 2000; 48(3): 849-52.

[18] Prasad R C, Herzog B, Boone B, Sims L, Waltner-Law M. An extract of Syzygium aromaticum represses genes encoding hepatic gluconeogenic enzymes. *J. Ethnopharmacol.* 2005; 96: 295-01.

[19] Gupta D, Raju J, Baquer N J. Modulation of some gluconeogenic enzyme activities in diabetic rat liver and kidney: effect of antidiabetic compounds. *Indian J. Exp. Biol.* 1999; 37(2): 196–9.

[20] Waltner-Law M E, Wang X L, Law B K, Hall R K, Nawano M, Granner D K.. Epigallocatechin Gallate, a Constituent of Green Tea, Represses Hepatic Glucose Production. *J. Biol. Chem.* 2002; 277(38): 34933-40.

[21] Prakasam A, Sethupathy S, Pugalendi KV. Influence of Casearia esculenta root extract on glycoprotein components in streptozotocin diabetic rats. *Pharmazie* 2005; 60(3): 229-32.

[22] Kumari K, Mathew B C, Augusti K T. Hypoglycemic and hypolipidemic effects of S-methyl cysteine sulfoxide isolated from Allium cepa Linn. *Indian J. Biochem. Biophys.* 1995; 32: 49–54.

[23] Sheela C G, Kumud K, Augusti K T. Antidiabetic effects of onion and garlic sulfoxide amino acids in rats. *Planta Med.* 1995; 61(4): 356-7.

[24] Punitha I S R, Rajendran K, Shirwaikar A, Shirwaikar A. Alcoholic stem extract of Coscinium fenestratum regulates carbohydrate metabolism and improves antioxidant status in streptozotocin-nicotinamide induced diabetic rats. *Evidence-based complementary and alternative medicine* 2005; 2(3): 375-81.

[25] Kar A, Choudhary B K, Bandyopadhyay N G. Comparative evaluation of hypoglycaemic activity of some Indian medicinal plants in alloxan diabetic rats. *J. Ethnopharmacol*. 2003; 84(1): 105-8.

[26] Babu P S, Stanely Mainzen Prince P. Antihyperglycaemic and antioxidant effect of hyponidd, an ayurvedic herbomineral formulation in streptozotocin-induced diabetic rats. *J. Pharm. Pharmacol.* 2004; 56(11): 1435-42.

[27] Che-Yi C, Ching-jang Huang. Bitter Gourd (*Momordica charantia*) Extract Activates Peroxisome Proliferator-Activated Receptors and upregulates the expression of the acyl CoA oxidase gene in H4IIEC3 hepatoma cells, *Journal of Biomedical Science* 2003; 10: 782–91.

[28] Grover J K, Vats V, Yadav S. Medicinal plants of India with antidiabetic properties. *J. Ethnopharmacol.* 2002; 81: 81-100.

[29] Hikino H, Kobayashi M, Suzuki Y, Konno C. Mechanisms of hypoglycemic activity of aconitan A, a glycan from Aconitum carmichaeli roots. *J. Ethnopharmacol.* 1989; 25(3): 295-04.

[30] Mukherjee K, Ghosh N C, Datta T. Coccinia indica Linn. as potential hypoglycemic agent. *Indian J. Exp. Biol.* 1972; 10(5): 347–9.

[31] Kumar G P, Sudheesh S, Vijayalakshmi NR. Hypoglycaemic effect of Coccinia indica: mechanism of action. *Planta med.* 1993; 59(4): 330-2.

[32] Grindley P B, Omoruyi F O, Asemota H N, Morrison EYSTA. Effect of yam (Dioscorea cayenensis) and dasheen (Colocassia esculenta) extracts on the kidney of streptozotocin-induced diabetic rats. *Int. J. Food Sci. Nutr.* 2001; 52(5): 429-33.

[33] Halder N S, Joshi S, Gupta S K. Lens aldose reductase inhibiting potential of some indigenous plants. *J. Ethnopharmacol.* 2003; 86(1): 113-6.

[34] Khan BA, Abraham A, Leelamma S. Hypoglycemic action of *Murraya koeingii* (curry leaf) and *Brassica juncea* (mustard): mechanism of action. Indian J Biochem Biophys 1995; **32**(2): 106–8.

[35] Santhakumari P, Prakasam A, Pugalendi K V. Antihyperglycemic activity of Piper betle leaf on streptozotocin-induced diabetic rats. *Journal of medicinal food* 2006; 9(1): 108-12.

[36] Kimura I, Nakashima N, Sugihara Y, Fu-jun C, Kimura M. The antihyperglycaemic blend effect of traditional Chinese medicine byakko-ka-ninjin-to on alloxan and diabetic KK-CA(y) mice. *Phytotherapy Research* 1999; 13(6): 484-8.

[37] Chattopadhyay R R. Possible mechanism of antihyperglycemic effect of *Azadirachta indica* leaf extract, Part IV, *Gen. Pharmacol.* 1996; **27**(3): 431–4.

[38] Puls W, Keup U, Krause H, Thomas P G, Hoffmeister F. *Glucosidase inhibition: a new approach to the treatment of diabetes, obesity and hyperlipoproteinemia.* Naturwissenschaften 1977; 64: 536–7.

[39] Anurakkun N J, Bhandari M R, Kawabata J. α-Glucosidase inhibitors from Devil tree (*Alstonia scholaris*). *Food Chemistry* 2007; 103: 1319–23.

[40] Jones P M, Persaud S J. Protein Kinases, Protein Phosphorylation, and the Regulation of Insulin Secretion from Pancreatic β-Cells. *Endocrine Reviews* 19(4): 429–61.

[41] Fernyhough M E, Okine E, Hausman G, Vierck J L, Dodson M V. PPARγ and GLUT-4 expression as developmental regulators/markers for preadipocyte differentiation into an adipocyte. *Domest. Anim. Endocrinol.*, Volume 2007; 33(4): 367-78.

[42] Mae T, Tsukagawa M, Kitahara M. Peroxisome proliferator activated receptor ligands containing prenyl flavonoid, related substances, or plant extracts containing the same, and process for producing the same. *PCT Int. Appl.* 2003; 74.

[43] Mimaki Y. New biologically active compounds from natural sources. *Journal of Japanese Cosmetic Science Society* 2006; 30(4): 256-60.

[44] Shishodia S, Sethi G, Aggarwal BB. Curcumin: getting back to the roots. *Ann. N Y Acad. Sc.* 2005; 1056: 206-17.

[45] Kitamura T, Kitamura Y, Kuroda S. Hino Y, Ando M, Kotani K, Konishi H, Matsuzaki H, Kikkawa U, Ogawa W, Kasuga M. Insulin-Induced Phosphorylation and Activation of Cyclic Nucleotide Phosphodiesterase 3B by the Serine-Threonine Kinase Akt. *Mol. Cell Biol.* 1999; 19(9): 6286–96.

[46] Ngamrojanavanich N, Manakit S, Pornpakakul S, Petsom A. Inhibitory effects of selected Thai medicinal plants on Na^+-K^+-ATPase. *Fitoterapia* 2006; 77(6): 481

[47] Dhanabal SP, Edwin JE, Kumar EP, Suresh EP. Hypoglycemic effects of Alcoholic extract of various species of Passiflora on alloxan induced diabetes mellitus in albino Rats. *Nigerian Journal of Natural Products and Medicine* 2004; 8: 19-21.

[48] Perez G R, Vargas S Y D, Ortiz H. Wound healing properties of *Hylocereus undatus* on diabetic rats. *Phytother. Res.* 2005; 19(8): 665-8.

[49] Minami Y. Chemical modifications of momordin-α and luffin- α, ribosome-inactivating proteins from the seeds of *Momordica charantia* and *Luffa cylindrica*: involvement of His140, Tyr165, and Lys231 in the protein-synthesis inhibitory activity. *Biosci. Biotech. Bioch.* 1998; 62(5): 959-64.

[50] Anandharajan R, Jaiganesh S, Shankernarayanan NP, Viswakarma RA, Balakrishnan A. In vitro glucose uptake activity of Aegles marmelos and *Syzygium*

cumini by activation of Glut-4, PI3 kinase and PPARgamma in L6 myotubes. *Phytomedicine* 2006; 13(6): 434-41.

[51] Purintrapiban J, Suttajit M, Forsberg NE. Differential activation of glucose transport in cultured muscle cells by polyphenolic compounds from *Canna indica* L. root. *Biol. Pharm. Bull.* 2006; 29(10): 1995-8.

[52] Klein G, Kim J, Himmeldirk K, Cao Y, Chen X. Antidiabetes and Anti-obesity Activity of Lagerstroemia speciosa. *Evid. Based Complement Altern. Med.* 2007; 4(4): 401-7.

[53] Xu H Q, Hao H P. Effects of iridoid total glycoside from *Cornus officinalis* on prevention of glomerular overexpression of transforming growth factor beta 1 and matrixes in an experimental diabetes model. *Biol. Pharm. Bull.* 2004; 27(7): 1014-8.

[54] Muniyappa R, Montagnani M, Koh K K, Quon M J. Cardiovascular Actions of Insulin. *Endocrine Reviews* 2007; 28 (5): 463-91.

[55] Chakrabarti R, Vikramadithyanm R K, Mullangi R, Sharma V M, Jagadheshan H, Rao Y N, Sairam P, Rajagopalan R. Antidiabetic and hypolipidemic activity of *Helicteres isora* in animal models. *J. Ethnopharmacol.* 2002; 81(3): 343-9.

[56] Wang J C, Hu S H, Wang J T, Chen K S, Chia Y C. Hypoglycemic effect of extract of *Hericium erinaceus. Journal of the Science of Food and Agriculture* 2004; 85(4): 641-6.

[57] Petlevski R, Hadzija M, Slijepcevic M, Juretic D, Petrik J. Glutathione S-transferases and malondialdehyde in the liver of NOD mice on short-term treatment with plant mixture extract P-9801091. *Phytotherapy Research* 2003; 17(4): 311-4.

[58] Singh SS, Pandey SC, Srivastava S, Gupta VS, Patro B, Ghosh AC.. Chemistry and medicinal properties of *Tinospora cordifolia* (Guduchi). *Ind. J. of Pharmacology* 2003; **35:** 83–91.

[59] Chattopadhyay R R. A comparative evaluation of some blood sugar lowering agents of plant origin. *J. Ethnopharmacol.* 1999; **67:** 367–72.

[60] Mukherjee P K, Maiti K, Mukherjee K, Houghton P J. Leads from Indian medicinal plants with hypoglycemic potentials. *J. Ethnopharmacol.* 2006; 106: 1–28.

[61] Ng T B, Wong C M, Li W W, Yeung H W. Insulin-like molecules in Momordica charantia seeds. *J. Ethnopharmacol.* 1986; **15:** 107–17.

[62] Yu B C, Hung C R, Chen W C, Cheng J T. Antihyperglycemic effect of andrographolide in streptozotocin-induced diabetic rats. *Planta Medica* 2003; **69:** 1075–9.

[63] Sugihara Y, Nojima H, Matsuda H, Murakami T, Yoshikawa M, Kimura I. Antihyperglycemic effects of gymnemic acid IV, a compound derived from *Gymnema sylvestre* leaves in streptozotocin-diabetic mice. *J. of Asian Natl. Product Res.* 2000; **2:** 321–7.

[64] Ohnishi M, Matuo T, Tsuno T, Hosoda A, Nomura E, Taniguchi H, Sasaki H, Morishita H. Antioxidant activity and hypoglycemic effect of ferulic acid in STZ-induced diabetic mice and KK-Ay mice. *Biofactors* 2004; 21: 315–9.

[65] Vessal M, Hemmati M, Vasei M. Hypoglycemic effects of quercetin in streptozocin-induced diabetic rats. *Comparative Biochemistry and Physiology C: Toxicology and Pharmacology* 2003; 135C: 357–64.

[66] Hii C S, Howell S L. Effects of flavonoids on insulin secretion and $45Ca^{2+}$ handling in rat islets of Langerhans. *J. Endocrinol.* 1985; 107: 1–8.

[67] Mezei O, Banz WJ, Steger RW, Peluso MR, Winters TA, Shay N. Soy isoflavones exert hypoglycemic and hypolipidemic effects through the PPAR pathways in obese Zucker rats and murine RAW 264.7 cells. *J. Nutri.* 2003; 133: 1238–43.

[68] Chakravarthy B K, Gupta S, Gambhir S S, Gode K D. The prophylactic action of (−)-epicatechin against alloxan induced diabetes in rats. *Life Sci.* 1981; 29**:** 2043–7.

[69] Rizvi SI, Zaid MA. Insulin-like effect of (−)-epicatechin on erythrocyte membrane acetylcholinesterase activity in type 2 diabetes mellitus. *Clin. Exp. Pharmacol. Physiol.* 2001; 28: 776–8.

[70] Cherian S, Augusti K T. Antidiabetic effects of a glycoside of leucopelargonidin isolated from *Ficus bengalensis* Linn. *Indian J. Exp. Bio.* 1993; 31(1): 26-9.

[71] Cooper E J, Hudson A L, Parker C A, Morgan N G. Effects of the beta-carbolines, harmane and pinoline, on insulin secretion from isolated human islets of Langerhans. *Euro. J. Pharmacol.* 2003; 482: 189–96.

[72] Sheela CG, Augusti KT. Antidiabetic effects of S-allyl cysteine sulphoxide isolated from garlic *Allium sativum* Linn. *Indian J. Exp. Biol.* 1992; 30: 523-6.

Index

A

adipokines, 155, 170, 171, 174
Albiglutide, 160, 162
alkaloids, 237, 260, 263, 273, 277, 278
alpha-glucosidase inhibitors (AGIs), 74, 90, 168
American College of Obstetricians and Gynecologists (ACOG), 53, 56, 59, 61
American Diabetes Association (ADA), 10, 11, 17, 53, 55, 56, 61, 96, 139, 142, 171, 280
Analogliptin, 166
animal insulin, 66
antidiabetic, vii, viii, 63, 105, 107, 109, 114, 117, 120, 122, 131, 133, 136, 141, 143, 144, 147, 148, 149, 150, 163, 168, 171, 172, 173, 176, 180, 187, 188, 189, 190, 192, 199, 203, 204, 206, 207, 210, 211, 213, 216, 218, 220, 222, 223, 224, 225, 226, 227, 232, 233,235, 237, 241, 242, 243, 249, 250, 252, 253, 254, 255, 256, 257, 258, 260, 261, 263, 266, 267, 268, 269, 270, 271, 273, 281, 282, 284, 285
antidiabetic activity, 148, 187, 190, 192, 199, 204, 225, 232, 235, 253, 260, 267
antidiabetic agents, vii, viii, 63, 105, 141, 147, 148, 150, 172, 173, 187, 188, 206, 210, 211, 213, 216, 220, 223, 233, 235, 237
antidiabetic drugs, 117, 133, 141, 147, 163, 171, 187, 203, 207, 216, 218, 261, 281

B

Banaba (*Lagerstroemia Speciosa*), 264
bitter gourd (*Momordica charantia*), 239, 255, 263, 267, 268, 274, 275, 276, 277, 278, 282, 283, 284
blood sugar, ix, 1, 2, 7, 8, 9, 10, 11, 12, 13, 15, 21, 54, 59, 63, 64, 71, 80, 86, 89, 103, 105, 106, 107, 108, 113, 114, 115, 121, 123, 124, 127, 135, 148, 150, 154, 159, 164, 175, 187, 207, 212, 217, 221, 239, 240, 241, 249, 250, 251, 262, 264, 272, 273, 279, 284
blood sugar level, ix, 1, 2, 8, 10, 11, 12, 13, 15, 21, 59, 64, 80, 86, 106, 107, 108, 113, 115, 121, 123, 124, 127, 135, 159, 164, 175, 187, 212, 217, 221, 239, 240, 241, 249, 250, 251, 262, 264, 279
brittle diabetes, 14, 19, 236, 237, 253

C

canagliflozin, 77, 135, 144, 160, 163, 175, 176, 177, 178, 179, 183, 184, 185
carbohydrates, 78, 86, 101, 120, 129, 130, 131, 132, 148, 152, 244, 260, 273, 275, 276, 277
chemical scaffolds, viii, 187, 188
combination drug therapy, 77
communities, ix, 41
Coptis Chinensis (Huanglian), 263
coumarins, 238, 249, 257

D

dapagliflozin, 77, 135, 136, 144, 163, 173, 175, 176, 179, 182, 184, 207, 213
diabetes insipidus, 14
diabetes mellitus (DM), vii, viii, ix, 1, 2, 7, 12, 14, 15, 16, 17, 18, 19, 21, 32, 33, 34, 35, 36, 37, 38, 39, 42, 46, 47, 48, 51, 52, 61, 62, 63, 80, 92, 94, 95, 96, 97, 98, 99,

100, 101, 102, 103, 105, 108, 135, 138, 140, 141, 143, 144, 147, 149, 169, 170, 171, 172, 173, 174, 175, 183, 184, 185, 187, 189, 224, 225, 228, 235, 236, 237, 238, 242, 252, 253, 259, 260, 265, 266, 267, 269, 271, 272, 276, 277, 280, 281, 283, 285
diabetic ketoacidosis (DKA), 6, 14, 77, 90, 182, 183, 185
diet, 2, 8, 9, 12, 13, 28, 43, 45, 56, 59, 60, 64, 74, 84, 86, 89, 90, 101, 111, 135, 137, 164, 179, 182, 202, 207, 242, 254, 260, 268, 275, 279
dipeptidyl peptidase-4 (DPP-4), 42, 76, 95, 96, 114, 125, 126, 129, 143, 153, 156, 162, 164, 165, 166, 172, 173, 179, 180, 196, 197, 202, 203, 213, 215, 218, 219, 220, 221, 222, 226, 227, 230, 231, 232
Dutogliptin, 166

E

EMPA REG Renal, 181
empagliflozin, 77, 135, 160, 163, 175, 176, 178, 179, 180, 182, 184, 185
EMPA-REG trial, 180
environmental factors, 9, 26, 43
European Society for the Research of Diabetes (EASD), 17, 96, 180
Exenatide, 96, 162
exercise, 8, 10, 11, 12, 13, 45, 73, 74, 84, 85, 90, 100, 111, 135, 155, 164, 179

F

fasting plasma glucose (A1C), 2, 10, 53, 55, 78, 89, 109, 115, 136, 137, 176, 178, 179, 180, 183, 262
Fenugreek (*Trigonella Foenum-Graecum*), 264, 269
ferulic acid, 278, 284
flavonoid(s), 238, 242, 243, 244, 254, 256, 266, 277, 278, 279, 283, 285
Food and Drug Administration (FDA), 56, 57, 72, 73, 75, 135, 136, 253

G

gastric inhibitory peptide (GIP), 76, 80, 125, 130, 156, 164, 166
gestational diabetes (GD), 8, 10, 12, 13, 19, 52, 53, 54, 55, 56, 57, 58, 59, 60, 61, 62, 124, 148, 232, 236
ginseng, 241, 253, 259, 262, 266, 267, 274, 277, 281
glomerular filtration rate (GFR), 108, 177, 179, 181, 182
glucagon-like peptide-1 (GLP-1), 76, 77, 125, 130, 137, 144, 153, 154, 156, 162, 164, 173, 180, 266
glyburide, 52, 56, 57, 58, 106, 112, 113, 133, 142, 272
glycogenolysis, 57, 85, 107, 160, 262, 275
Gymnema, 264, 269, 270, 278, 284

H

herbal medicines, 259, 260, 261
human insulin, 33, 65, 66, 81, 83, 91, 92, 94
hyperglycemia, 1, 2, 9, 10, 11, 14, 17, 52, 53, 54, 55, 60, 61, 63, 67, 81, 83, 87, 96, 105, 106, 114, 117, 118, 119, 126, 127, 129, 130, 131, 132, 133, 148, 160, 165, 167, 168, 170, 173, 176, 177, 225, 236, 237, 239, 242, 249, 250, 251, 252, 255, 256, 259, 260, 262, 267, 271, 272, 276
Hyperglycemia and Adverse Pregnancy Outcomes (HAPO) study, 53, 61
hyperglycemic condition (HHS), 6, 10, 84

I

imidazoline compounds, 279
immunological factors, 24
insulin pump, 8, 10, 70, 71, 73, 74, 92, 93
insulin secretion, 10, 53, 57, 58, 75, 76, 81, 95, 115, 116, 117, 126, 130, 140, 141, 155, 162, 164, 170, 172, 176, 236, 239, 240, 244, 246, 252, 253, 255, 259, 261,

262, 263, 267, 268, 269, 276, 279, 283, 285
insulin-dependent diabetes mellitus (IDDM), 2, 32, 33, 34, 38, 97, 101, 260, 269
intramuscular, 68, 69, 93
intraperitoneal, 70, 93
islet transplantation, 77, 97

K

ketogenesis, 181, 182

L

lignans, 249
Linagliptin, 166, 174

M

major histocompatibility complex (MHC), 22, 26, 31, 33, 37
Mature Onset Diabetes of the Young (MODY), 14, 236, 237, 253
Metformin, 15, 54, 57, 58, 62, 75, 95, 107, 108, 109, 110, 111, 132, 133, 139, 140, 166
microbiota, 28, 37
molecular targets, vii, 147, 148, 149, 156, 158, 160, 171, 172, 187, 225

N

National Institutes of Health (NIH), 53
natural killer lymphocyte type (NKT) cells, 22, 29, 30, 32, 37, 38, 39
natural products, viii, ix, 235, 255, 258, 259, 261, 283
N-glucosyl indole(s), 207, 228
non-insulin-dependent diabetes mellitus (NIDDM), 2, 74, 93, 94, 100, 132, 139, 141, 143, 260, 270, 273
nutraceuticals, 88, 102, 265, 280

O

oral glucose tolerance test (OGTT), 2, 10, 13, 53, 165, 189, 217, 218, 219

P

pathophysiology, vii, 18, 21, 22, 23, 46, 88, 175
peroxisome proliferator-activated receptors (PPARs), 169, 170, 189, 190, 268, 276, 282
phenolics, 238, 250
phytoconstituents, viii, 235, 277
polysaccharides, 260, 273, 277, 278
pregnancy, vii, 4, 5, 12, 19, 51, 52, 53, 54, 55, 56, 57, 59, 61, 62, 128, 138, 148, 236
protein tyrosine phosphatase 1B (PTP1B), 156, 167, 172, 193, 194, 200, 202, 210, 212, 225, 226, 227, 229, 247

S

saponins, 238, 239, 240, 241, 242, 254, 278
saxagliptin, 125, 165, 179, 184
sitagliptin, 125, 126, 127, 128, 133, 143, 156, 164, 173, 178, 180, 183, 184, 222
social determinants, vii, 41, 45, 46, 49
sodium-glucose co-transporter, vii, 76, 162, 173, 175, 176, 184, 185
Sodium-Glucose Co-Transporter 2 Inhibitors (SGLT2), vii, 76, 77, 96, 135, 136, 144, 154, 162, 163, 164, 173, 185, 207, 213, 230
subcutaneous, 8, 10, 67, 68, 69, 70, 72, 78, 91, 92, 93, 94, 114, 124

T

teneligliptin, 156, 165, 197
terpenes, 238, 248, 249
therapy, 2, 3, 8, 10, 13, 14, 15, 21, 25, 28, 51, 52, 55, 56, 58, 63, 65, 69, 71, 73, 74,

75, 77, 78, 80, 81, 82, 83, 90, 91, 92, 93, 94, 96, 97, 98, 99, 105, 109, 110, 112, 114, 123, 124, 127, 128, 132, 133, 136, 137, 139, 141, 142, 143, 144, 148, 149, 150, 168,172, 173, 176, 178, 179, 181, 182, 183, 184, 225, 243, 281
thiadiazole derivatives, 198
Type 1 Diabetes Mellitus (T1DM), 5, 6, 7, 8, 9, 10, 11, 12, 13, 14, 21, 22, 23, 24, 25, 26, 27, 28, 29, 30, 31, 42, 52, 53, 55, 56, 59, 63, 67, 77, 84, 90, 135, 148, 176, 236, 250
Type 2 Diabetes Mellitus (T2DM), 5, 6, 7, 8, 10, 11, 12, 13, 14, 30, 42, 44, 52, 53, 54, 55, 56, 57, 59, 60, 67, 72, 74, 75, 76, 78, 83, 84, 85, 86, 87, 88, 89, 105, 108, 110, 111, 112, 114, 115, 116, 117, 122, 125, 127, 130, 131, 132, 135, 136, 138, 148, 149, 162, 163, 164, 165, 166, 168, 169, 176, 177, 179, 182, 183, 189, 207, 236, 242, 246, 251, 262, 263, 264, 279

U

US Food and Drug Administration (FDA), 57, 72, 73, 75, 135, 136, 177, 253

V

vildagliptin, 125, 126, 127, 128, 129, 143, 165, 174, 203
vitamins, 87, 102, 160

W

World Health Organization (WHO), 4, 11, 15, 23, 32, 46, 47, 49, 53, 61, 236, 280

Y

yoga, 85, 86, 101

About the Editors

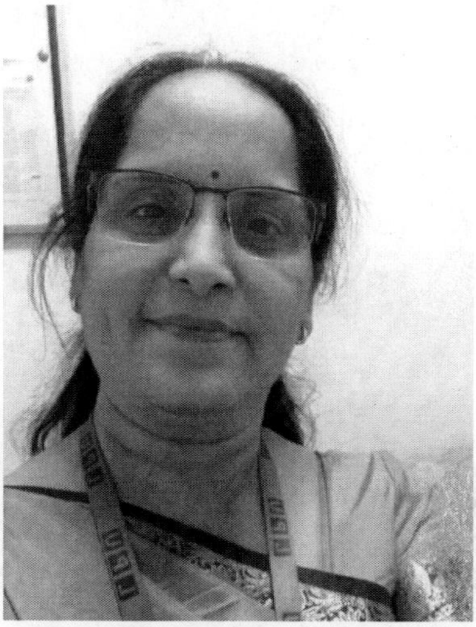

Yachana Mishra, PhD
Associate Professor
School of Bioengineering and Biosciences
Lovely Professional University, Phagwara, (Punjab), India
Email: yachanamishra@gmail.com

Dr. Yachana Mishra is working as an Associate Professor at the School of Bioengineering and Biosciences, Lovely Professional University, (Phagwara), Punjab, India. She received her PhD degree from Indian Grassland and Fodder Research Institute (IGFRI), Bundelkhand University, Jhansi (U.P.), India. She has published 25 research and review articles, 15 International book chapters, 1 International book, and 2 Indian patents (Filed). She is a life member of different reputed organizations like Indian Science Congress Association, Kolkata (India), and Society of Pharmaceutical Education and Research

(SPER), India. Her research areas include nanomedicine, cancer, diabetes and nanocarriers.

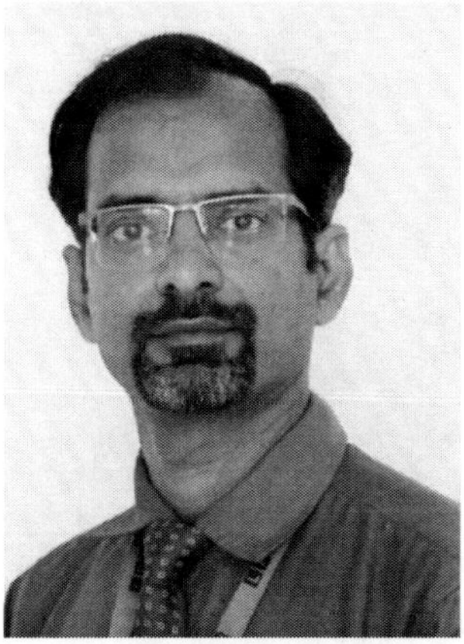

Vijay Mishra, PhD
Professor, School of Pharmaceutical Sciences
Lovely Professional University, Phagwara, (Punjab), India
Email: vijaymishra2@gmail.com

Dr. Vijay Mishra is working as a Professor at the School of Pharmaceutical Sciences, Lovely Professional University, Phagwara (Punjab), India. He earned his doctoral degree from Dr. H.S. Gour Central University, Sagar (MP), India. He has authored more than 130 international publications in reputed journals, 20 International book chapters, 5 books, 10 Indian patents (filed and published), 1 Australian and 1 Indian patent (granted). He is a life member of Indian Science Congress Association, Kolkata, India. He is an Editorial board member of Anti-Cancer Agents in Medicinal Chemistry, and Recent Patents on Anti-Cancer Drug Discovery (Bentham). Dr. Mishra has been selected as World's Top 2% scientist in 2021 and 2022 as per Stanford University, USA report. His current research interests encompass nanomedicine, cancer, dendrimers, carbon nanotubes, gold nanoparticles, graphene oxide, and novel drug delivery systems.